Pharmaceutical Coating Technology

Pharmaceutical Coating Technology

edited by

Graham Cole

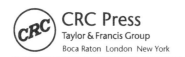

CRC Press
Taylor & Francis Group
Boca Raton London New York

CRC Press is an imprint of the
Taylor & Francis Group, an **informa** business

Contents

8. Coating pans and coating columns
Graham C. Cole

9. Environmental considerations: treatment of exhaust gases from film-coating processes
Graham C. Cole

10. Automation of coating processes
Graham C. Cole

1

Introduction and overview of pharmaceutical coating

Graham C. Cole

> 'Would you tell me, please,' said Alice, a little timidly, 'why you are painting those roses?'
>
> Five and Seven said nothing, but looked at Two. Two began, in a low voice, 'Why, the fact is, you see Miss, this here ought to have been a red rose-tree, and we put a white one in by mistake; and if the Queen was to find it out, we should all have our heads cut off, you know?'
>
> Lewis Carroll, *Alice in Wonderland*

This would appear to be a very good reason for painting anything (film coating is a painting process) and while the penalty for coating tablets the wrong colour is unlikely to be so extreme, the Queen (FDA, MCA, etc.) is likely to extract very costly and damaging retribution. No doubt 'heads would roll' metaphorically. So why are tablets coated? After all, it is a messy, complicated and expensive process.

> 'Look out now, Five! Don't go splashing paint over me like that!'
> 'I couldn't help it,' said Five, in a sulky tone. 'Seven jogged my elbow.'

It adds a degree of risk to the production process that could result in the whole batch being rejected. The costs in terms of space, personnel, equipment, Quality Control and Validation are considerable.

The modern coating technique has developed over the years from the use of sugar to provide a pleasant taste and attractive appearance to tablets which were unpleasant to swallow due to their bitterness. There are, of course, many forms of coating which have a special function (such as enteric coating to delay the release of the drug until it reaches the intestine), but here the simple case will be examined. First of all to answer the question 'Why are tablets coated?' A number of reasons can be suggested, some not quite so obvious as others:

- The core contains a substance which imparts a bitter taste in the mouth or has an unpleasant odour.
- The core contains a substance which is unstable in the presence of light and subject to atmospheric oxidation, i.e. a coating is added to improve stability.
- The core is pharmaceutically inelegant.
- The active substance is coloured and migrates easily to stain patient's clothes and hands.
- The coated tablet is packed on a high-speed packaging unit. The coating reduces friction and increases the production rate.
- To modify the drug release profile, e.g. enteric coating, sustained release coating, osmotic pumps, etc.
- To separate incompatible substances by using the coat to contain one of them or to coat a pellet which was previously compressed into a core.

This is not an exhaustive list but suggests several good reasons for coating tablets.

This book contains sections on modern pharmaceutical coating materials and processes and these can be broken down into three main groups and one minor section:

- Sugar coating
- Film coating
- Particulate/pellet coating
- Compression coating.

These processes and the selection and evaluation of equipment will be discussed in detail. Some chemical engineering unit operations will also be used to illustrate the differences between types of equipment.

There are several other historical coating processes such as pearl coating and pill coating which will not be discussed here.

In addition, some of the more fundamental aspects of film coating are covered, for example, an examination of the properties of coating solutions and suspensions, a detailed examination of the atomization stage, an explanation of surface interactions occurring between the coating liquid and the substrate (essential for an understanding of wetting and film adhesion), and a discussion on the mechanical properties and overall quality (with respect to roughness and defects, particularly) of the resulting coats.

HISTORICAL PERSPECTIVE

Sugar coating was largely borrowed from the confectionery industry which had developed this technique over the ages and is still widely used today. The pharmaceutical industry concentrated on using the open, copper, bowl-shaped pan, which has been largely replaced by stainless steel. It was not uncommon for as many as one hundred of these pans to be installed in a coating department. The sugar-coating process was a skilled manipulative operation and could last five days. The operator was highly skilled and jealously guarded his knowledge. In one operation the installation of temperature gauges on the inlet air duct almost caused a strike. This was only averted by some modification to the bonus scheme to increase payments for improved productivity!

This type of pan was used for batches of up to 150–200 kg and there was pressure to increase the batch sizes. Some pans were developed subsequently which improved handling, particularly in the way the drying air was introduced and extracted.

The Pelligrini pan, which was a large cylinder mounted on rollers with dished ends, was widely used in Europe, as was the doughnut-shaped pan in the United States. This enabled batches of 500–600 kg to be coated. It should be remembered that these sugar-coating processes double the weight of the core and, therefore, batch sizes have to be calculated on the finished tablet weight (i.e. after coating). Also, material was applied from ladles by hand and the operator 'worked' the batch. The air flow and temperature were very critical in achieving an elegant finish.

Generally, today, the pharmaceutical industry does not develop new sugar-coated tablets due to the lengthy process, the high degree of operator skill required and the fact that identification of the product is difficult. Printing of individual tablets with the house logo and product name and identification is another messy, slow and expensive process, and produces additional reject material. It is a process to be avoided if at all possible. The last major sugar-coated tablet to be developed was Brufen (Boots).

Film coating has the advantage that logo, identification numbers and names can be engraved on the tablet core, and these intagliations, as they are known in some companies, are clearly legible after coating.

The pressure to develop alternative methods was considerable. In the last twenty-five years tablet coating has undergone several fundamental changes. Although the sugar-coating process produced a very elegant product, its main disadvantage was the processing time, which could last up to five days. Many modifications were advocated to improve the basic process, such as air suspension techniques in a fluidized bed, the use of atomizing systems to spray on the sugar coating, the use of aluminium lakes of dyes to improve the evenness of colour, and more efficient drying systems. However, the process remained complicated. Generally the sugar-coating process resulted in the weight of the tablet being doubled but the use of modern spraying systems enabled this increase to be dramatically reduced.

Compression coating was one of these alternative techniques. Two methods enjoyed some popularity in the 1950s and 1960s. The process was designed to replace the long lead time of sugar coating by, in one case, compressing the core and then compressing the core-coating material around the core. This technique was favoured by Manesty Machines in the design of their Drycota machine. Two rotary machines were combined on a common base. The core was compressed on the first machine and then transferred to the second machine where coating was applied. However, the process relies on a number of very important effects.

1. The drug to be coated can be incorporated into a core of probably no more than 12 mm in diameter and no greater weight than 150 mg.
2. The coat bonds onto the substrate.
3. The total tablet size is not greater than 15 mm in diameter.
4. The total tablet weight is not greater than 900 mg.

The disadvantages of this process are:

1. It is difficult to bond the coat and core satisfactorily.
2. The core expansion causes the coat to split.
3. It is impossible to recover cores coated with this method.
4. The process is relatively slow, i.e. 1000 tablets per minute maximum, compared to compressing outputs of up to 10 000 tablets per minute.

One of the main advantages of the Drycota process is that incompatible drugs can be separated into core and coat. However, layered tablets achieve the same result and can be produced at a faster rate.

Killian, on the other hand, favoured feeding precompressed cores into a Prescota machine which applied the coat. This process, it was reasoned, enabled the core to expand overnight (or longer) and did not result in splitting of the coated tablet, the main disadvantage of both of these processes.

Many of the products developed for this equipment used drugs that were moisture sensitive, e.g. aspirin, but other methods of protecting these materials eliminated even this advantage. Some machines are still in use around the world but the development of the film-coating process sealed their fate as a viable coating option. Currently renewed interest has been shown in this technique as a means of blinding Clinical Trials.

MODERN PROCESSES

The first reference to tablet film coating appeared in 1930 but it was not until 1954 that Abbott Laboratories produced the first commercially available film-coated tablet. This was made possible by the development of a wide variety of materials — for example, the cellulose derivatives. One of the most important of these is hydroxypropyl methylcellulose which is prepared by the reaction of methyl chloride and propylene oxide with alkali cellulose (*Remington Pharmaceutical Sciences*, 1990). It was generally applied in solution in organic solvents at a concentration of between 2 and 4%w/v: the molecular weight fraction chosen gives a solution viscosity of 5×10^{-2} Pas at these concentrations.

When Abbott introduced this process into production they used a fluidized bed-coating column based on the Wurster principle (Wurster, 1953) and this process was developed a stage further by Merck in their plants in the US and the UK. The plant in the UK had a design capacity of 1000 million coated tablets per annum. However, the advent of aqueous film coating and the development of side-vented pans heralded the demise of the coating column for tablets. It is still probably the system of choice for coating particulates and pellets.

During the period 1954–1975 the lower molecular weight polymers of hydroxypropyl methylcellulose with a solution viscosity of $3-15 \times 10^{-3}$ Pas did not receive much attention because of the cheapness of organic solvents and the ease with which the coating could be applied. There was also a belief that the lower viscosity grades produced weaker films which would not meet the formulation requirement for stability and patient acceptability. However, there is now a very significant move towards aqueous film coating for the following reasons:

1. The cost of organic solvents has escalated.
2. A number of regulatory authorities have banned chlorinated hydrocarbons altogether because of environmental pollution.
3. The development of improved coating pans and spraying systems has enabled these more difficult coating materials to be applied.
4. Flameproof equipment is not required. This reduces capital outlay and a less hazardous working environment is provided for the operator.
5. Solvent recovery systems are not required resulting in less capital outlay.

Most of the early development work for aqueous film coating concentrated on the use of existing conventional coating pans and tapered cylindrical pans such as the Pellegrini, largely because models already existed in production departments. This pan is open at the front and rear, and the spray guns are mounted on an arm positioned through the front opening. The drying air and exhaust air are both fed in and extracted from the rear. The drying air is blown onto the surface of the tablets, but because of the power of the extraction fan most of the heat is lost with the exhaust air. Very poor thermal contact results and a poor coating finish is obtained. The perforated rotary coating pan, which permits the drying air to be drawn co-current with the spray through the tablet bed and pan wall during film coating, offers better heat and mass transfer and results in a more efficient coating process and a more elegantly finished product.

There are several companies which offer equipment of this type; the Manesty Accelacota, the Driam Driacoater and the Glatt Coater are three well-known models. There are significant differences between them.

In this book the authors will show how materials can be controlled, selected and used in the current available equipment to produce a pharmaceutically elegant product so that we do not have to resort to the solutions used by Two, Five and Seven.

REFERENCES

Remington Pharmaceutical Sciences, 18th edn, 1990.
Wurster, D. E. (1953) Winsconsin (Alumini Research Foundation), US Patent 2,648,609.

2

Film-coating materials and their properties

John E. Hogan

SUMMARY

The chapter commences by reviewing the properties of the broad classes of materials used in film coating, polymers, plasticizers, pigments and solvents (or vehicles).

An initial consideration of the polymers shows that while processing is most commonly performed using these materials in solution, there are systems which utilize polymers in suspension in water. The mechanism of coalescence and film formation for these types of materials are discussed.

The individual polymers are dealt with in some detail and an attempt is made to divide them into functional and non-functional coating polymers. Functional polymers being defined as those which modify the pharmaceutical function of the compressed tablet, for instance an enteric or modified releae film. However, this distinction is sometimes blurred as one coating polymer can fall into both groups. The essential polymer characteristics of solubility, solution viscosity, film permeability and mechanical properties are described in terms of ultimate film requirements.

In the treatment and description of plasticizers, some prominence is given to their effect on the mechanical properties of the film and its permeability characteristics, especially to water vapour. A section is provided on the assessment of plasticizer activity on film-coating polymers.

The section on pigments describes how they function as opacifiers and also their ability to modify the permeability of a film to gases.

In considering the solvents and vehicles used in film-coating techniques a discussion is provided of the respective merits of aqueous and non-aqueous processing.

The chapter is concluded by some examples of formulae of film-coating systems which illustrate several of the principles described previously.

2.1 INTRODUCTION

A film coating is a thin polymer-based coat applied to a solid dosage form such as a tablet, granule or other particle. The thickness of such a coating is usually between 20 and 100 μm. Under close examination the film structure can be seen to be relatively non-homogeneous and quite distinct in appearance, for example, from a film resulting from casting a polymer solution on a flat surface. This non-homogeneous character results from the deliberate addition of insoluble ingredients such as pigments and by virtue of the fact that the film itself is built up in an intermittent fashion during the coating process. This is because most coating processes rely on a single tablet or granule passing through a spray zone, after which the adherent material is dried before the next portion of coating is received. This activity will of course be repeated many times until the coating is complete.

Film-coating formulations usually contain the following components:

- Polymer.
- Plasticizer.
- Pigment/opacifier.
- Vehicle.

However, while plasticizers have an established place in film-coating formulae they are by no means universally used. Likewise, in clear coating, pigments and opacifiers are deliberately omitted. Consideration must also be given to minor components in a film-coating formula such as flavours, surfactants and waxes and, in rare instances, the film coat itself may contain active material.

2.2 POLYMERS

The vast majority of the polymers used in film coating are either cellulose derivatives, such as the cellulose ethers, or acrylic polymers and copolymers. Occasionally encountered are high molecular weight polyethylene glycols, polyvinyl pyrrolidone, polyvinyl alcohol and waxy materials.

The characteristics of the individual polymers and the essential properties of polymers used for film coating will be covered in subsequent sections.

Frequently, the polymer is dissolved in an appropriate solvent either water or a non-aqueous solvent for application of the coating to the solid dosage form. However, some of the water-insoluble polymers are available in a form which renders them usable from aqueous systems. These materials find considerable application in the area of modified release coatings. Basically there are two classes of such material depending upon the method of preparation; true latexes and pseudolatexes.

2.2.1 True latexes

These are very fine dispersions of polymer in an aqueous phase and particle size is crucial in the stability and use of these materials. They are characterized by a particle size range of between 10 and 1000 nm. Their tendency to sediment is counterbalanced by the Brownian movement of the particles aided by microconvection currents found in the body of the liquid. The Stokes equation can be used to determine the greatest particle diameter that can be tolerated in the system without sedimentation. At the other end of the size range the characteristic of colloidal particles is approached where such dispersions are barely opaque to light and are almost clear. One of the chief ways of producing latex dispersions is by emulsion polymerization. Characteristically the process starts with the monomer which after purification is emulsified as the internal phase with a suitable surfactant (Lehmann, 1972). Polymerization is activated by addition of an initiator. Commonly the system is purged with nitrogen to remove atmospheric oxygen which would lead to side reactions. As with any polymerization process, the initiator controls the rate and extent of the reaction. The reaction is quenched when the particle size is in the range 50–200 nm. Using this process the following acrylate polymers are produced: Eudragit L100-55 and NE30D (Lehmann, 1989a).

2.2.2   Psuedolatexes

Commercially there are two main products which fall into this category, both of them utilize ethylcellulose as the film former but are manufactured in quite a different way and their method of application also differs significantly. Characteristically pseudolatexes are manufactured starting with the polymer itself and not the monomer. By a physical process the polymer particle size is reduced thereby producing a dispersion in water; the characteristics of this dispersion need not differ significantly from a true latex, including particle size considerations. The pseudolatex is also free of monomer residue and traces of initiator, etc.

The earliest of the two ethylcellulose products (Aquacoat) is manufactured by dissolving ethylcellulose in an organic solvent and emulsifying the solution in an aqueous continuous phase. The organic solvent is eventually removed by vacuum distillation, leaving a fine dispersion of polymer particles in water. Steuernagel (1989) has defined the composition of Aquacoat to have a solids content of 30% w/w and a moisture content of 70%w/w, the solids being composed of ethylcellulose 87%, cetyl alcohol 9% and sodium lauryl sulphate 4%. A food grade antifoam is also present. The cetyl alcohol and sodium lauryl sulphate act as surfactants/stabilizers during the later stages of production.

The newer of the ethylcellulose products is Surelease. This is manufactured using a patented process based on phase inversion technology (Warner, 1978). The ethylcellulose is heated in the presence of dibutyl sebacate and oleic acid, and this mixture is then introduced into a quantity of ammoniated water. The resulting phase inversion produces a fine dispersion of ethylcellulose particles in an aqueous continuous phase. The dibutyl sebacate (fractionated coconut oil can also be used) is to be found in the ethylcellulose fraction while the oleic acid and the ammonia together effectively stabilize the dispersed phase in water. This siting of the dibutyl sebacate and oleic acid is important for the use of this material as an effective coating agent. Both materials act as plasticizers and with the Surelease system are physically situated where they are able to function most effectively, that is, in intimate contact with the polymer. Surelease, unlike Aquacoat, does not require the further addition of plasticizer. Surelease also contains a quantity of fumed silica which acts as an antitack agent during the coating process. Its total nominal solids content is 25% w/w.

Aqueous dispersions have significant advantages, enabling processing of water-insoluble polymers from an aqueous media (see Chapter 14).

2.2.3 Mechanism of film formation

Film formation from an aqueous polymeric dispersion is a complex matter and has been examined by several authors (Bindschaedler *et al.*, 1983; Zhang *et al.*, 1988, 1989). In the wet state the polymer is present as a number of discrete particles, and these have to come together in close contact, deform, coalesce and ultimately fuse together to form a discrete film. During processing, the substrate surface will be wetted with the diluted dispersion. Under the prevailing processing conditions water will be lost as water vapour and the polymer particles will increase in proximity to each other—a process which is greatly aided by the capillary action of the film of water surrounding the particles. Complete coalescence occurs when the adjacent particles are able to mutually diffuse into one another, as shown in Fig. 2.1.

Minimum film-forming temperature (MFT)

This is the minimum temperature above which film formation will take place using individual defined conditions. It is largely dependent on the glass transition temperature (T_g) of the polymer, an attribute which is capable of several definitions but can be considered as that temperature at which the hard glassy form of an amorphous or largely amorphous polymer changes to a softer, more rubbery, consistency. Lehmann (1992) states that the concept of MFT includes the plasticizing effect of water on the film-forming process. With aqueous dispersions Lehmann recommends to keep the coating temperature 10–20°C above the MFT to ensure that optimal conditions for film formation are achieved. Examples of MFTs of Eudragit RL and RS aqueous dispersions are given by Lehmann (1989a).

2.3 POLYMERS FOR CONVENTIONAL FILM COATING

The term conventional film coating has been used here to describe film coatings applied for reasons of improved product appearance, improved handling, and prevention of dusting, etc. This is to make a distinction with functional film coats, which will be described in a later section, and where the purpose of the coating is to confer a modified release aspect on the dosage form. An alternative term for conventional film coating, therefore, would be non-functional film coating.

2.3.1 Cellulose ethers

The majority of the cellulose derivatives used in film coating are in fact ethers of cellulose. Broadly they are manufactured by reacting cellulose in alkaline solution with, for example, methyl chloride, to obtain methylcellulose. Hydroxypropoxyl substitution is obtained by similar reaction with propylene oxide. The product is

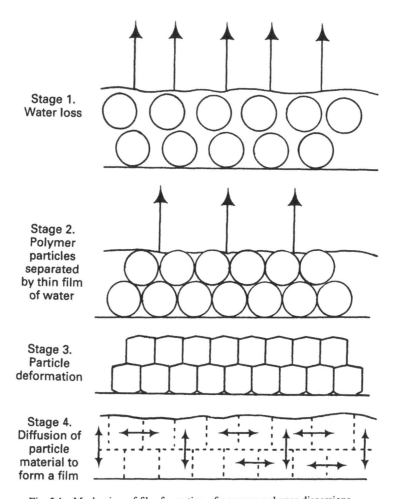

Stage 1.
Water loss

Stage 2.
Polymer
particles
separated
by thin film
of water

Stage 3.
Particle
deformation

Stage 4.
Diffusion of
particle
material to
form a film

Fig. 2.1   Mechanism of film formation of aqueous polymer dispersions

thoroughly washed with hot water to remove impurities, dried and finally milled prior to packaging.

The structure of cellulose permits three hydroxyl groups per repeating anhydroglucose unit to be replaced, in such a fashion. If all three hydroxyl groups are replaced the degree of substitution (DS) is designated as 3, and so on for lower degrees of substitution. The term molar substitution (MS) covers the situation where a side chain carries hydroxyl groups capable of substitution and takes into account the total moles of a group whether on the backbone or side chain. Both DS and MS profoundly affect the polymer properties with respect to solubility and thermal gel point.

The polymer chain length, together with the size and extent of branching, will of course determine the viscosity of the polymer in solution. As a generality, film coating demands polymers at the lower end of the viscosity scale.

Table 2.1   Substitution data of some cellulose ethers (after Rowe, 1984c)

Polymer	Methoxyl substitution		Hydroxypropoxyl substitution		
	%w/w	DS	%w/w	DS	MS
Methylcellulose	27.5–31.5	1.64–1.92	—	—	—
Hydroxypropyl methylcellulose	28.0–30.0	1.67–1.81	7.0–12.0	0.15–0.25	0.22–0.25
Hydroxypropyl cellulose	—	—	≤ 80.5	—	≤ 4.6

Individual cellulose ethers
Various groups are capable of substitution into the cellulose structure, as shown in Fig. 2.2.

Hydroxypropyl methylcellulose (HPMC)
Substituent groups: $-CH_3$, $-CH_2-CH(OH)-CH_3$

This polymer provides the mainstay of coating with the cellulose ethers and its usage dates back to the early days of film coating. It is soluble in both aqueous media and the organic solvent systems normally used for film coating. HPMC provides aqueously soluble films which can be coloured by the use of pigments or used in the absence of pigments to form clear films. The polymer affords relatively easy processing due to its non-tacky nature. A typical low-viscosity polymer can be sprayed from an aqueous solution containing around 10–15%w/w polymer solids. From the regulatory aspect, in addition to its use in pharmaceutical products, HPMC has a long history of safe use as a thickener and emulsifier in the food industry.

Table 2.2 shows that the USP and JP recognize definite substitution types in separate monographs. The first two digits of the four-digit designation specify the nominal percentage of methoxyl groups while the final two specify the nominal

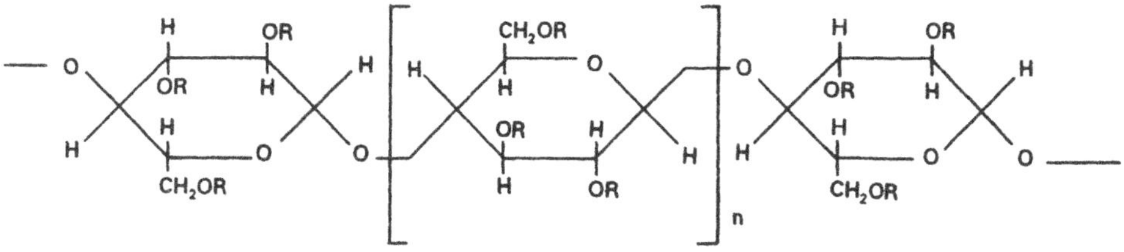

Fig. 2.2   The structure of a substituted cellulose. (R can be represented as –H or, as in the text, under individual polymers.)

Table 2.2 Compendial designations of HPMC typess in the USP and JP

	2910	2208	2906	1828[a]
% Methoxyl	7–12	4–12	4–7.5	16–20
% Hydroxypropoxyl	28–20	19–24	27–30	23–32

[a] Monograph only in the USP.

percentage of hydroxypropoxyl groups. The EP has no specified ranges for substitution. Significant differences exist between the USP and EP monographs. These relate to tighter requirements for ash, chloride for the EP which also possesses tests on solution colour, clarity and pH. Methodology differences also exist, particularly with regard to solution viscosity. The JP has a very low limit on chloride content.

Methylcellulose (MC)
Substituent group: $—CH_3$
This polymer is used rarely in film coating possibly because of the lack of commercial availability of low viscosity material meeting the appropriate compendial requirements. As a distinction from the USP and the JP the EP has no required limits on the content of methoxyl substitution. However, the USP and JP have slightly different limits, which are 27.5–31.5% against 26.0–33.0% respectively.

Hydroxyethyl cellulose (HEC)
Substituent group: $—CH(OH)—CH_3$
This water-soluble cellulose ether is generally insoluble in organic solvents. The USNF is the sole pharmacopoeial specification; there is no requirement on the quantity of hydroxyethyl groups to be present. The USNF allows the presence of additives to promote dispersion of the powder in water and to prevent caking on storage.

Hydroxypropyl cellulose (HPC)
Substituent group: $—CH_2—CH(OH)—CH_3$
HPC has the property of being soluble in both aqueous and alcoholic media. Its films unfortunately tend to be rather tacky, which possess restraints on rapid coating; HPC films also suffer from being weak. Currently this polymer is very often used in combination with other polymers to provide additional adhesion to the substrate. The EB/BP has no requirements on hydroxypropoxyl content. The USNF states this must be less than 80.5% while the JP has two monographs differing in substitution requirements. The monograph most closely corresponding to the USNF material has a substitution specification of 53.4–77.5%. The other monograph relates to material of much lower substitution content and is used for purposes other than film coating, e.g. direct compression.

2.3.2 Acrylic polymers
These comprise a group of synthetic polymers with diverse functionalities.

Methacrylate aminoester copolymer
This polymer is basically insoluble in water but dissolves in acidic media below pH 4. In neutral or alkaline environments, its films achieve solubility by swelling and increased permeability to aqueous media. Formulations intended for conventional film coating can be further modified to enhance swelling and permeability by the incorporation of materials such as water soluble cellulose ethers, and starches in order to ensure complete disintegration/dissolution of the film.

This material is supplied in both powder form or as a concentrated solution in isopropanol/acetone, which can be further diluted with solvents such as ethanol, methanol, acetone and methylene chloride. Talc, magnesium stearate or similar materials are useful additions to the coating formula as they assist in decreasing the sticky or tacky nature of the polymer. In general, the polymer does not require the addition of a plasticizer.

2.4 POLYMERS FOR MODIFIED RELEASE APPLICATION

Despite the considerable difference in application between a polymer intended for a simple conventional (non-functional) coating and one intended to confer a modified release performance on the dosage form, the categorizing of the polymers themselves into these divisions is not such an exact process. Several examples exist of polymers fulfilling both needs, hence there is a considerable overlap of use. However, the divisions used here represent perhaps the majority practice.

Table 2.3 Methacrylate aminoester copolymers (after Lehmann & Dreher, 1981)

$$\left[CH_2 - \underset{\underset{\displaystyle OC_4H_9}{\overset{\displaystyle |}{C}}}{\overset{\overset{\displaystyle CH_3}{|}}{C}} \!\!\diagup\!\!\!{}^O \right]_{n_1} \!\!\!-\!-\!- \left[CH_2 - \underset{\underset{\displaystyle OR}{\overset{\displaystyle |}{C}}}{\overset{\overset{\displaystyle CH_3}{|}}{C}} \!\!\diagup\!\!\!{}^O \right]_{n_2} \!\!\!-\!-\!- \left[CH_2 - \underset{\underset{\displaystyle OCH_3}{\overset{\displaystyle |}{C}}}{\overset{\overset{\displaystyle CH_3}{|}}{C}} \!\!\diagup\!\!\!{}^O \right]_{n_3}$$

Scientific name	$n_1{:}n_2{:}n_3$	MW	USNF designation	Eudragit type	Marketed form
Poly(butylmethacrylate), (2-dimethylaminoethyl) methacrylate, methylmethacrylate	1:2:1	150 000	None	E12.5	12.5% solution in isopropanol/ acetone
$R = -CH_2-CH_2-N(CH_3)_2$			None	E100	Granulate

2.4.1 Methacrylate ester copolymers

Structurally these polymers bear a resemblance to the methacrylic acid copolymers but are totally esterified with no free carboxylic acid groups. Thus these materals are neutral in character and are insoluble over the entire physiological pH range. However they do possess the ability to swell and become permeable to water and dissolved substances so that they find application in the coating of modified release dosage forms. The two polymers Eudragit RS and RL, can be mixed and blended to achieve a desired release profile. The addition of hydrophilic materials such as the soluble cellulose ethers, polyethylene glycol (PEG), etc., will also enable modifications to be achieved with the final formulation. The polymer Eudragit RL is strongly permeable and thus only slightly retardant. Its films are therefore also indicated for use in quickly disintegrating coatings. The polymers themselves have solubility characteristics similar to the methacrylic acid copolymers.

For aqueous spraying a latex form of each polymer is available. In addition the polymer Eudragit NE30D has been made for this purpose. This materal is also used as an immediate-release non-functional coating in film coat formulations where relatively large quantities of water-soluble materials are added to ensure efficient disruption of the coat.

2.4.2 Ethylcellulose (EC)

Substituent group (Fig. 2.2): $—CH_2—CH_3$

Ethylcellulose is a cellulose ether produced by the reaction of ethyl chloride with the appropriate alkaline solution of cellulose. Apart from its extensive use in controlled release coatings, ethylcellulose has found a use in organic solvent-based coatings in a mixture with other cellulosic polymers, notably HPMC. The ethylcellulose component optimizes film toughness in that surface marking due to handling is minimized. Ethylcellulose also conveys additional gloss and shine to the tablet surface.

In many ways ethylcellulose is an ideal polymer for modified release coatings. It is odourless, tasteless and it exhibits a high degree of stability not only under physiological conditions but also under normal storage conditions, being stable to light and heat at least up to its softening point of c. 135°C (Rowe, 1985). Commercially, ethylcellulose is available in a wide range of viscosity and substitution types giving a good range of possibilities for the formulator. It also possesses good solubility in common solvents used for film coating but this feature is nowadays of lesser importance with the advent of water-dispersible presentations of ethylcellulose which have been especially designed for modified release coatings. The polymer is not usually used on its own but normally in combination with secondary polymers such as HPMC or polyethylene glycols which convey a more hydrophilic nature to the film by altering its structure by virtue of pores and channels through which drug solution can more easily diffuse. Only the USNF contains a monograph, an ethoxy group content of between 44.0 and 51.0% is specified. The USNF also contains a monograph 'Ethylcellulose Aqueous Dispersion' which defines one type of such material which finds a use in aqueous processing. The monograph permits the presence of cetyl alcohol and sodium lauryl sulphate which are necessary to stabilize the dispersion.

Table 2.4 Methacrylate ester copolymers (after Lehmann
& Dreher, 1981)

$$\left[\begin{array}{c} H \\ | \\ CH_2 - C - \\ | \quad \diagup O \\ C \diagdown OC_2H_5 \end{array} \right]_{n_1} ---- \left[\begin{array}{c} CH_3 \\ | \\ CH_2 - C - \\ | \quad \diagup O \\ C \diagdown OCH_3 \end{array} \right]_{n_2} ---- \left[\begin{array}{c} CH_3 \\ | \\ CH_2 - C - \\ | \quad \diagup O \\ C \diagdown OR \end{array} \right]_{n_3}$$

Scientific name	n_1:n_2:n_3	MW	USNF designation[a]	Eudragit type	Marketed form
Poly(ethylacrylate, methylmethacrylate	2:1	800 000	None	NE30D	30% aqueous dispersion
Poly(ethylacrylate, methylmethacrylate) trimethylammonioethylmethacrylate chloride	1:2:0.2	150 000	Type A	RL12.5	12.5% solution in isopropanol/acetone
				RL100	Granulate
R = CH$_2$—CH$_2$—N$^+$(CH$_3$)$_3$Cl$^-$				RL30D	30% aqueous dispersion
Poly(ethylacrylate, methylmethacrylate) trimethylammonioethylmethacrylate chloride	1:2:0.1	150 000	Type B	RS12.5	12.5% solution in isopropanol/acetone
				RS100	Granulate
R = CH$_2$—CH$_2$—N$^+$(CH$_3$)$_3$Cl$^-$				RS30D	30% aqueous dispersion

[a] Ammoniomethacrylate co-polymer

2.5 ENTERIC POLYMERS

As will be seen later, enteric polymers are designed to resist the acidic nature of the stomach contents, yet dissolve readily in the duodenum.

2.5.1 Cellulose acetate phthalate (CAP)

Substituent groups (Fig. 2.2):   —CO—CH$_3$, —CO—C$_6$H$_4$—COOH

This is the oldest and most widely used synthetic enteric coating polymer patented as an enteric agent by Eastman Kodak in 1940. It is manufactured by reacting a partial acetate ester of cellulose with phthalic anhydride. In the resulting polymer, of the free hydroxyl groups contributed by each glucose unit of the cellulose chain, approximately half are acylated and one-quarter esterified with one of the two carboxylic acid groups of the phthalate moiety. The second carboxylic acid group being free to form salts and thus serves as the basis of its enteric character.

CAP is a white free-flowing powder usually with a slightly odour of acetic acid. Among the pharmacopoeias it is found in the EP, JP and USNF. The USNF and JP impose specifications for the percentage content of the substituent groups. The JP has requirements for the content of acetyl and phthalyl to be respectively 17–22 and 30–40% while the USNF requires 21.5–26 and 30–36% respectively. The JP is alone in not specifying any viscosity control on a standard solution. All three pharmacopoeias require a maximum limit on the quantity of free acid (JP specifies phthalic acid) and loss on drying (EP specifies water content). The last two parameters are important as CAP is somewhat prone to hydrolysis.

Of the generally accepted solvents used for tablet coating, CAP is insoluble in water, alcohols and chlorinated hydrocarbons. In the following solvents or solvent mixtures (data from the *Handbook of Pharmaceutical Excipients*, 1986) it possesses greater than 10% solubility:

acetone
    ethyl acetate:isopropanol   1:1
    acetone:ethanol   1:1
    acetone:methanol   1:1 and 1:3
    acetone:methylene chloride   1:3

A pseudolatex version of CAP is available (Aquateric) as a dry powder for reconstitution in water and offers the convenience of aqueous-based processing.

Owing to their chemical constitution, most of the phthalate-based enteric coating agents are to a greater or lesser degree unstable. This important aspect is dealt with in more detail in Chapter 14, along with the implications this has on the use of the materal in practice.

2.5.2   Polyvinyl acetate phthalate (PVAP)

PVAP was first patented by the Charles E. Frost Company of Canada and was subsequently investigated by Millar (1957) who studied the effect that the phthalyl content of the polymer had upon the pH of disintegration of tablets coated with the material. He found the optimal phthalyl content to be between 60 and 70%. However, given the characteristics of the polymer commercially available nowadays, this range has been revised and now forms part of the USNF monograph. It is manufactured by reacting polyvinyl alcohol with acetic acid and phthalic anhydride.

The USNF contains a monograph specifying a total phthalate content of between 55 and 62%. The polymer characteristics are further controlled by imposition of a viscosity specification. The extent of hydrolysis, while much less likely than CAP for instance, is controlled with a limit on free phthalic acid and other free acids. As the final separation process is from water, a limit of 5% of water is specified.

Polyvinyl acetate phthalate possesses the following solubility characteristics, with the extent of solubility given in parentheses:

methanol (50%)
methanol/methylene chloride (30%)

ethanol 95% (25%)
ethanol/water 85:15 (30%)

An aqueous dispersible form (Sureteric) is available for water-based spraying.

2.5.3 Shellac

This is a purified resinous secretion of the insect *Laccifer lacca*, indigenous to India and other parts of the Far East. Shellacs can be modified to suit specialized needs. For instance, bleached shellac is produced by dissolving crude shellac in warm soda solution followed by bleaching with hypochlorite. Various grades of dewaxed material can be produced by removing some or all of the approximately 5% of wax in the final shellac.

Shellac is insoluble in water but shows solubility in aqueous alkalis; it is moderately soluble in warm ethanol.

Over the years, shellac has been used for a variety of applications, which have included.

- A seal coat for tablet cores prior to sugar coating.
- An enteric-coating material. This application is really of historic interest only as shellac has a relatively high apparent pK_a of between 6.9 and 7.5 and leads to poor solubility of the film in the duodenum (Chambliss, 1983).
- A modified release coating.

For all these applications, shellac suffers from the general drawback that it is a material of natural origin and consequently suffers from occasional supply problems and quality variation. As will be described later, there are also stability problems associated with increased disintegration and dissolution times on storage.

2.5.4 Methacrylic acid copolymers

Because these polymers possess free carboxylic acid groups they find use as enteric-coating materials, forming salts with alkalis and having an appreciable solubility at pH in excess of 5.5

Of the two organic solvent soluble polymers, Eudragit S100 has a lower degree of substitution with carboxyl groups and consequently dissolves at higher pH than Eudragit L100. Used in combination, these materials are capable of providing films with a useful range of pH over which solubility will occur.

All the polymers shown in Table 2.5 are recommended to be used with plasticizers. Pigments and opacifiers are useful additions as they counteract the sticky nature of the polymers. A feature of these polymers is their ability to bind large quantities of pigments—approximately two or three times the quantity of polymer used. Polyethylene glycols are frequently added as they provide a measure of gloss to the final product. They also assist in stabilizing the water-dispersible form, Eudragit L30D. Pigment and other additions to the water-dispersible forms Eudragit, L30D and L100-55, should be performed according to the manufacturer's recommendations to prevent coagulation of the coating dispersion.

Table 2.5   Methacrylic acid copolymers (after Lehmann
& Dreher, 1981)

$$\left[\begin{array}{c} CH_3 \\ | \\ -CH_2-C- \\ | \quad O \\ C \diagdown \\ \qquad OH \end{array}\right]_{n_1} \quad ---- \quad \left[\begin{array}{c} R_1 \\ | \\ -CH_2-C- \\ | \quad O \\ C \diagdown \\ \qquad OR_2 \end{array}\right]_{n_2}$$

Scientific name	$n_1{:}n_2$	MW	R_1	R_2	USNF designation[a]	Eudragit type	Marketed form
Polymethylacrylate, ethylacrylate)	1:1	250 000	H	C_2H_5	Type C	L30D	30% aqueous dispersion
						L100–55	Powder
Poly(methacrylic acid, methylmethacrylate)	1:1	135 000	CH_3	CH_3	Type A	L12.5	12.5% solution in isopropanol
						L100	Powder
Poly(methacrylic acid, methylmethacrylate)	1:2	135 000	CH_3	CH_3	Type B	S12.5	12.5% solution in isopropanol
						S100	Powder

[a] Methacrylic acid copolymer

These polymers comply with the USNF requirements for methacrylic acid copolymer as outlined in Table 2.5. Both Eudragit L100 and S100 are available in powder form and for convenience purposes they are also available as concentrates in organic solvent solution, which are capable of further dilution in the common processing solvents used in organic solvent-based film coating. As previously indicated, two further commercial forms are available, first, a 30% aqueous dispersion, Eudragit L30D, and, secondly, a water-dispersible powder, Eudragit L100-55.

The Eudragit acrylate polymers can be described using a generic type nomenclature as given below. Reference can also be made to the corresponding parts of Tables 2.3, 2.4 and 2.5.

Monomers
MMA   methylmethacrylate
MA   methacrylic acid
EA   ethylacrylate
TAMCl   trimethylammonioethylmethacrylate chloride

Copolymers
poly(MA-EA) 1:1   copolymer of MA and EA in a molar ratio of 1:1 (Eudragit L30D, Eudragit L100-55)
poly(MA-MMA) 1:1   copolymer of MA and MMA in a molar ratio of 1:1 (Eudragit L100)

poly(MA-MMA) 1:2	copolymer of MA and MMA in a molar ratio of 1:2 (Eudragit S100)
poly(EA-MMA-TAMCl) 1:2:0.1	copolymer of EA, MMA and TAMCl in a molar ratio of 1:2:0.1 (Eudragit RS30D, Eudragit RS100)
poly(EA-MMA-TAMCl) 1:2:0.2	copolymer of EA, MMA and TAMCl in a molar ratio of 1:2:0.2 (Eudragit RL30D Eudragit RL100)

2.5.5 Cellulose acetate trimellitate (CAT)

Substituent groups (Fig. 2.2): $-CO-CH_3$, $CO-C_6H_3-(COOH)_2$

Chemically this polymer bears a strong resemblance to cellulose acetate phthalate but possesses an additional carboxylic acid group on the aromatic ring. Manufacturer's quoted typical values for timellityl and acetyl percentages are 29 and 22% respectively. The useful property of this polymer is its ability to start to dissolve at the relatively low pH of 5.5 (Anon., 1988) which would help ensure efficient dissolution of the coated dosage form in the upper small intestine.

As yet, CAT does not appear in any pharmacopoeia but is the subject of a US FDA Drug Master File.

The solubility of CAT in organic solvents is similar to that for CAP. For aqueous processing, the manufacturers recommend the use of ammoniacal solutions of CAT in water, and fully enteric results are claimed. The recommended plasticizers for aqueous use are triacetin, acetylated monoglyceride or diethyl phthalate.

2.5.6 Hydroxypropyl methylcellulose phthalate (HPMCP)

Substituent groups: $-CH_3$, $-CH_2CH(OH)CH_3$, $-CO-C_6H_4-COOH$

HPMCP is prepared by treating hydroxypropyl methylcellulose with phthalic acid. The degree of substitution of the three possible substituents determines the polymer characteristics, in particular the pH of dissolution.

HPMCP may be plasticized with diethylphthalate, acetylated monoglyceride or triacetin. Mechanically it is a more flexible polymer and on a weight basis will not require as much plasticizer as CAP or CAT.

HPMCP is a white powder or granular material; monographs can be found in both the USNF and JP. Both pharmacopoeias describe two substitution types, namely HPMCP 200731 and 220824. The six-digit nomenclature refers to the percentages of the respective substituent methoxyl, hydroxypropoxyl and carboxybenzoyl groups. For example, HPMCP 200731 has a nominal methoxyl content of 20% and so on for the other two substituents. Substitution requirements are the same in both pharmacopoeias. Commercial designations such as '50' or '55' refer to the pH ($\times$10) of the aqueous buffer solubility. Fine particle size grades designated with a suffix 'F' are intended for suspension in aqueous systems, with suitable plasticizers prior to spray application.

HPMCP is insoluble in water but soluble in aqueous alkalis and acetone/water 95:5 mixtures. The following summarizes the solubility of HPMCP in common non-aqueous processing solvents:

	HP55	HP50
Acetone/methanol 1:1	+	+
Acetone/ethanol 1:1	+	*
Methylene chloride/ethanol 1:1	+	+

+ = soluble, clear solution
* = slightly soluble, cloudy solution
(data from the *Handbook of Pharmaceutical Excipients*, 1986)

2.6 POLYMER CHARACTERISTICS

2.6.1 Solubility

Inspection of the solubility characteristics of the film-coating polymers show that the following have a good solubility in water: HPMC, HPC, MC, PVP, PEG plus gastrointestinal fluids and the common organic solvents used in coating.

Acrylic polymers used for conventional film coating include methacrylate amino ester copolymers. These bcome water soluble by swelling, increasing permeability in aqueous media. The polymer in its unmodified form is however soluble only in organic solvents.

Where it is proposed to use an aqueous solvent for film coating it is necessary to consider, first, the need to minimize contact between the tablet core and water and, secondly, the need to achieve a reasonable process time. Both can be achieved by using the highest possible polymer concentration (i.e. the lowest possible water content). The limiting factor here is one of coating suspension viscosity.

2.6.2 Viscosity

HPMC coating polymers, for example, are available in a number of viscosity designations defined as the nominal viscosity of a 2%w/w aqueous solution at 20°C. Thus a 5mPa s grade will have a nominal viscosity of 5 mPa s in 2% aqueous solution in water at 20°C and similarly with 6 mPa s, 15 mPa s and 50 mPa s grades. Commercial nomenclature for these grades may still describe them as '5 cP' etc. Commercial designations such as E5 (Methocel) or 606 (Pharmacoat) also correspond with the viscosity designation, such that for example Methocel E5 has a nominal viscosity of 5mPa s under the previously described standard conditions. While Pharmacoat 606 would have a nominal viscosity of 6 mPa s under the same conditions.

Considering the final polymer solution to be sprayed, a normal HPMC-based system would have a viscosity of approximately 500 mPa s. Inspection of Fig. 2.3 shows that if, for instance, a 5 mPa s grade is used (E5) a solids concentration of about 15%w/w can be achieved. This has the advantage over, for example, a coating solution prepared from a 50 mPa s grade (E50) where only a 5%w/w solids concentration could be achieved. The lower viscosity grade polymer permits a higher solids concentration to be used, with consequent reduction in solvent content of the solution. The practical advantage to be gained is that the lower the solvent content of the solution, the shorter will be the processing time as less solvent has to be removed

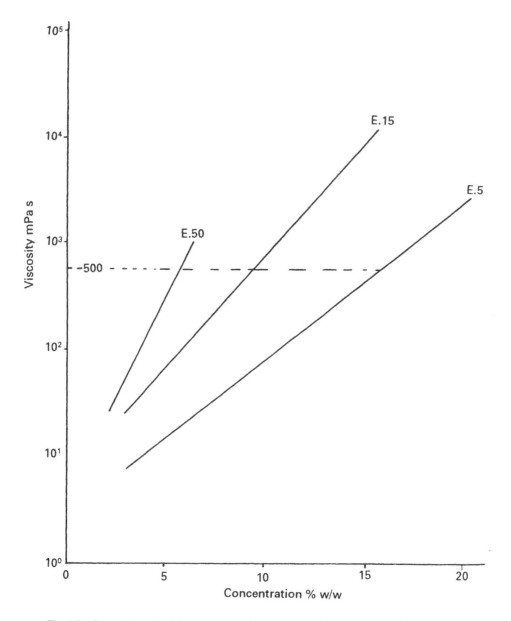

Fig. 2.3   Comparison of solution viscosity of three commercially available HPMC grades.

during the coating procedure. This beneficial interaction between polymer viscosity and possible coating solids is self-limiting in that very low viscosity polymers will suffer from poor film strength due to low molecular weight composition. Delporte (1980) has examined polymer solution viscosities in the 250–300 mPa s range and has concluded that 5 mPa s HPMC is preferable to the use of 15 mPa s material.

Furthermore, Delporte advocated the use of elevated temperature coating media in order to additionally increase solids loadings via a decrease in viscosity.

2.6.2   Permeability

One of the reasons for coating tablets is to provide a protection from the elements of the atmosphere such that a shelf-life advantage for the product may be gained.

With the continuing change from sugar- to film-based coating has come associated problems of stability due to sugar-coating techniques providing a better moisture barrier than that offered by simple non-functional cellulosics or acrylics. Usually the moisture permeability of a simple film may be decreased by the incorporation of water-insoluble polymers, however disintegration and dissolution characteristics of the dosage form must be carefully checked.

Permeability effects can be assessed practically by a technique of sealing a sample of cast film over a small container of desiccant or saturated salt solution, the permeability to water vapour being followed by successive weighings to determine respectively weight gain or weight loss (Hawes, 1978). In addition to being tedious to perform, the results are only comparable when performed under identical conditions. Using similar techniques Higuchi & Aguiar (1959) demonstrated that water vapour permeability of a polymer is dependent on the relative polarity of the polymer. Both Hawes (1978) and Delporte (1980) have seen little difference in water vapour permeability between two commercial grades of HPMC (E5 and E15) which differ only in molecular weight. Okhamafe & York (1983) have used an alternative method of assessing water vapour permeability, and that is a sorption-desorption technique to evaluate the performance of two film-forming polymers, HPMC (606) and polyvinyl alcohol (PVA). Addition of PVA to the HPMC was seen to enhance very effectively the moisture barrier effect of the HPMC. The authors ascribe this behaviour to the possible potentiation of the crystallinity of the HPMC by the PVA.

Sometimes permeability of other atmospheric gases is of concern, particularly that of oxygen. This area has been studied by Prater et al. (1982) who examined the permeability of oxygen through films of HPMC. These workers used a specially constructed cell which held a 21 mm diameter sample of the film. The passage of gas into the acceptor portion of the cell was monitored by using a mass spectrometer detection system. Earlier, Munden et al. (1964) had also determined oxygen permeability through free films of HPMC. They concluded that there was an inverse relationship between oxygen permeation and water vapour transmission. These results were obtained using a technique of sealing the films across a container of alkaline pyrogallol and measuring the consequent solution darkening. As Prater et al. (1982) point out, this method is not only tedious but water vapour from the pyrogallol is capable of plasticizing the film and modifying the result.

2.6.4   Mechanical properties

Some of the film mechanical properties of concern are:

- tensile strength
- modulus of elasticity

- work of failure
- strain.

To perform any function a film coat must be mechanically adequate so that in use it does not crack, split or generally fail. Also, during the rigours of the coating process itself the film is often relied upon for the provision of some mechanical strength to protect the tablet core from undue attrition.

These attributes may be conveniently measured by tensile tests on isolated films although other techniques such as indentation tests have a part to play. Much discussion has also taken place in the literature on the merits and validity of examining isolated films as opposed to examination of a film produced under the actual conditions of coating. Both arguments have been reviewed by Aulton (1982). Suffice it to say that much useful data can be obtained relatively easily from isolated films which, in practice, has demonstrated the validity of such techniques.

A typical stress–strain curve for a coating polymer is shown in Fig. 2.4. From this, several definitions become apparent:

- *Tensile strength*: The most important parameter here is the ultimate tensile strength, which is the maximum stress applied at the point at which the film breaks.

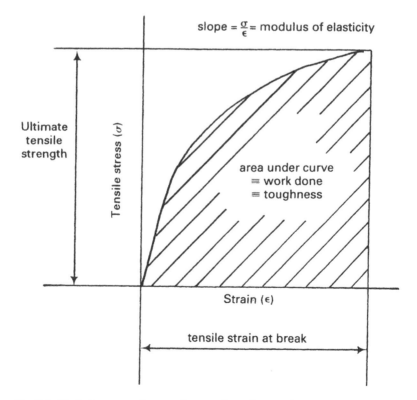

Fig. 2.4 Typical stress–strain curve for a coating polymer (after Aulton *et al.*, 1982).

- *Tensile strain at break*: A measure of how far the sample elongates prior to break.
- *Modulus (elastic modulus)*: This is applied stress divided by the corresponding strain in the region of linear elastic deformation. It can be regarded as an index of stiffness and rigidity of a film.
- *Work of failure*: This is numerically equivalent to the area under the curve and equates to the work done in breaking the film. It is an index of the toughness of a film and is a better measure of the film's ability to withstand a mechanical challenge than is a simple consideration of tensile strength.

Table 2.6 gives a comparison of some simple mechanical properties of a selection of film coating materials. All these properties of a polymer film are related to its molecular weight which, in turn, affects the viscosity of the polymer in solution. In general, apart from the acrylics, the different types of individual polymers are available in various commercial viscosity designations. These designations rely on the description of a standard solution in a specified solvent, as previously indicated.

The relationship between molecular weight and apparent viscosity of a polymer in solution can be summarized as follows:

$$MWT = K \, (\eta_{app})^k \tag{2.1}$$

where K and k are constants and η_{app} is the apparent viscosity. This equation, although useful, is empirical as the necessarily high concentrations needed for viscosity determination mean that significant molecular interaction will be taking place. Other equations can be used which take into account this interaction (Okhamafe & York, 1987).

Some techniques used for molecular weight determination rely on molecular mass for the result (M_w) while others provide data based on molecular numbers (M_n). An approximate index of molecular weight distribution can be obtained by dividing M_w by M_n—the higher the value, the wider the distribution.

It should be realized that polymer manufacturers achieve the correct viscosity for the specification by blending different polymer batches together. It therefore follows that different batches of the same viscosity grade of polymer may have substantially different ranges of molecular weights. Rowe (1980) quotes examples (Fig. 2.5) of how polymer grades of differing apparent viscosity have very similar peak molecular weights; the viscosity difference being accounted for by the fact that the higher viscosity grades possess rather more of a very high molecular weight fraction.

The effect of molecular weight on polymer mechanical properties is a well-understood phenomenon in polymer science and is not confined to tablet-coating polymers. Generally, as molecular weight increases so does the strength of the film. Ultimately a limiting value is reached, and Rowe (1980) has quoted this molecular weight value as $7-8 \times 10^4$ for the commonly used tablet-coating polymers. In addition, increases in polymer molecular weight result in the polymer film becoming successively more rigid owing to associated increases in the modulus of elasticity.

Table 2.6   Mechanical properties of polymers for film coating of drugs

	σ_R (N/mm^2)	ϵ_R (%)
Cellulose derivative		
HP-50	39	12
HP-55	33	6
CMEC (Duodcell)[d]	11	5
CAP + 25% DEP	16	14
Pharmacoat 606	44	13
Pharmacoat 603[e]	22	3
Methocel E5[e]	24	4
Poly(meth)acrylate		
MA-MMA 1:2 = Eudragit S100	52	3
MA-MMA 1:1 = Eudragit L100	24	1
MA-EA 1:1 = Eudragit L100-55[a]	10	14
Eudragit RS100[b]	5	40
Eudragit RL100[b]	5	22
Eudragit E100[b]	2	200
EA-MMA 1:1 = Eudragit E30D	8	600
Eudragit E30D/L30D 1:1	17	75
Eudragit E30D/L100 7:3[c]	7	410
Eudragit E30D/S100 7:3[c]	2	620
Eudragit E30D/E100-citrat 4:1	4	400
Eudragit E30D/E100-phosphat 4:1	5	360
Other polymers		
Polyvinylacetate phthalate[f]	31	5

Note: σ_R = tensile strength at break (after DIN 53455; ϵ_R = elongation at break).

[a] 10% PEG.   [d] 30% Glycerylmonocaprylate.
[b] 10% Triacetin   [e] 20% PEG.
[c] 10% Tween 80   [f] 10% Diethylphthalate.

2.6.5 Tackiness

In a film-coating sense, tack is a property of a polymer solution related to the forces necessary to separate two parallel surfaces joined by a thin film of the solution. It is a property responsible for processing difficulties and is a limitation on the use of some polymers, e.g. hydroxypropyl cellulose (Porter & Bruno, 1990) and certain polymers intended for enteric use, e.g. Eudragit L30D and PVAP. Kovacs & Merenyi (1990) examined several polymers using a technique combining measure-

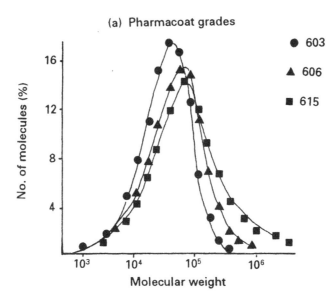

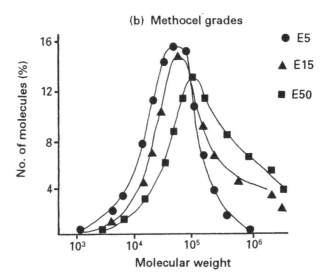

Fig. 2.5   Molecular weight distribution for various grades of HPMC.

ment of the force necessary to remove a probe from a film together with a time element. On changing from Pharmacoat 603 to the 606 grade, the tack value was seen to change by an order of magnitude. For a series of hydroxy ethylcelluloses the tack was seen to increase greatly for small increases in concentration. Eudragit L100-55 was demonstrated to have a low order of tack.

2.7 PLASTICIZERS

Plasticizers are simply relatively low molecular weight materials which have the capacity to alter the physical properties of a polymer to render it more useful in performing its function as a film-coating material. Generally the effect will be to make it softer and more pliable. There are often chemical similarities between a polymer and its plasticizer—for instance, glycerol and propylene glycol, which are plasticizers for several cellulosic systems, possess —OH groups, a feature in common with the polymer.

It is generally considered that the mechanism of action for a plasticizer is for the plasticizer molecules to interpose themselves between the individual polymer strands thus breaking down to a large extent polymer–polymer interactions. This action is facilitated as the polymer–plasticizer interaction is considered to be stronger than the polymer–polymer interaction. Hence, the polymer strands now have a greater opportunity to move past each other. Using this model it can be visualized how a plasticizer is able to transform a polymer into a more pliable material.

Most of the polymers used in film coating are either amorphous or have very little crystallinity. Strongly crystalline polymers are difficult to plasticize in this fashion as disruption of their intermolecular structure is not an easy matter. Experimentally, the effect of a plasticizer on a polymeric system can be demonstrated in many ways; for instance, isolated film work using tensile or indentation methods will reveal significant changes in mechanical properties between the plasticized and unplasticized states.

One fundamental property of a polymer which can be determined by several techniques is the glass transition temperature (T_g). This is the temperature at which a polymer changes from a hard glassy material to a softer rubbery material. The action of a plasticizer is to lower the glass transition temperature. The transition can be followed by examining the temperature dependence of such properties as modulus of elasticity, film hardness, specific heat, etc. These properties will be expanded on later. Sakellariou *et al.* (1986a) have utilized a dynamic mechanical method, namely torsion braid analysis, to characterize the effect of PEGs on HPMC and ethylcellulose.

2.7.1 Classification

The commonly used plasticizers can be categorized into three groups:

1. *Polyols*
   (a) glycerol (glycerin);
   (b) propylene glycol;
   (c) polyethylene glycols PEG (generally the 200–6000 grades).

2. *Organic esters*
   (a) phthalate esters (diethyl, dibutyl);
   (b) dibutyl sebacete;
   (c) citrate esters (triethyl, acetyl triethyl, acetyl tributyl);
   (d) triacetin.

3. *Oils/glycerides*
   (a) castor oil;
   (b) acetylated monoglycerides;
   (c) fractionated coconut oil.

2.7.2   Compatibility and permanence
It follows from what has been described above regarding plasticizer–polymer inter-actions that one attribute of an efficient platicizer could be that it acts as a good solvent for the polymer in question. Indeed, Entwistle & Rowe (1979) have used this as a measure of plasticizer efficiency. They found a correlation between the intrin-sic viscosity of the polymer/plasticizer solutions and the mechanical attributes of polymer films plasticized with the specified plasticizers—the mechanical properties of tensile strength, elongation at rupture and work of failure being at a minimum when the intrinsic viscosity of the polymer/plasticizer solution was at a maximum.

With the predominance today of aqueous-based film coating there is a concentra-tion on those plastizers with an appreciable water miscibility. This includes the polyols and, to a lesser extent, triacetin and triethylcitrate. Glycerol has the added advantage that its regulatory acceptance for food supplement products (e.g. vitamin and mineral tablets) is greater than for other plasticizers in those parts of the world where this type of product is covered by food legislation. Permanence of the more volatile plasticizers, e.g. diethylphthalate (DEP), can be a problem with organic solvent-based processing and likewise in the aqueous field utilizing propylene glycol as the plasticizer. Permanence is an attribute to be taken into consideration as loss of plasticizer, for instance during storage of the coated tablets, could have serious consequences on the integrity of the dosage form. One such consequence could lead to the cracking of the coating under inappropriate storage. These considerations are of much greater significance in the realm of functional coatings. Permanence is obviously related to plasticizer volatility, however a change to a more non volatile plasticizer by changing to a higher molecular weight plasticizer is not always an advantageous move. An example here would be the change from a low molecular PEG to a high molecular PEG such as the 6000 grade. This move has unfortunately brought with it a change to a less effective plasticizer. Regarding losses during processing, Skultety & Sims (1987) have shown that, in a statistically based study to determine the factors involved in the loss of propylene glycol during the coating process, values of 81–96% of theoretical were shown. The only independent variable in the study having an effect was the initial concentration of propylene glycol. On the other hand, no loss was seen when either glycerol or PEG was used as the plasticizer.

The possibility of plasticizer migration should also be considered. Conceivably this can occur in two ways:

● migration into the tablet core.
● migration into packaging materials.

A related phenomena is the migration of materials from the tablet core into the film coating which may themselves have a plasticizer-like action on the polymer used. Abdul-Razzak (1983) demonstrated the migration of several salicylic acid derivatives into an ethylcellulose film coating where the derivatives concerned possessed plasticizer activity for ethylcellulose. Later, Okhamafe & York (1989) examined the effect of ephedrine hydrochloride on both HPMC and PVA. This drug was shown to display strong plasticizer characteristics for both polymers, namely a decrease in softening temperature T_g, crystallinity and melting point. Again, the consequences of this are rather more serious with functional than non-functional coatings, as the pharmaceutical performance of the film could be compromised.

2.7.3 Effect of plasticizers on the mechanical properties of the film
This can be quite profound and capable of making significant alterations to its properties, either advantageously or adversely. These have been well documented in the literature.

With reference to Fig. 2.6, these changes in relation to tensile properties can be summarized as follows:

- Increase in strain or film elongation
- Decrease in elastic modulus
- Decrease in tensile strength.

Returning to the earlier proposed mechanism of plasticizer action, it can be seen that as a plasticizer interacts with a polymer the structure of that polymer will be modified so as to permit increased segmental movement. The tertiary structure of the polymer will therefore be altered in such a way as to give a more porous, flexible and less cohesive structure. When a plasticized polymer is subjected to a tensile force it can be seen that this structure would be less resilient and would deform at a lower force than without the plasticizer.

Aulton *et al.* (1981) have utilized an 'Instron' materials tester to evaluate the effect of a series of plasticisers on the mechanical properties of cast films of HPMC (Methocel E5). Of particular interest was the finding that low molecular weight PEG was a more efficient plasticizer for this polymer than corresponding high molecular weight grades (Fig. 2.7). The authors also examined films using the technique of indentation. This showed that the introduction of plasticizer to the polymer film promoted increasing viscoelastic behaviour in the polymer. Indentation studies at low and high humidity also provided experimental evidence for the plasticizing effect of water on HPMC films. Porter (1980) and Delporte (1981) are in general agreement with the findings of Aulton *et al.* (1981) and, interestingly, Porter used a technique whereby the film for investigation was obtained by spraying and not by casting. Okhamafe & York (1983) have also studied the effects of PEG and HPMC films. Again they are in agreement with the findings of Aulton *et al.* (1981) in that PEG 400 was preferable to PEG 1000. This view was also held by Entwistle & Rowe (1979) using their technique involving polymer/plasticizer solution viscosity determination. Okhamafe & York (1983) also showed that polyvinyl alcohol (PVA) had a quantitatively different effect on HPMC to that displayed by the PEGs. PVA decreases to a lesser degree, the decrease seen in tensile strength and the increase seen in elongation compared with the PEGs. The authors postulate an increasing crystallinity as a result of PVA addition to the film. It is also noted from the results

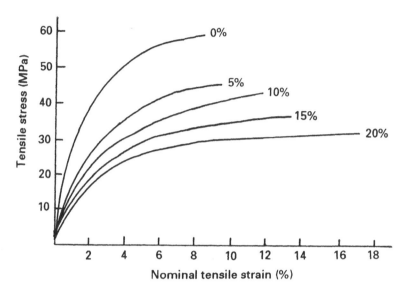

Fig. 2.6   Stress–strain curves for HPMC films containing different concentrations of
glycerol (0–20%) (after Aulton *et al.*, 1981).

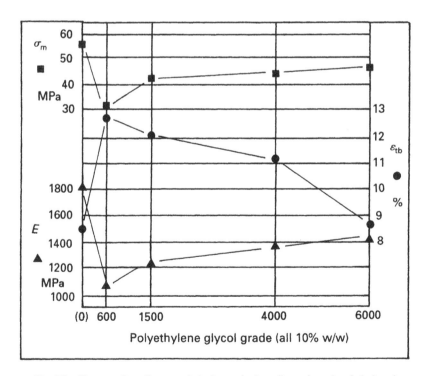

Fig. 2.7   Changes of tensile strength (σ_m), nominal tensile strain at break (ε_{tb}) and
modulus of elasticity (E) of HPMC films with change in grade of added polyethyleneglycol.

that the elongation effect obtained by the addition of PEG and PVA to the films exhibits anisotropy. The authors speculate as to whether this is a real effect or whether it is due to the experimental protocol.

Dechesne and Jaminet (1985) have studied the mechanical properties of cellulose acetate phthalate when plasticized by triacetin, DEP and Citroflex A2 in a statistically designed study. One interesting feature was that triacetin was shown to be a very potent plasticizer for CAP. A practical point of significance is the ability of plasticizers to lower the residual internal stress within a film coating. This is accomplished by the effect of the plasticizer on the modulus of elasticity of the film (Rowe, 1981). This aspect will be dealt with in greater detail in the problem-solving section, Chapter 13.

Another important point is that film coatings which confer a modified release effect on the dosage form need to be mechanically tough in order that the coating is not inadvertently damaged during normal handling. Dechesne et al. (1982) emphasized the activity of plasticizers in their investigation of the effect that different plasticizers have on the diametral crushing strength of, in this case, sodium fluoride tablets. At an application level of 10 mg of Eudragit L30D/cm^2 for example, considerable differences were evident in the behaviour of six different plasticizers. Crushing strengths of approximately 4.75 kg were recorded employing dibutyl phthalate compared with a value of almost 10 kg when propylene glycol was used.

2.7.4 Effect of plasticizers on permeability of film coatings

Occasionally it is required to optimize the permeability characteristics of a film in order to use the film coat to retard the entry of water vapour or other gases into the dosage form. This is another area in which plasticizers have a part to play. The transport of a permeant across a barrier is defined by Crank's relationship (see Okhamafe & York, 1983)

$$P = D{\cdot}S \tag{2.2}$$

where P, D and S are the permeability, diffusion and solubility coefficients respectively of the film coating. It can be envisaged that the passage of a permeant across the film is governed by two steps:

1. Dissolution of the permeant in the film material.
2. Diffusion of the permeant across the film.

In turn, this later process can take place by the permeant diffusing through the polymer matrix itself and/or diffusion through voids containing either true liquids or vapours. It follows, therefore, that as a plasticizer has the capacity to alter the structure of a polymer, these materials will have the ability to alter the permeability characteristics of a film coating. The above authors have determined the diffusion coefficients for water through HPMC films plasticized with PEG 400 and 1000, and in both cases an increase was observed. Previously Porter (1980) and Delporte (1981) had been unable to demonstrate any significant effect with PEG.

2.7.5   Measurement and characterization of plasticizer activity

Thermal method

This method has proved ideally suited to investigate plasticizer activity, in particular determination of the glass transition temperature, T_g. This attribute of a polymer is readily detected as an endotherm prior to the endotherm resulting from melting or decomposition. Other endotherms may be seen usually at lower temperatures, resulting from loss of solvent from the polymer.

Using these techniques several authors have demonstrated correlations between plasticizer concentration and degree of lowering of T_g (Porter & Ridgway, 1983; Dechesne *et al.*, 1984).

Thermomechanical analysis

Like DSC this method has the useful feature that actual plasticized films can be used for the determination. Using the technique (Fig. 2.8) a film sample is placed in a holder, and at the commencement of the experiment a weighted stylus is brought into contact with the specimen. Indentation of the stylus into the specimen as the temperature is gradually raised is followed by an LVDT. The temperature rise of the specimen is accompanied by changes in the polymer structure, which are reflected by movement of the LVDT trace. Hence changes due to softening, melting decomposition and glass transitions can be readily followed (Fig. 2.9) (see also Masilungan & Lordi 1984; Majeed, 1984).

Mechanical methods

Mention has already been made of tensile and indentation methods. Depending on the area of interest, such parameters as decrease in tensile strength, increase in strain (elongation) or changes in the modulus of elasticity with changes in plasticizer concentration can be followed. Sinko & Amidon (1989) have used low strain elongational creep compliance to analyse the intrinsic mechanical response of films of Eudragit S100 with different plasticizers. They studied plasticizer-induced changes on the rate of mechanical response as solvent leaves the film and the polymer passes through a rubber to glass transition. Using a free volume analysis, a plasticizing effectiveness term was calculated for the plasticizers used in this study. This showed, for instance, that for Eudragit S100 films, dibutyl phthalate is a more efficient plasticizer than PEG 200.

Solubility methods

These methods usually rely on a consideration of the solubility parameter.

In order for a polymer to dissolve in a solvent (plasticizer) the Gibbs free energy of mixing, ΔG, must be negative:

$$\Delta G = \Delta H - T \cdot \Delta S \qquad (2.3)$$

where ΔH is the heat of mixing, T the absolute temperature and ΔS the entropy of mixing.

Okhamafe & York (1987) have demonstrated how ΔH may be obtained from the following relationship due to Hildebrand and Scott (1950):

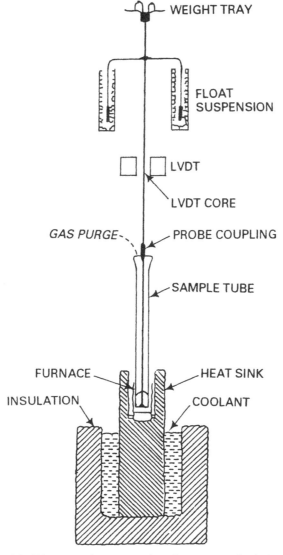

Fig. 2.8   Diagrammatic representation of a thermomechanical analyser
(after Majeed, 1984).

$$\Delta H = V_m \left[\left(\frac{\Delta E_1}{V_1} \right)^{1/2} - \left(\frac{\Delta E_2}{V_2} \right)^{1/2} \right]^2 \phi_1 . \phi_2$$

(2.4)

where V_m is the total volume of the mixture, ΔE the energy of vaporization of component 1 or 2, V the molar volume of component 1 or 2 and ϕ the volume fraction of component 1 or 2. The term $\Delta E/V$ is generally referred to as the cohesive

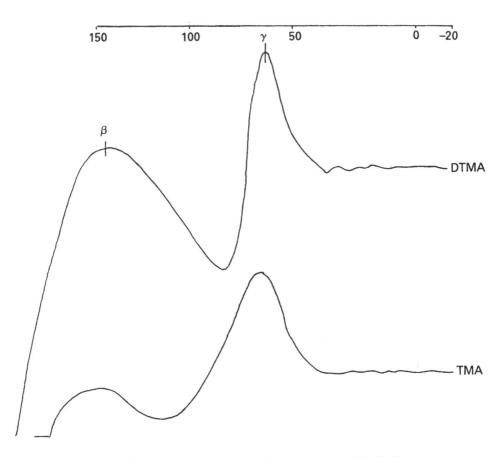

Fig. 2.9   Typical trace of thermomechanical analyser on an HPMC film
(after Majeed, 1984).

energy density (CED) and its square-root as the solubility parameter, δ. Equation (2.4) can then take the following form:

$$\Delta H = V_{\mathrm{m}}\,(\delta_1 - \delta_2)^2\,\phi_1 \cdot \phi_2 \tag{2.5}$$

From equation (2.5), if δ_1 and δ_2 are the same, the heat of mixing will be zero, which will be a state of maximum compatibility between polymer and plasticizer (see also Sakellariou *et al.*, 1986b). This approach, of course, can be used not only for polymer compatibility with plasticizers but also with solvents.

2.8   COLOURANTS/OPACIFIERS

This group of materials are commonly used as ingredients in film-coating formulae. They obviously contribute to the aesthetic appeal of the product, but they also enhance the product in other ways:

● Identification of the product by the manufacturer and therefore act as an aid (not a replacement) for existing GMP procedures. Colourants also aid in the identification of individual products by patients, particularly those taking multiple medication.

● They reinforce brand imaging by a manufacturer and thereby decrease the risk of counterfeiting.

● Colourants for film-coated tablets have to a greater or lesser extent opacifying properties which are useful when it is desired to optimize the ability of the coating to protect the active ingredient against the action of light.

2.8.1 Classification

Organic dyes and their lakes
This group would include such materials as Sunset Yellow, Patent Blue V, Quinoline Yellow, etc. As water solubles their use is extremely restricted regarding the colouring of any form of coated tablet. However, their water-insoluble complexes with hydrated alumina, known as lakes, are in widespread use as colours for coated tablets. The reason for this will be considered in the appropriate section below.

In the laking process a substratum of hydrated alumina is produced by reacting aluminium chloride with sodium carbonate. The appropriate dye in aqueous solution is then adsorbed onto the prepared alumina hydrate. Finally additional aluminium chloride is added to ensure complete formation of the aluminium salt of the dye. Filtration and washing of the product complete the process.

Inorganic colours
Stability towards light is an important characteristic displayed by these materials, some of which have a useful opacifying capacity, e.g. titanium dioxide. Another great advantage of inorganic colours is their wide regulatory acceptance, making them most useful for multinational companies wishing to standardize international formulae. One drawback to their use is that the range of colours that can be achieved is rather limited.

Natural colours
This is a chemically and physically diverse group of materials. The description 'natural' is of necessity loose, as some of these colours are the products of chemical synthesis rather than extraction from a natural source, e.g. β-carotene of commerce is regularly synthetic in origin. The term frequently applies to such materials is 'nature identical', which in many ways is more descriptive. Some would even make the case that any product which is not a constituent of the normal diet should not be called 'natural'. This viewpoint would remove colours such as cochineal and annatto from consideration. As a generalization, natural colours are not as stable to light as the other groups of colours; their tinctorial powers are not high and they tend to be more expensive than other forms of colour. They do, however, possess a regulatory advantage in that they have a wide acceptability. Even with these advantages their penetration into the pharmaceutical area has not been great.

Examples of colours:

Organic dyes and their lakes
* Sunset Yellow
* Tartrazine
* Erythrosine.

Inorganic colours
* Titanium dioxide
* Iron oxide yellow, red and black
* Talc.

Natural colours
* Riboflavine
* Carmine
* Anthocyanins.

2.8.2   Regulatory aspects and specifications

Pharmaceutical colours are unusual in that, in most parts of the world, they are subject to requirements over and above normal pharmacopoeial specifications. For example, within the EU they must meet certain purity requirements laid down by current European Union Directives. Likewise, in the United States, the Code of Federal Regulations imposes its own set of purity criteria. Countries can and frequently do differ in the colours that are permitted in pharmaceutical preparations. Specialist publications exist which should be consulted in case of doubt (e.g. Anon., 1993).

2.8.3   Advantages of pigments over dyes

Previously it had been indicated that water-soluble colours were technically inferior to water-insoluble (pigments) colours. The reasons for this are given below.

Migration

Drying is an integral part of the coating process and, as a consequence, water will leave the film coat continuously as the coat is formed. If the colour is in the form of insoluble particles, then no migration takes place. However, a water-soluble colour tends to follow the escaping water molecules to the tablet surface and produce a mottled finish to the coating.

Opacity

Pigments are much more opaque than dyes, hence they offer a much greater measure of protection against light than dye-coloured film coats.

Colour stability

Edible colours for medicinal products have an established use by virtue of their low order of toxicity. Some of their technical attributes, for example colour stability, can represent somewhat of a compromise. In general the inorganic pigments, e.g. iron oxides, have an excellent stability while the synthetic organic dyes are much less satisfactory in this respect. The lake forms of many of the synthetic organic dyes, however, provide a degree of improvement in this respect.

Permeability
Pigments decrease the permeability of films to water vapour and oxygen thereby offering the possibilities of increased shelf-life.

Coating solids
Pigments contribute to the total solids of a coating suspension without significantly contributing to the viscosity of the system. Thus faster processing times by virtue of more rapid drying is possible. This is particularly significant with aqueous-based processes.

Anti-tack activity
Tack is a concept that is widely used to describe the forces involved in the separation of two parallel surfaces separated by a thin film of liquid. Such considerations are important during the coating process as excess tack can cause troublesome adhesion of tablets to each other or to the coating vessel. Since the early days of film coating it has been appreciated that solid inclusions, including pigments, in the formula have a part to play in combating the effects of tack. Chopra & Tawashi (1985) have quantified the action of titanium dioxide, talc and indigo carmine lake on the tackiness of coating polymer solutions. They have shown that, at high polymer concentrations, increasing the pigment concentration and decreasing the pigment particle size, reduced the effect of tack, whereas at low polymer concentration only talc was effective in reducing tack. Alternative methods of tack evaluation have been utilized by other workers such as Massoud & Bauer (1989) and Wan & Lai (1992).

2.8.4   Effects of pigments on film-coating systems
Because of their very diverse nature it can be expected that the effects of pigments on film-coating systems can be rather complex.

Mechanical effects
In general, the presence of pigments will reduce the tensile strength of a film, increase the elastic modulus and decrease the extension of the film under a tensile load. All of these are, of course, negative effects. However, as pigments consist of discrete individual particles the need for efficient pigment dispersion should be emphasized. Another generalization is that the lower the particle size of the pigment concerned, the smaller will be the deleterious effect on film properties. These effects are of some importance in the consideration of stress-related film-coating defects. Lehmann & Dreher (1981) describe the property displayed by several of the acrylic film-coating polymers, that of being able to bind substantially higher quantities of pigment than is possible for example with the cellulosics. The authors point to the advantages of mechanical stability and resistance to attrition achieved.

Aulton *et al.* (1984) have examined the effect of a wide range of pigments on the mechanical properties of cast films of HPMC (Methocel E5). In addition to confirming the general effects above, they emphasized the need to consider the whole stress–strain diagram and not to merely one feature in isolation. For instance, a pigmented film may well show very little decrease in tensile strength compared with the unpigmented film; however, a consideration of the area under the curve could show significant differences (Fig. 2.10). The term 'work of rupture' was coined by the authors for this particular parameter. In comparing the effects of different pigments the authors concluded that there were pigment-specific effects and that the pigment was not merely occupying space in an inert manner or behaving as an inert diluent. The pigment effect has also been discussed by Rowe (1982) in a study on the effect of pigments on edge splitting of tablet film coats. Talc was seen to be an exception to the general behaviour of pigments. The reason postulated was that as talc exists as flakes it orientates itself parallel to the surface of the substrate in a restraint on volume shrinkage of the film parallel to the plane of coating (Fig. 2.11).

In another study, Okhamafe & York (1985a) have looked at the mechanical properties stated above for free films in combination with PVA or PEG 1000 and loaded with talc or titanium dioxide. Broadly, the results were in agreement with the findings of Aulton *et al.* (1984). The results were presented not only in mechanical terms but polymer–pigment interactions were also taken into account in either rein-

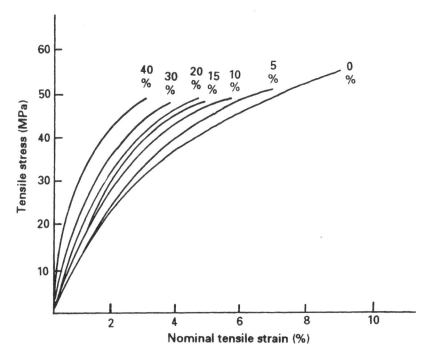

Fig. 2.10   Stress–strain curves for cast HPMC films loaded with titanium dioxide. The figures on the curves refer to the TiO_2 concentration (%w/w) in the dried films.

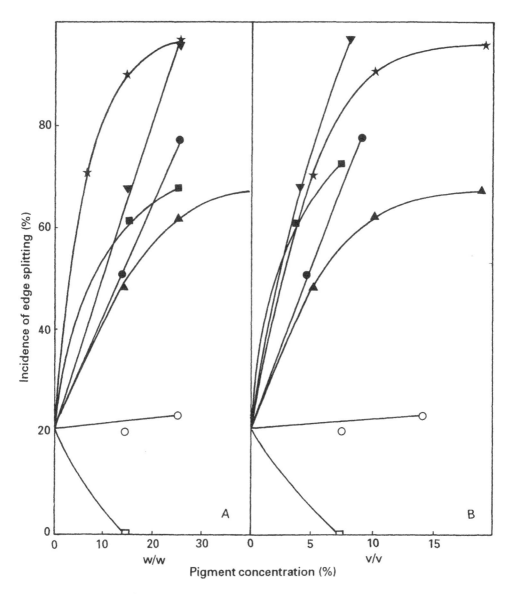

Fig. 2.11   The effect of both pigment weight and volume concentration on the incidence of edge splitting. ★ Carmosine lake; ▼ black iron oxide; ■ red iron oxide; ● yellow iron oxide; ▲ titanium dioxide; ○ calcium carbonate; □ talc.

forcing the mechanical effect or working against it. For example, in the case of high pigment–polymer interaction, the loss of film elongation was greatly potentiated.

The same authors, in further work (1985b), have examined the effect of pigmented and unpigmented films on the adhesion of those films to the surfaces of aspirin tablets. They found that pigments incorporated in an applied film can exert two opposing effects on adhesion: one decreases adhesion by increasing internal stress and the other increases adhesion by strengthening the film–tablet surface interation. From the results obtained, the adhesion of HPMC films was initially increased in the presence of talc because of a stronger film–tablet interface and a smaller increase in the internal stress of the film, but above 10% by weight of the pigment, the internal stress factor began to dominate and adhesion fell.

In a large comparative study (Gibson *et al.*, 1988), the effect of the iron oxide pigments titanium dioxide, talc, erythrosine lake, and sunset yellow lake were examined upon HPMC (Pharmacoat 606) films plasticized with PEG 200. The authors concluded that the Young's modulus of the films is raised by the pigments to an extent that largely depends upon pigment shape and can be predicted by existing theories. The exceptions are titanium dioxide and the lake pigments which have less of an effect on the modulus than expected due to polymer–pigment interactions or, in the case of the lake pigments, to a loose particle structure. The ultimate tensile properties of the films depend mainly on the concentration of the particles added. Pigments cause a large decrease in tensile strength except in the cases of yellow or black iron oxides which are not weakened to such an extent because the shape of the particles allows the growth of flaws to be retarded. If the thermal expansion coefficients of the matrix and filler promote premature cracking on cooling from the fabrication temperature, then the introduction of filler in any concentration is detrimental to the tensile strength of the system.

Considerations of opacity

One of the main functions of a pigment in a film is to provide opacity. This may be for aesthetic reasons where there is a need to cover possible batch to batch variations in visual appearance, or there may be reasons of stability where an opaque film coating is required to prevent degradation of an active substance by light. If Fig. 2.12 is considered, it can be seen that there are several ways in which light can interact with a pigmented film coating, and of greatest interest are

- light reflected at the film/pigment boundary
- light absorbed by the pigment particles.

Regarding the amount of light reflected at pigment–polymer interface, the refractive indices of both materials have a fundamental part to play in that the magnitude of the difference largely determines the film's ability to reflect light. Rowe (1983) quotes the following equation linking the two

$$R = \left[\frac{\eta_1 - \eta_2}{\eta_1 + \eta_2} \right]^2 \tag{2.6}$$

where R is the amount of light reflected and η_1 and η_2 are the refractive indices of the pigment and the polymer respectively. It can be seen that if $\eta_1 = \eta_2$, then R will be zero and the film will have no opacity. However, if $\eta_1 \neq \eta_2$ then the greater this difference, the greater will be the opacity of the film. Rowe (1984a) provides an in-depth treatment on the theory of opacity by utilizing the Mie theory and the Kubelka-Munk equation.

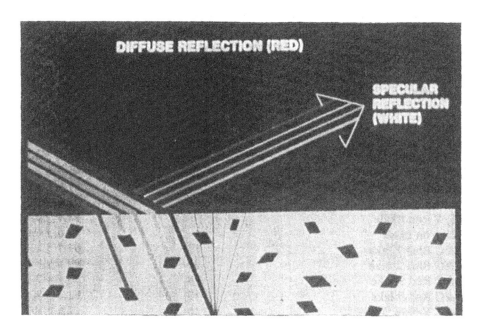

Fig. 2.12   The interaction of incident light with a tablet film coating.

The wavelength of the light absorbed by a pigment, of course, gives rise to its characteristic colour. For example, red pigment reflects predominantly in the red part of the visible spectrum and absorbs the remainder of the incident light. The quantity of light actually absorbed is determined by the index of absorption. An ideal black pigment will have a very high index of absorption and will function as an extremely efficient opacifying agent by virtue of the fact that it will be a near perfect absorber of light.

Contrast ratio
This function is practically used to quantify the opacifying efficiency of an opaque film. It may be defined as the ratio of light reflected when the test film is placed over a black background compared to the situation where the film is placed over a white background multiplied by 100.

Inspection of Table 2.7 shows considerable variation in the contrast ratios of the commonly used pigments. For instance, talc with a value of 46.4 is shown to be relatively poor in comparison with the iron oxide pigments and titanium dioxide. As would be expected, there is a relationship linking contrast ratio and thickness of film. The Fell relationship states that the logarithm of the contrast ratio is proportional to the reciprocal of film thickness. Rowe (1984a) has pointed out the usefulness of this as a Fell plot can be extrapolated to 100% opacity and the requisite thickness so obtained. The information shown in Table 2.8 actually expresses opacity in terms of 'hiding power', which is the difference of the two reflective terms defined above rather than their ratio.

Table 2.7   The effect of pigment and filler type on the opacity of tablet film coatings (pigment/filler concentration 16% w/w dry film) (after Rowe, 1984b).

Pigment/filler	Dye content	Contrast ratio (%)
No filler	—	33.3 ± 3.8
Calcium carbonate	—	46.7 ± 3.3
Calcium sulphate	—	46.8 ± 3.2
Talc	—	46.4 ± 2.2
Titanium dioxide	—	91.6 ± 1.2
Red iron oxide	—	99.5 ± 0.2
Yellow iron oxide	—	98.4 ± 0.8
Black iron oxide	—	99.6 ± 0.6
FD&C Blue 2 lake	13	97.5 ± 1.1
FD&C Blue 2 lake	30	99.5 ± 0.3
FD&C Red 3 lake	18	70.1 ± 3.3
FD&C Red 3 lake	39	81.3 ± 4.1
FD&C Yellow 5 lake	16	62.9 ± 3.5
FD&C Yellow 5 lake	25	65.2 ± 3.8
FD&C Yellow 5 lake	37	66.7 ± 3.3
FD&C Yellow 6 lake	17	73.2 ± 3.6
FD&C Yellow 6 lake	39	78.1 ± 3.1

An example of contrast ratio theory providing an explanation of expermental results is demonstrated by the findings of Nyqvist *et al.* (1982). These workers showed that the sensitivity towards light of research compound FLA 336(+) was more effectively combated by a coating containing yellow iron oxide compared with one containing titanium dioxide; in other words, by using a pigment with the higher contrast ratio.

Permeability effects
It has long been appreciated that pigments have a significant part to play in the modification of the permeability of a film. Chatfield (1962) propounded a theory to account for the passage of water vapour through films containing increasing loadings of pigments. At low pigment volume concentrations the passage of permeant through the film is decreased with increasing pigment volume concentration. At a point known as the critical pigment volume concentration, a limiting value is reached and for increasing quantities of pigment, an increase in permeability is observed (see Fig. 2.13). Chatfield ascribed this behaviour to the fact that at low pigment volume concentrations the presence of pigment particles acted as a barrier to permeation. This effect would increase with increasing content of pigment until the point was reached when there was insufficient polymer to bind the pigment particles. This situation would be characterized by a film where poor interaction

Table 2.8   Relative hiding power of coloured film coatings

Colour classification	Colour	TiO$_2$:colourant volume ratio	Colourants used[a]	Relative hiding power (DL values at stated film thickness		
				9.5 μm	19.1 μm	38.1 μm
Dark	Brown	1:10	Y6,B2,R3	−0.82	−0.23	−0.16
	Orange	1:7	Y6,R40	−14.79	−12.53	−2.99
Medium	Maroon	1:3.5	B1,R3,R40, Y6	−0.23	−0.18	−0.01
Dark	Purple	1:5	R3,B1	0.09	0.06	0.00
	Red	1:5.5	Y6,B2,R3	−5.63	—	−1.49
	Yellow	1:4.5	Y10,Y6	−11.61	−3.13	−1.79
Medium	Green	1:1	B1,Y5	−0.01	0.05	0.10
	Green	2:1	B1,Y10,Y6	−2.18	−0.51	−0.29
	Purple	1.5:1	B2,R7	−2.17	0.46	0.12
	Orange	1.5:1	Y10,Y6	−1.47	−1.16	−1.38
	Blue	1:1.5	B2	—	0.07	0.16
Light	Beige	6:1	Y2,B2	−1.06	−0.78	−0.48
	Blue	10:1	B2	−0.95	−0.44	−0.26
	Pink	20:1	R7	−0.61	−0.50	−0.10
Oxide	Beige	6.5:1	R10,Y10, B10	−0.10	−0.00	0.47
	Beige	18.5:1	R10,Y10	−0.37	0.08	0.16

[a] *Key:*   B1 – FD&C Blue #1 Lake   Y10 – D&C Yellow #10 Lake
              B2 – FD&C Blue #2 Lake   R40 – FD&C Red #40 Lake
              R3 – FD&C Red #3 Lake   R10 – Red iron oxide
              Y5 – FD&C Yellow #5 Lake   Y10 – Yellow iron oxide
              Y6 – FD&C Yellow #6 Lake   B10 – Brown iron oxide
              R7 – D&C Red #7 Lake

existed between polymer and pigment, resulting in many cracks; fissures and discontinuities. Such a film would readily permit the transmission of water vapour and other gases.

Several authors have pointed out that as the Chatfield theory assumes perfect spheres for the pigment particles then it has its limitations for predicting behaviour in pigmented films. Nielsen (1967) has proposed a tortuosity factor which would take into account the shape of the particles.

Okhamafe & York (1985a) propose that the Chatfield and Nielsen hypotheses will be unsuitable for predicting moisture permeation because both hypotheses assume perfect polymer–filler interaction, a situation rarely achieved. The lower the

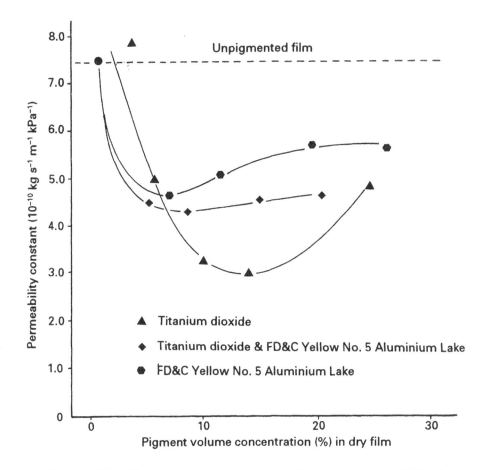

Fig. 2.13   Effect of pigment volume concentration on the water-vapour permeability of
HPMC E5 films at 30°C, 75% r. h. (after Porter, 1980).

degree of polymer–filler interaction, the larger and more numerous will be the voids
at the interface. They illustrate this point by considerng talcs of different surface
area and a titanium dioxide grade which had been surface treated.

2.9   SOLVENTS/VEHICLES

These materials perform a necessary function in that they provide the means of
conveying the coating materials to the surface of the tablet or particle. The major
classes of solvents capable of being used are:

- water
- alcohols
- ketones
- esters
- chlorinated hydrocarbons.

A prerequisite for a solvent would be that it has to interact well with the chosen polymer; this is needed as high polymer solvent interaction permits film properties such as adhesion and mechanical strength to be optimized. Selection of the correct solvent can be predicted by a thermodynamic approach as described in section 2.7.5.

Kent & Rowe (1978) utilized the solubility parameter approach in evaluating the use of ethylcellulose in various solvents for film coating. By evaluating the effect of solubility parameter on intrinsic viscosity for a range of solvents graded as to the extent of hydrogen bonding, they were able to determine not only which was the best class of solvent to use but also what was the optimum solvent solubility parameter. Rowe (1986) has pointed out that ideally for this use the solubility parameter needs modification to take into account components due to van der Waals' forces, hydrogen bonding and polarity. Thus, using a modification proposed by Hansen (1967), Rowe has produced solubility parameter maps to evaluate the compatibility of ethylcellulose in admixture with methylcellulose and HPMC.

Considering polymer solvents in a wider sense, a thermodynamically based compatibility is not the only practical requirement. Kinetic considerations of the ability of the solvent to penetrate the polymer mass effectively and solvate the polymer in such a way that polymer swelling and dissolution take place effectively are also very important. Thermodynamically good solvents do not always make kinetically good solvents, and vice-versa. Hence the choice of a suitable solvent selected on the above criteria is likely to be a process of compromise.

Another practical feature is that the chosen solvent should not pose volatility problems. Besides causing processing difficulties, the controlled deposition of coating materials to form a coherent film coat could be compromised.

The use of solvent mixtures should be fully validated. The problem here is that during the coating process preferential evaporation of solvents from the mixture is liable to take place (unless, of course, a constant boiling mixture is used). An extreme example would be that as a result, polymer precipitation would occur with no film-formation. At the least, polymer solubility could be affected to the extent that film-forming ability would suffer. This problem has been described by Spitael & Kinget (1977) in considering the effect of processing solvent on the film-forming property of cellulose acetate phthalate. Using three different methods of preparing films they demonstrated that entire films were formed only with certain solvents or combinations. For example, only two solvents gave consistently good results, namely acetone and the azeotropic mixture of 77% ethyl acetate and 23% isopropanol. The other solvents, which were 1:1 mixtures of ethyl acetate with isopropanol and acetone with ethanol, gave opaque, brittle films which lacked cohesiveness. Less than optimal film-forming conditions for a functional film such as this would have serious consequences.

2.10 AUXILIARY SUBSTANCES IN THE FILM-COATING FORMULAE

Mention has already been made of the occasional addition of substances such as flavours and waxes to film-coating formulae. In recent times there has emerged a new class of auxiliary substances which, when combined with the traditional ingredients of a film-coating formula, show advantageous properties. These are saccharide materals such as polydextrose, maltodextrin and lactose. Perhaps their most remarkable property is to increase the adhesion of cellulosic systems to substrates. Jordan *et al.* (1992) have quoted examples where lactose–HPMC combinations under defined conditions demonstrated an adhesive force of 40 kN/m^2 for a waxy tablet core where an HPMC–HPC combination measured only 26 kN/m^2 and a simple HPMC coating failed to show any measurable adhesion to the core. These saccharide–cellulosic combinations have also been shown to improve the stability towards light of several unstable colours used as film-coating colourants. As yet, the mechanism of action of these auxiliary materials is not totally understood.

2.11   THE CHOICE BETWEEN AQUEOUS AND ORGANIC SOLVENT-BASED COATING

Since the 1970s there has been a steady move away from the originally used organic solvents to the use of water as the coating medium (Hogan, 1982). The reasons for this change are not hard to find. Considerations of environmental pollution enforced by local legislation have made it impossible to operate in the same manner as in the early days of the technology. This, coupled with safety and health-related issues of people in the workplace, has meant that there is an increasing number of companies who are willing to consider aqueous processing. Only since the advent of the aqueous dispersed forms of the original acrylic polymers has it been possible to utilize aqueous processing for these materials. However, the commonly used cellulosic polymers, with the exception of ethylcellulose, have an appreciable water solubility which has always made them theoretically available for aqueous processing.

It must be remembered that in the early 1970s the sophistication of processing equipment was inferior to the situation today. In particular, drying ability was deficient, thus placing a necessary emphasis on the use of as low a boiling point solvent as practically possible. In addition, the cellulose derivatives in common use, although water soluble, were not ideally suited to aqueous use as the grades available had an excessively high viscosity in water, thus rendering their solutions difficult to atomize.

Gradually the introduction of new purpose-built coating equipment and lower viscosity cellulosic polymers enabled the interest in aqueous processing to be translated into activity. During this period several of the misconceptions of aqueous processing were removed from the minds of workers in this area—notably that aqueous processing would mean overly long coating processes or that the use of water was bound to pose severe stability problems. As a generalization there are very few tablet formulations that cannot be aqueously film coated (Tonadachie *et al.*, 1977). It is also true to say that the requirement for water-based processing is now so strong in certain parts of the world that film-coating systems and polymers are specifically designed with this requirement in mind. For modified release coatings, where water-insoluble polymers have traditionally been used, special water-dispersible forms have been developed by manufacturers.

2.12 FILM-COATING FORMULAE EXAMPLES

The following are intended as examples of formulae utilizing some of the principles described in previous sections relating to the properties of the materials concerned. Thus, they represent starting formulae which may need optimization for individual needs.

Basic cellulosic formula

	% w/w	Function
HPMC 5 mPa s	7.5	Polymer
PEG 400	0.8	Plasticizer
Iron oxide yellow	0.6	Pigment/opacifier
Titanium dioxide	3.1	Pigment/opacifier
Purified water	88.0	Polymer solvent and coating medium vehicle
Total	100.0	

Comments: For the polymer specified, 12% represents a good compromise between adequate polymer concentration and the ability of most spray systems to atomize the formulation. The plasticizer is present as 10% by weight of the polymer. Should coating defects such as logo bridging or poor adhesion be apparent with individual tablet core formulations, then alteration of plasticizer content, and possibly type, may be indicated (see Chapter 13).

The iron oxide yellow/titanium dioxide mixture in addition to providing colour to the dosage form will act as an opacifier. Should formula optimization be required regarding moisture vapour permeability, the concentration of pigments/opacifiers will have to be reviewed.

Increased plasticizer formula

	% w/w
HPMC 5 mPa s	7.5
Propylene glycol	1.6
Iron oxide yellow	0.6
Titanium dioxide	3.0
Purified water	87.3
Total	100.0

Comments: The higher plasticizer level in this formula reflects the greater volatility of propylene glycol over PEG 400. An increased plasticizer concentration may be beneficial in overcoming adhesion, bridging and cracking problems (see Chapter 13).

High opacity formula

	% w/w
HPMC 5 mPa s	6.9
PEG 400	0.7
Iron oxide red	4.4
Purified water	88.0
Total	100.0

Comments: The sole pigment used is iron oxide red, taking advantage of this pigment's high contrast ratio and, hence, high opacity. Owing to its higher pigment content, this formula is also likely to prove beneficial where lower moisture transmission is sought.

Alternative colour formula

	% w/w
HPMC 5 mPa s	7.5
PEG 400	0.8
Indigo carmine lake	0.4
Titanium dioxide	3.3
Purified water	88.0
Total	100.0

Comments: The shade produced by this combination will not have the colour stability of the iron oxide formulae. Pale shades from non oxide formula will require careful assessment on stability trials in the final pack.

Talc-containing formula

	% w/w
HPMC 5 mPa s	6.5
PEG 400	0.7
Iron oxide yellow	0.5
Talc	4.3
Purified water	88.0
Total	100.0

Comments: Talc is an interesting addition to a film-coating formula. Nearly all pigments have an adverse effect on film cracking, the exception being talc which is beneficial in this respect. Other potential advantages of talc are its anti-tack ability and the pleasing lustrous appearance it imparts on film coating. Its disadvantages are that its opacity is poor and coating formulations have to be carefully stirred otherwise the talc will settle out quickly to the bottom of the vessel.

Typical aqueous acrylic formula (Lehmann, 1989b)

Pigment suspension 30%	% w/w	Function
Talc	15.0	Anti-tack agent
Titanium dioxide	8.0	Pigment/opacifier
Quinoline yellow lake	4.0	Pigment/opacifier
Antifoam emulsion	0.1	Process aid
PEG 6000	3.0	Stabilizer
Water	69.9	Vehicle
Total	100.0	

Final formulation	% w/w	Function
Eudragit RL30D (as 30% w/w dispersion)	5.5	Polymer
Pigment suspension (as 30 % w/w)	16.4	
Citroflex 2	1.1	Plasticizer
Water	77.0	Vehicle
Total	100.0	

Comments: This formula utilizes an aqueous latex form of the acrylic copolymer in a non-functional, rapid disintegrating film. The very high quantity of pigment that can be applied using this system compared with a typical cellulosic formulation should also be noted.

Basic acrylic formula using organic solvents (Lehmann, 1989b)

Pigment Suspension 30%	% w/w	Function
Talc	14.0	Anti-tack agent and glidant
Magnesium stearate	2.0	Anti-tack agent and glidant
Titanium dioxide	6.0	Pigment/opacifier
Quinoline yellow lake	6.0	Pigment/opacifier
PEG 6000	2.0	Polish
Water	4.0	Vehicle
Isopropanol	66.0	Vehicle
Total	100.0	

Final Formulation	% w/w	Function
Eudragit E100	2.0	Polymer
Pigment suspension (as 30% w/w)	6.0	
Isopropanol	53.6	Polymer solvent
Acetone	37.6	Polymer solvent
Water	0.8	Polymer solvent
Total	100.0	

Comments: This methacrylate aminoester copolymer produces pliable flexible films, hence there is no need to add plasticizers to the formulation.

GLOSSARY OF CHEMICAL SUBSTANCES AND POLYMERS

Abbreviation	*Name*	*Tradename*
CAP	Cellulose acetate phthalate aqueously dispersible form	Aquateric (FMC)
CAT	Cellulose acetate trimellitate	
DEP	Diethylphthalate	
EC	Ethylcellulose	
	Ethylcellulose Aqueous Dispersion	Aquacoat (FMC) Surelease (Colorcon)
HPC	Hydroxypropyl cellulose	
HPMC	Hydroxypropyl methylcellulose	Methocel (Dow) Pharmacoat (Shin-Etsu)
HPMCP	Hydroxypropyl methylcellulose phthalate	
MC	Methylcellulose	
PEG	Polyethylene glycol	
PVA	Polyvinyl alcohol	
PVP	Polyvinyl pyrrolidone	
PVAP	Polyvinyl acetate phthalate aqueously dispersible form	Opadry-A, Sureteric (Colorcon)
	Various acrylic polymers/ copolymers	Eudragit (Rohm Pharma)
	Triethylcitrate	Citroflex (Pfizer)
	Polysorbate	Span, Tween (ICI)

REFERENCES

Abdul-Razzak, M.H. (1983) Ph.D Thesis, C.N.A.A., Leicester Polytechnic.
Anon. (1988) *Manufacturing Chem.* June, 33, 35.
Anon. (1993) *Colour Kit and International Pharmaceutical Colour Regulation Chart*, Colorcon Limited, Orpington (GB).
Aulton, M.E. (1982) *Int. J. Pharm. Tech. Prod. Mfr* **3**, 9–16.
Aulton, M.E., Abdul-Razzak, M.H. & Hogan, J.E. (1981) *Drug Dev. Ind. Pharm.* **7**, 649–648.
Aulton, M.E., Abdul-Razzak, M.H. & Hogan, J.E. (1984) *Drug Dev. Ind. Pharm.* **10**, 541–561.
Bindschaedler, C., Gurney, R. & Doelker, E. (1983) *Labo-Pharma Probl. Tech.* **31**, 389–394.
Chambliss, W.G. (1983) *Pharm. Tech.* **8(9)**, 124, 126, 128, 130, 132, 138, 140.

Chatfield, H.W. (1962) In *The science of surface coatings*, Van Nostrand, New York.

Chopra, S.K. & Tawashi, R. (1985) *J. Pharm. Sci.* **74**, 746–749.

Dechesne, J.P. & Jaminet, F. (1985) *J. Pharm. Belg.* **40**, 5–13.

Dechesne, J.P., Delporte, J.P., Jaminet, F. & Venturas, K. (1982) *J. Pharm. Belg.* **37**, 283–286.

Dechesne, J.P., Vanderschueren, J. & Jaminet, F. (1984) *J. Pharm. Belg.* **39**, 341–347.

Delporte, J.P. (1980) *J. Pharm. Belg.* **35**, 417–426.

Delporte, J.P. (1981) *J. Pharm. Belg.* **36**, 27–37.

Entwistle, C.A. & Rowe, R.C. (1979) *J. Pharm. Pharmacol.* **31**, 269–272.

Gibson, S.H.M., Rowe, R.C. & White, E.F.T. (1988) *Int. J. Pharm.* **48**, 63–77.

Handbook of Pharmaceutical Excipients (1986) American Pharmaceutical Association, Washington and Royal Pharmaceutical Society, London.

Hansen, C.M. (1967) *J. Paint Technol.* **39**, 104–117.

Hawes, M.R. (1978) R.P. Scherer Award Submission.

Higuchi, T. & Aguiar, A. (1959) *J. Am. Pharm. Soc. Sci. Ed* **48**, 574–583.

Hildebrand, J.H. & Scott, R.I. (1950) In *Solubility of non-electrolytes*, 3rd edn, Rheinhold, New York.

Hogan, J.E. (1982) *Int. J. Pharm. Tech. Prod. Mfr* **3**, 17–20.

Jordan, M.P., Easterbrook, M.G. & Hogan, J.E. (1992) *Proc. 11th Int. Pharmaceutical Technology Conf., Manchester*.

Kent, D.J. & Rowe, R.C. (1978) *J. Pharm. Pharmacol.* **30**, 808–810.

Kovacs, B. & Merenyi, G. (1990) *Drug Dev. Ind. Pharm.* **16**, 2302–2323.

Lehmann, K. (1972) *APV-Informationsdienst* **18**, 48–60.

Lehmann, K. (1989a) In *Aqueous polymeric coatings for pharmaceutical dosage forms* (ed. McGinity, J.W.), Marcel Dekker, New York, 153–247.

Lehmann, K. (1989b) In *A practical course in lacquer coating*, Rohma Pharma., Weiterstadt (Germany).

Lehmann, K. (1992) In *Microcapsules and nanoparticles in medicine and pharmacy* (ed. Donbrow, M.), CRC Press, Boca Raton, 74–96.

Lehmann, K. & Dreher, D. (1981) *Int. J. Pharm. Tech. Prod. Mfr* **2**, 31–43.

Majeed, S.S. (1984) M.Phil. Thesis, C.N.A.A., Leicester Polytechnic.

Masilungan, F.C. & Lordi, N.G. (1984) *Int. J. Pharm.* **20**, 295–305.

Massoud, A. & Bauer, K.H. (1989) *Pharm. Ind.* **51**, 203–209.

Millar, J. (1957) US Patent 2, 897, 122.

Munden, B.J., DeKay, H.G. & Banker, G.S. (1964) *J. Pharm. Sci.* **53**, 394–401.

Nielsen, L.E. (1967) *J. Macromol. Sci.-Chem.* **A1**, 929.

Nyqvist, H., Nicklasson, M. & Lundgren, P. (1982) *Acta Pharm. Suec.* **19**, 1–6.

Okhamafe, A.O. & York, P. (1983) *J. Pharm. Pharmacol.* **35**, 409–415.

Okhamafe, A.O. & York, P. (1985a) *Pharm. Acta Helv.* **60**, 92–96.

Okhamafe, A.O. & York, P. (1985b) *J. Pharm. Pharmacol.* **37**, 849–853.

Okhamafe, A.O. & York, P. (1987) *Int. J. Pharm.* **39**, 1–21.

Okhamafe, A.O. & York, P. (1989) *J. Pharm. Pharmacol.* **41**, 1–6.

Porter, S.C. (1980) *Pharm. Tech.* **4**(3), 67–76.

Porter, S.C. & Bruno, C. (1990) In *Pharmaceutical dosage forms: Tablets*, Vol. 3, Chap. 2, 2nd edn (Eds Lieberman, H.A., Lachman, L. & Schwartz, J.), Marcel Dekker, New York.

Porter, S.C. & Ridgway, K. (1983) *J. Pharm. Pharmacol.* **35**, 341–344.

Prater, D.A., Meakin, B.J. & Wilde, J.S. (1982) *Int. J. Pharm. Tech. Prod. Mfr* **3**, 33–41.

Rowe, R.C. (1980) *J. Pharm. Pharmacol.* **32**, 116–119.

Rowe, R.C. (1981) *J. Pharm. Pharmacol.* **33**, 423–426.

Rowe, R.C. (1982) *Pharm. Acta Helv.* **57**, 221–225.

Rowe, R.C. (1983) *J. Pharm. Pharmacol.* **35**, 43–44.

Rowe, R.C. (1984a) *Int. J. Pharm.* **22**, 17–23.

Rowe, R.C. (1984b) *J. Pharm. Pharmacol.* **36**, 569–572

Rowe, R.C. (1984c) Materials used in the film coating of oral solid dosage forms, in *Materials used in pharmaceutical formulation* (ed. Florence, A.T.), *Critical Reports on Applied Chemistry* **6**, Soc. Chem. Ind., Blackwell Scientific Publications

Rowe, R.C. (1985) *Pharm. Int.* Jan., 14–17.

Rowe, R.C. (1986) *J. Pharm. Pharmacol.* **38**, 214–215.

Sakellariou, P., Rowe, R.C. & White, E.F.T. (1986a) *Int. J. Pharm.* **31**, 55–64.

Sakellariou, P., Rowe, R.C. & White, E.F.T. (1986b) *Int. J. Pharm.* **31**, 175–77.

Sinko, C.M. & Amidon, G.M. (1989) *Int. J. Pharm.* **55**, 247–256.

Skultety, P.F. & Sims, S. (1987) *Drug Dev. Ind. Pharm.* **13**, 2209–2219.

Spitael, J. & Kinget, R. (1977) *J. Pharm. Belg.* **32**, 569–577.

Steuernagel, C.R. (1989) In *Aqueous polymeric coatings for pharmaceutical dosage forms* (ed. McGinity, J.W.), Marcel Dekker, New York, pp. 1–63.

Tonadachie, M., Hoshi, N. & Sekigawa, F. (1977) *Drug Dev. Ind. Pharm.* **3**, 227–240.

Wan, L.S.C. & Lai, W.F. (1992) *S.T.P. Pharma Sci.* **2**, 174–180.

Warner, G.L. (1978) US Patent 4,123,403.

Zhang, G., Schwartz, J.B. & Schnaare, R.L. (1988) *Proc. 15th Int. Symp. Controlled Release of Bioactive Materials, Basel.*

Zhang, G., Schwartz, J.B. & Schnaare, R.L. (1989) *Proc. 16th Int. Symp. Controlled Release of Bioactive Materials, Chicago.*

3

Sugar coating

John E. Hogan

SUMMARY

The chapter commences with a brief introduction to the technique of sugar coating, which includes a note on the advantages and disadvantages of this method of coating. The various sequential steps involved in sugar coating are covered in some detail, i.e. sealing, subcoating, smoothing, colour coating, polishing and printing.

In the section dealing with subcoating several suitable formulations are provided with details regarding application. Traditionally the colour-coating step in sugar coating has received much attention as the aesthetics of this dosage form are most important. Accordingly this section provides considerable depth, including a comparison of previously utilized water-soluble colour systems with modern pigment coloured systems.

A description of sugar coating faults emphasizes the need for adequate drying conditions during the process to prevent a build up of residual moisture within the tablet. Problems of sucrose inversion and difficulties in polishing are also covered.

The chapter concludes with a consideration of how the process of sugar coating can affect the dissolution and stability behaviour of the dosage form.

3.1 INTRODUCTION

The pharmaceutical process of sugar coating remains a widely practised technology despite the interest arising from film-coating techniques since the 1950s. However, it is true to say, as has been indicated in Chapter 1, that the technology of sugar coating has remained relatively static while attention has been focused increasingly on film coating.

3.2   BASIC PROCESS REVIEW

Unlike film coating, sugar coating is still a multistep process. Its use of labour is more intensive than in film coating and process operators require a fair degree of skill but less than in former days when more traditional methods prevailed.

In suitable sugar-coating equipment the tablet cores are successively treated with aqueous sucrose solutions which, depending on the stage of coating reached, may contain other functional ingredients, e.g. fillers, colours, etc. The build up of coating material is due to a transference of coating medium from one tablet to another. Typically a single liquid application will be made which will be allowed to spread over the entire tablet bed utilizing the mixing capability of the particular equipment. At this point, drying, usually in the form of heated air, will be used to dry the application. The whole cycle will then be successively repeated.

In this respect sugar coating differs from film coating as in this process each tablet passes through a zone of application which is subject to rapid and continuous drying.

3.3   ADVANTAGES OF SUGAR COATING

Despite the undoubted disadvantages of the sugar-coating process in terms of process length, intensive operator attention and so forth, it is important to be aware that sugar coating can have certain advantages:

- It utilizes inexpensive and readily available raw materials.
- Constituent raw materials are widely accepted—no regulatory problems.
- Modern, simplified techniques have greatly reduced coating times over traditional sugar-coating methods.
- No complex equipment or services are required.
- The process is capable of being controlled and documented to meet modern GMP standards.
- Simplicity of equipment and ready availability of raw materials make sugar coating an ideal coating method for developing countries.
- The process is generally not as critical as film coating; recovering and reworking procedures are usually possible.
- For high humidity climates, it generally offers a stability advantage over film-coated tablets.
- Results are aesthetically pleasing and have wide consumer acceptability.
- Tablet cores may generally be softer than those demanded by film coating, especially those for aqueous film coating.

3.4   THE STAGES IN SUGAR COATING

3.4.1   Sealing

It is necessary to protect the tablet core from the aqueous nature of sucrose applications to follow. Sealing also prevents certain types of materials from migrating to

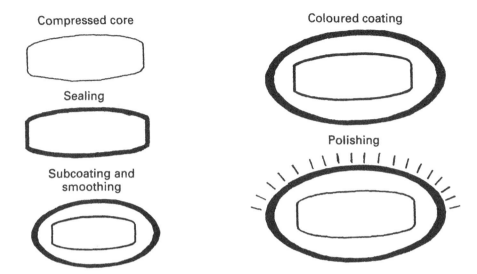

Fig. 3.1 The stages in sugar coating.

the tablet surface and spoiling the appearance, e.g. oils, acids, etc. This is unfortunately an organic solvent-dependent step in an otherwise aqueous process.

A film of water-impervious polymer is built up using materials such as:

● Shellac
● CAP
● PVAP
● Zein.

Shellac has all the disadvantages of a natural material (see Chapter 2 for a more detailed description), the other polymers used tend to be those which have an additional use as enteric-coating materials so that they should be applied only in sufficient quantity to form an efficient seal. A lamination process, whereby an application of sealant is followed by an application of dusting power, e.g. talc, is nearly always used.

3.4.2 Subcoating

During the sugar-coating process the increase in weight achieved can be 30–50% of the weight of the original tablet core. Much of the added weight is applied at the subcoating stage. Subcoating serves to confer on the tablet core a perfectly rounded aspect.

The ideal shape for sugar coating is a deeply convex core with minimal edges (Fig. 3.2). This condition will obviously require less coating material than where the tablet edge is comparatively thick. Seager *et al.* (1985) have cautioned that deeply convex tablet cores may not be exactly ideal as their crowns tend to be soft. Basically there are two methods:

Lamination process

Below are illustrated two typical examples of binder solution formulations for subcoating, together with their corresponding dusting powder formulations. The principle of the process is that a volume of binder solution is applied to the sealed cores in the coating pan. Once this has spread over the tablet bed an application of powder is dusted into the pan, and when this has evenly distributed itself over the contents, drying air is applied. The drying air process needs to be carefully controlled to prevent too rapid evaporation of the water. The objective should be to create as smooth a coat as possible in order to reduce the time for smoothing the coat in the final stages of process. Excessively rapid drying results in a very uneven surface. Too low an evaporation rate gives rise to a lengthy process and the danger of cores adhering together.

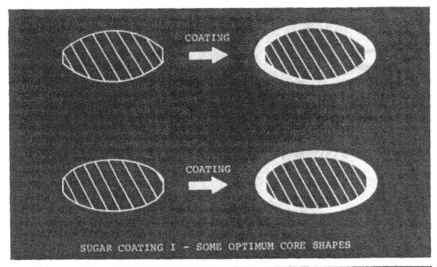

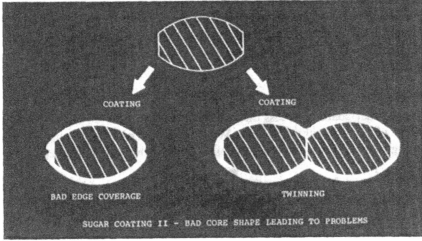

Fig. 3.2   Ideal and non-ideal tablet core shapes for sugar coating.

Binder solution formulation:

	I(% w/w)	II(% w/w)
Gelatin	3.3	6.0
Gum acacia (powdered)	8.7	8.0
Sucrose	55.3	45.0
Water	to 100.0	to 100.0

Dusting powder formulation:

	I(% w/w)	II(% w/w)
Calcium carbonate	40.0	—
Titanium dioxide	5.0	1.0
Talc	25.0	61.0
Sucrose (powdered)	28.0	38.0
Gum acacia (powdered)	2.0	—

Features of the lamination process

- The use of a binder solution with gum binds the powder application on the tablet.
- Utilizes inexpensive ingredients with high opacity.
- In skilled hands a very fast build up to the required shape is obtained.

Disadvantages of the lamination process

- The use of free dusted powders tends to create clean-up problems.
- Difficult to control in documentary terms as frequently volumes not weights of powders are specified.
- Difficult to automate as both powders and liquids are involved.

Suspension process

In recent years, automation in the sugar-coating process has required the use of a liquid subcoat. These are generally suspensions of the filler materials, e.g. calcium carbonate, talc, sucrose in the gum solutions. The example quoted below is suitable for hand panning or automatic methods with a little modification. A description of a typical sugar-coating pan is given and the latest type of side-vented coating pans is given in Chapter 8. The system contains only approximately 23% water and consequently dries quickly.

Formulae

Quantities are for a batch of 250 000 tablets having an average weight of 200 mg and providing a batch weight of 50 kg in a 4 ft diameter pan.

Coating powder: Calcium carbonate, light   6.8 kg
                    Talc   1.8 kg

Starch, pulverized	1.0 kg
Titanium dioxide	0.4 kg

The powders are mixed in a simple blender (e.g. V-section type) and sifted through a 60 mesh screen.

Subcoat Syrup:	Water	10.0 kg
	Dextrin	0.5 kg
	Sucrose	22.5 kg

The dextrin is dissolved in the water and the resultant solution boiled; the sucrose is then added and stirred until dissolved. Two applications of this clear syrup are made prior to adding 8 kg of coating powder to the remaining syrup before commencing the subcoating.

3.4.3 Smoothing

The product at the end of the subcoating will be too rough to continue with colour coating. Smoothing is usually achieved by applications of plain 70% w/w syrup. However large degrees of unevenness will require some subcoating solids in the initial smoothing coats. Typically, however, if subcoating is carried out well, then approximately ten applications of 70% syrup will be required for tablets that are suitable for the next stage.

3.4.4 Colour coating

This is one of the most important steps in the sugar-coating process as it has immediate visual impact. During this step the coating syrup contains the colour solids necessary to achieve the desire shade. Water-soluble dyes were used previously as colouring agents for sugar-coated tablets. This has largely been superseded by the use of modern water-insoluble pigment forms including the aluminium lakes of the water-soluble colours. Here, the water-soluble dye is adsorbed onto a hydrated alumina surface, filtered, washed and dried. By careful processing, the optimum particle size profile is achieved. The smaller and more even the particle size, the greater the colouring power and hence the smaller the quantity that need be used to achieve the same result. These lake pigments are essentially insoluble in aqueous systems between pH 3.5 and 9.0 and find important uses in tablet coatings both using the sugar- and film-coating processes. The advantages of lakes over soluble dyes, including the soluble natural colours, are multi-fold.

Advantages of lakes over dyes

The following arguments apply not only to lakes as insoluble forms but to all other pigments, e.g. iron oxides, titanium dioxide, etc. During the sugar-coating process with soluble dyes specific dye concentrations are used in the applied coating syrups. Very often this is performed sequentially with increasing dye concentration to achieve maximum colour. The process must be carefully controlled to ensure that the finished tablets are not over-coloured or under-coloured. However, if insoluble pigments are employed as colourants, especially when used in conjunction with an opacifier such as titanium dioxide, a single colour concentration can be used, and since the colouring system is opaque, only one shade of colour will result. In order to obtain a different shade, the ratio of pigment to titanium dioxide must be altered. Thus, when employed in this manner, titanium dioxide serves both as an extender to reduce colourant costs and as an opacifier to yield only one shade of colour in a given situation.

The use of soluble dyes in coating solutions requires that the subcoated core must be perfectly smooth prior to the colouring stage. This is essential in order to achieve a final uniform colour. The presence of any surface irregularity before colour coating will result in an uneven colour, since it must be remembered that the final colour seen is an in-depth one resulting from light being reflected from the opaque underlayer of the subcoat. Irregularities in the surface of this layer result in a variation in length of the path of reflected light, which manifests itself as a series of colour concentration differences, and hence an irregular colour (Fig. 3.3).

Common examples of this are shown in the case of poorly subcoated tablets where the sharp edge of the core has not been properly covered, resulting in a pale ring being visible around the edge of the tablet after colouring.

Since a pigment-coloured system is opaque, the resultant colour is not dependent on the depth (or thickness) of the colour layer, and the observed colour results from light which is reflected from the surface of the colour layer. Provided that sufficient colour has been applied to cover the tablets uniformly, the resultant colour will be completely even (Fig. 3.4).

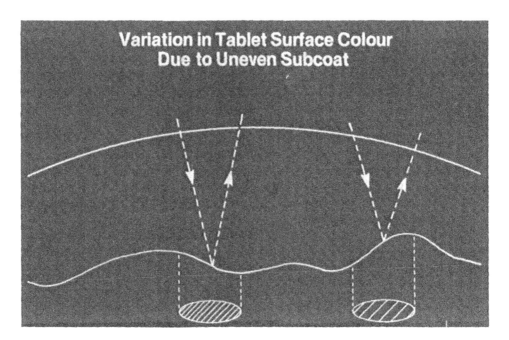

Fig. 3.3 Shade irregularities with a dye-colour coat caused by uneven subcoat surface.

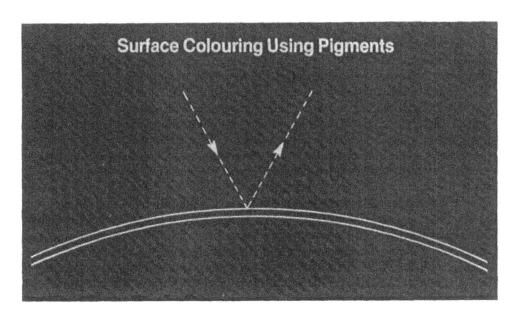

Fig. 3.4   Uniform shade obtained from pigment-coloured coat.

The typical dye-colouring process employs relatively low concentrations of colourants, and relies for its final colour on a substantially thick colour coat being applied. This process takes time, with 30–50 colour applications being made. If the process is rushed, and drying between each application is allowed to proceed too quickly, colour migration becomes a problem since there is a tendency for the soluble dye to 'move' with the moisture as it leaves the tablet. This disrupts the uniformity of the colour layer, and results in an uneven final colour being achieved (Mattocks, 1958). Conversely, if the tablets are under-dried between each colour application, the final colour achieved might initially be uniform, but there is a tendency for the tablets to 'sweat' on storage, that is to say the excess moisture leaves the tablet and again causes migration of the colour resulting in final colour unevenness.

On the other hand, a typical pigment-colouring process employs a relatively high concentration of colour. Since this is opaque and is not subject to colour migration problems, it can be applied and dried rapidly, resulting in an overall time-saving process without having a detrimental effect on the uniformity of the final colour.

The soluble dye-colouring system can pose a problem from a batchwise colour control point of view. This is a transparent system, and if the number of colour applications varies from batch to batch either from carelessness, or desire to maintain a strict control over the final product weight, this will result in a variation in the thickness of the colour layer and, consequently, a batchwise variation in final colour.

Again it can only be stressed that as the pigment system is opaque, once complete colour coverage has been achieved, no variation in colour can occur.

To summarize, a pigment system is superior to a water-soluble dye for colouring sugar-coated tablets due to:

1. maintenance of evenness of colour because
   (a) the colour is not water soluble and thus is not prone to colour migration problems;
   (b) the colour is opaque, and thus is not affected by any minor unevenness in the subcoat layer;
2. maintenance of colour uniformity from batch to batch, which results from the fact that, again because the colourant is opaque, the final colour is not affected by small fluctuations in the quantity of colour solution applied;
3. reduction in overall processing time;
4. reduction in the thickness of the colour-coating layer (see Anon., 1969).

3.4.5 Polishing
After the colour-coating process the tablets have a somewhat dull, matt appearance which requires a separate polishing step to give them the high degree of gloss traditionally associated with sugar-coated tablets. Methods vary considerably, but it is generally important that the tablets are dry prior to polishing. Preferably they should be at least trayed overnight in a suitable atmosphere.

Some examples of polishing methods which are currently in use include:

- Application of an organic solvent solution/suspension of waxes, e.g. carnauba and beeswax. A recently available variant on this theme provides an emulsion of both waxes in an aqueous continuous phase stabilized by a food and pharmaceutically acceptable surfactant. The results obtained are equivalent to traditional methods utilizing organic solvent solutions but, of course, with the big bonus of aqueous processing.
- Use of wax-lined pan.
- Use of canvas-lined pan with wax solution/suspension.
- Finely powdered wax application.
- Mineral oil application.

In addition, there are polishing techniques reliant upon the use of glazes containing shellac in alcohol with or without waxes. The use of these materials is rather more dependable, and is not so reliant on atmospheric conditions of temperature and humidity to obtain the optimum result. This comment does not apply, however, to the aqueous material, which has a high degree of dependability in use.

3.4.6 Printing
Some regulatory authorities demand that tablets, be they coated or uncoated, should possess some detailed identifying mark. Those authorities who do not actually require this actively encourage it as part of the overall GMP and product acceptability requirements. Unfortunately, unlike film-coated tablets, sugar-coated tablets cannot be monogrammed by engraving the punch tooling. Instead a printing process is used.

A typical edible pharmaceutical ink formulation is: shellac, alcohol, pigment, lecithin, antifoam and other organic solvents.

The printing process suitable for a formulation such as this is a modified offset gravure. Shellac still has a traditionally dominant position as the lacquer most commonly encountered,but is slowly giving ground to cellulose derivatives in newer formulations as it can pose severe stability problems in some formulae. Lecithin is frequently included to maximize the quantity of pigment that can be utilized. Antifoam is a necessary ingredient to prevent the nuisance of foam build up in the ink container during a print run.

Careful formulation of solvent blends are necessary in order to achieve the correct drying time demanded by the particular application. As in so many facets of coating in general, pharmaceutical ink formulation trends are to maximize the aqueous content of formulae. The offset gravure process, while capable of producing impressive results, is sensitive to minor changes in procedure. Attempts are being made to utilize more robust technology, for example ink-jet printing, in this process step.

3.5   SUGAR-COATING FAULTS

Because the sugar coating itself is deliberately isolated from the tablet core there is the possibility of much more standardization here than in the area of film-coating formulae, which are in intimate contact with the tablet surface and hence subject to faults arising from core–coating interactions.

A common fault is cracking and splitting of the sugar coat which is caused by excess residual moisture from the processing. The remedy, of course, is to allow sufficient drying time between individual applications of syrup. Reich & Gstirnir (1969), using a mercury porosimetry technique, have demonstrated that coating powders with high porosity lose moisture most easily during the coating process and showed the converse is also true for powders of low porosity, Wakimoto & Otsuka (1980) have developed a technique for measuring the distortion of a sugar coating which itself is a precurser to cracking. Previous to this point, distortion had been difficult to measure. The authors' method utilized laser holographic interferometry and has the advantage that it is a non-invasive technique.

Inversion and stickiness are caused by the presence of inverted sugar which is difficult to dry adequately. It can be encountered if slightly acidic colour-coating suspensions are maintained at too high a temperature for too long. Sugar coatings are unfortunately brittle and are prone to chipping if subjected to an inappropriate mechanical stress. The difficulties that can arise during the colour-coating step have been dealt with under the appropriate section. Several problems can be encountered during the polishing stage. One common fault is to attempt to polish tablets which are not quite smooth. Under these conditions, wax will collect in the depressions on the tablet surface and remain as tiny white spots at the end of the process.

3.6 DISSOLUTION AND STABILITY BEHAVIOUR

Many authors have pointed out the crucial nature of the sealing step of the sugar-coating process and its ability to affect the disintegration and dissolution properties of the dosage form as a whole, for example Gross & Endicott (1960). Other authors have detailed instances of impaired dissolution characteristics of sugar-coated tablets and ascribed the behaviour to delayed break up of the sugar coating. In a comprehensive study of fourteen batches of chlorpromazine sugar-coated tablets, Sawsan & Khalil (1984) reinforce this general point. Other reports have suggested an incompatibility between the gelatin and calcium carbonate used in the subcoat (Barrett & Fell, 1975; Chapman *et al.*, 1980) as a cause of impaired dissolution.

Sandell & Mellstrom (1975) report finding considerable variation in the disintegration time of batches of coated tablets, including sugar-coated tablets. Romero *et al.* (1988) have examined the stability of Ibuprofen coated tablets at elevated temperature and humidity storage. They found the sugar-coated tablets to be especially sensitive to the storage conditions and suggest that this may be a general phenomena of the dosage form.

3.7 INCORPORATION OF DRUGS IN THE SUGAR COATING

This is a feasible practice with sugar-coated tablets and is usually performed for reasons of separating incompatible active substances. Carstensen *et al.* (1970), in a statistical study of the process, have deduced that tablet to tablet variation in drug content is inversely proportional to the number of coats applied to the tablets. The larger the core the better the drug distribution will be compared to smaller core tablets.

REFERENCES

Anon. (1969) *Drug Cosm. Ind.* Aug., 63, 64, 144.
Barrett, D. & Fell, J.T. (1975) *J. Pharm. Sci.* **64**, 335–337.
Carstensen, J.T., Koff, A., Johnson, J.B. & Rubin, S.H. (1970) *J. Pharm. Sci.* **59**, 553–555.
Chapman, S.R., Rubinstein, M.H., Duffey, T.D. & Ireland, D.S. (1980) *J. Pharm. Pharmacol.* **32**, 20P.
Gross, H.M. & Endicott, C.J. (1960) *Drug Cosm. Ind.* **86(2)**, 170, 171, 264, 288–291.
Mattocks, A.M. (1958) *Am. Pharm. Mfg. Assoc., Proc. Prod. Conf.*, 196.
Reich, B. & Gstirnir, F. (1969) *Cesk. Farm.* **18**, 112–113.
Romero, A.J., Grady, L.T. & Rhodes, C.T. (1988) **14**, 1549–1586.
Sandell, E. & Mellstrom, G. (1975) *Acta Pharm. Suec.* **12**, 293–296.
Sawsan, A.E. & Khalil, A.H. (1984) *Int. J. Pharm.* **18**, 225–234.
Seager, H., Rue, P.J., Burt, I., Ryder, J., Warrack, J.K. & Gamlen, M.J. (1985) *Int. J. Pharm. Tech. Prod. Mfr* **6**, 1–20.
Wakimoto, T. & Otsuka, A. (1980) *Drug Dev. Ind. Pharm.* **12**, 641–650.

4

Solution properties and atomization in film coating

Michael E. Aulton and Andrew M. Twitchell

SUMMARY

A little-considered stage of the film-coating process is the atomization of the coating solution by the spray gun. This chapter will show how formulation and process factors can cause marked changes in the characteristics of the spray, which may have important consequences for film formation and film properties.

The chapter begins by describing how film-coating solution or suspension properties, such as density, surface tension and viscosity, alter with changing formulation and then continues by presenting predictions of how these properties could influence spray droplet size. The chapter then discusses various techniques for measuring and representing mean droplet size and size distribution.

The influence of formulation and atomization conditions on spray characteristics is discussed and data are presented for aqueous HPMC droplets produced under a wide range of conditions. Parameters examined include concentration of polymer in solution, atomizing air pressure, liquid flow rate (spray rate), gun-to-substrate distance, spray-gun design, spray shape, liquid nozzle diameter and atomizing air velocity.

4.1 INTRODUCTION

The overall process of film coating comprises a number of important stages:

- Solution or suspension preparation.
- Droplet generation.

● Droplet travel from the spray gun to the substrate bed. The substrate in question will usually be either a tumbling bed of tablets or a fluidized bed of multiparticulates, i.e. beadlets or pellets.

● Impingement, wetting, spreading and coalescence of the droplets at the surface of the tablet or multiparticulate.

● Subsequent drying, gelation and adhesion of the film.

All the above are important stages that need to be understood and, where possible, controlled. These stages are outlined schematically in Fig. 4.1.

Atomization has been found to be a particularly important stage in the overall process of film coating. This chapter will discuss the factors which influence the atomization stage—i.e. formulation variables and process variables. The ways in which these factors affect the quality of the film coat in terms of visual examination (both macroscopically and by scanning electron microscopy), film thickness (by light-section microscopy) and surface roughness (by profilimetry) are discussed in Chapter 13.

4.2 SOLUTION PROPERTIES

4.2.1 Introduction
The physical properties of film-coating solutions or suspensions can potentially

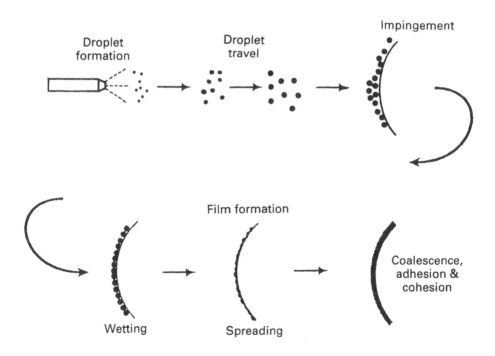

Fig. 4.1   Schematic representation of the stages in spray film coating.

exert an influence at many stages during the film-coating process. These stages include delivery to and droplet production at the atomizing device, travel to the tablet or multiparticulate surface and the wetting, spreading, penetration, evaporation and adhesion of the atomized formulation at the substrate surface.

It is important, therefore, to quantify the physical properties of the coating solutions and suspensions that are to be used in the film-coating process in order that their influence on the appearance and properties of the final film coat can be appreciated.

The following discussion reviews the areas where the physical properties of the coating solution or suspension may be of importance during the atomization of the droplets and their travel to the tablet or multiparticulate bed. The way in which solution properties influence the wetting, spreading and adhesion of these droplets is discussed in Chapter 5. How, in turn, these properties influence the quality of the resulting coat is described in Chapter 13.

Little work has been published to date on the effect of solution physical properties on the droplet size distribution or spray shape produced during atomization of film-coating solutions. Schæfer and Wørts (1977), when studying the fluidized-bed granulation process, found with aqueous granulating fluids based on gelatin, methylcellulose, carboxymethylcellulose and polyvinylpyrollidone (PVP), that the higher the solution viscosity, the larger were the droplets formed on atomization. Banks (1981), however, found that with aqueous solutions of PVP K30, increasing the concentration from 5 %w/v to 10 %w/v did not produce a significant change in droplet size, the effect of the viscosity increase being overridden by other factors. The same author also demonstrated that the addition of sodium lauryl sulphate in increasing quantities to PVP-based granulating fluids caused both an increase in the diameter of the spray cone produced on atomization and a reduction in the distance from the spray gun at which the spray maintained its integrity in terms of general shape and pattern. These effects were attributed to the lower surface tension produced by the addition of the surfactant.

Work carried out with a variety of other (i.e. non-film-coating) materials and processes has yielded various predictive equations describing how changes in viscosity, surface tension and density affect the quality of the spray. These equations illustrate a wide divergence of findings on the relative importance of these variables. This is due presumably to the wide range of atomizer designs used in the experiments, probably indicating that each equation is valid for the test conditions studied but fails when extrapolated to other systems.

The process of airless (hydraulic) atomization (which is used for organic coating systems) is not complicated by the volume, velocity and density of the atomizing gas, as is airborne (pneumatic) atomization. For airless atomization, Fair (1974) suggested the use of equation (4.1) as a guide to the effect of solution properties on the average droplet diameter produced during atomization.

$$\frac{D_{\text{VM soln}}}{D_{\text{VM solvent}}} = \left[\frac{\gamma_{\text{soln}}}{\gamma_{\text{solvent}}}\right]^{0.5} \times \left[\frac{\mu_{\text{soln}}}{\mu_{\text{solvent}}}\right]^{0.2} \times \left[\frac{\rho_{\text{solvent}}}{\rho_{\text{soln}}}\right]^{0.3} \qquad (4.1)$$

In this equation D_{VM} is the volume mean droplet diameter (see section 4.3.2) and γ, μ and ρ the surface tension, viscosity and density, respectively.

More complex equations have been developed for predicting droplet sizes produced by pneumatic atomization. An often-quoted example is that of Nukiyama & Tanasawa (1939), an adapted form of which is:

$$D_s = \left[\frac{585 \times 10^3}{v}\right] \times \left[\frac{\gamma}{\rho}\right]^{0.5} + 1683\mu^{0.45}\left[\gamma \times \rho\right]^{-0.225}\left[\frac{1000}{J}\right]^{1.5} \tag{4.2}$$

Here D_s is the surface mean diameter of the droplets (μm), v is the velocity of air relative to liquid at the atomizer nozzle exit (m/s), γ is the liquid surface tension (N/m), ρ is the liquid density (kg/m³), μ is the liquid viscosity (Pa s) and J is the air/liquid volume ratio at the air and liquid orifices.

Both these equations indicate that the solution physical properties of viscosity, surface tension and density will influence the atomization process and therefore potentially could affect the quality of the final film coat.

Once atomized, the physical properties of the droplets may influence their behaviour during passage to the substrate to be coated. The viscosity of the droplet may affect solvent evaporation rate, with droplets of higher viscosity exhibiting reduced evaporation. Similarly, any surface-active components may form a layer on the surface of the droplets which could retard evaporation. The surface tension and viscosity of the droplet may also affect the tendency of the airborne droplets to coalesce.

Thus, of the solution properties which could exert an influence, the following are most likely to have the greatest effect during the atomization of film coat formulations:

1. density
2. surface tension
3. viscosity.

These properties of solutions have been investigated in some detail for aqueous hydroxypropyl methylcellulose (HPMC E5) (Methocel E5) solutions (Aulton *et al.*, 1986; Twitchell, 1990). The results of some of this work are discussed below. Unless stated otherwise, all data presented are the result of these studies. In examining these data for HPMC E5 it could be considered that many of these relationships will probably also be applicable to other grades and types of polymer.

4.2.2 Density

Table 4.1 shows the density values for a range of HPMC E5 formulations at 20°C and 40°C. Density is found to vary little between these formulations and over the temperature range used in practice, and thus is likely to contribute little to any changes in droplet size distribution. Again it is possible that a similar situation occurs with other grades of HPMC and for dispersion systems, although there is little published data to support this.

Table 4.1   The density of a range of aqueous film-coating formulations based on HPMC E5

HPMC E5 concentration (%w/w)	Additive	Additive concentration (%w/w)	Temperature (°C)	Formulation density (kg/m³)
5	—	—	20	1010
9	—	—	20	1021
9	—	—	40	1014
12	—	—	20	1029
12	—	—	40	1022
9	Opaspray	15	20	1044
9	Opaspray	15	40	1038
9	PEG 200	3	20	1025
9	PEG 200	3	40	1019
9	Glycerol	3	20	1028
9	Glycerol	3	40	1020

4.2.3   Surface tension

The surface tension of coating solutions is likely to have a profound effect on the process of film coating. It will influence droplet generation from bulk solution, behaviour during travel to the substrate and the fate of the droplets once they hit the tablet or multiparticulate substrate. The latter will also be influenced by the interfacial tension between the atomized droplet and either the naked tablet or pellet core or the partially coated substrate. Changes in surface tension will influence wetting, spreading, coalescence and thus the adhesion of the dried film, and these points are discussed in Chapter 5. The specific case of the surface tension of aqueous HPMC solutions is discussed below.

The surface tension of HPMC solutions

HPMC is itself surface active and reduces the surface tension of water; this reduction occurs at very low concentrations. Fig. 4.2 illustrates the surface tension/concentration profile exhibited by very dilute HPMC E5 solutions at equilibrium.

There is a linear decrease in equilibrium surface tension with increasing concentration from 72.8 mN/m (at 20°C) for water alone up to a concentration of approximately 2×10^{-5} %w/w. After this point there is an abrupt change in the gradient of the line and the surface tension falls far less steeply with increasing concentration. The point of intersection between the extrapolated straight lines on either side of the break in the curve is analogous to the critical micelle concentration commonly shown by surface-active materials.

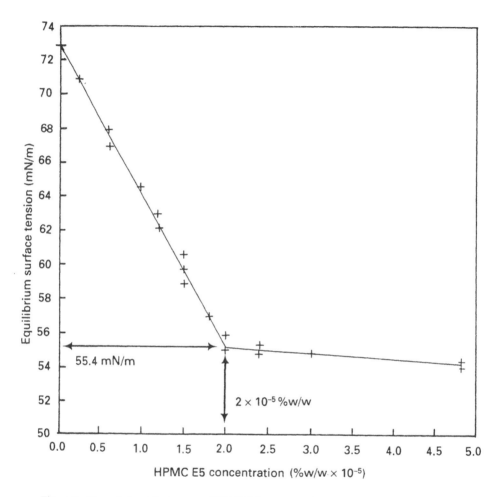

Fig. 4.2   The relationship between HPMC E5 concentration and equilibrium solution surface tension at low HPMC concentrations.

Table 4.2 shows the surface tension of much more concentrated HPMC E5 solutions at various temperatures.

It illustrates that with HPMC E5 solutions of concentrations between 1 and 12 %w/w (i.e. encompassing those likely to be used in practice for aqueous film coating) there is very little variation in surface tension, its value reducing with increasing concentration from 46.8 to 44.5 mN/m at 20°C. Thus, although a considerable reduction in surface tension occurs up to 1 %w/w HPMC E5, minimal further reduction occurs between 1 and 12 %w/w HPMC E5.

Table 4.2 also shows that increasing solution temperature has minimal effect on its surface tension. Increasing the temperature of a 9 %w/w solution of HPMC E5 from 20 to 40°C was found to result in a reduction in surface tension of only about

Table 4.2   The effect of polymer concentration and solution temperature on the surface tension of a range of aqueous HPMC E5 solutions

HPMC E5 concentration (%w/w)	Temperature (°C)	Surface tension (mN/m)
1	20	46.8
1	30	46.3
1	40	46.0
5	20	46.2
5	30	45.8
5	40	45.6
9	20	45.7
9	30	44.8
9	40	44.5
12	20	44.5
12	30	44.1
12	40	43.9

1 mN/m. Water over the same temperature range would be expected to exhibit a reduction in surface tension of about 4 mN/m (Bikerman, 1970), this being due to the gradual reduction in intermolecular cohesive forces as the temperature increases (surface tension will be zero at some finite temperature). The difference in behaviour between HPMC E5 solutions and water probably results from the non-volatile nature of HPMC, with the situation being complicated by the differing levels of solvation of HPMC at different temperatures.

Any reduction in surface tension, in the absence of other changes in physical properties, would be expected to favour droplet formation and influence solution spreading on a tablet or multiparticulate surface. The data in Table 4.2 would appear, however, to indicate that any effects caused by the reduction in surface tension with increasing concentration or temperature are likely to be minimal.

Surface ageing
The data presented above are for equilibrium situations in which migration of the surface-active HPMC molecules to the surface of the liquid is complete and a dynamic equilibrium has been reached.

However, in practical situations enormous areas of fresh liquid surface are produced during atomization. The large HPMC molecules will take a finite time to migrate to the surface, and thus there will be a time-dependent reduction in the observed surface tension (see section 5.2.2). This phenomenon is known as *surface ageing*. It is quite possible that the actual surface tension of HPMC droplets is far higher than the values measured in an equilibrium situation. The consequences of this are discussed in Chapter 5.

The effect of formulation additives on the surface tension of HPMC E5 solutions at different temperatures
The inclusion of additives (such as plasticizers, opacifiers, etc.) also has little effect on surface tension over a range of concentrations and temperatures (Table 4.3). The surfactants sodium lauryl sulphate and polysorbate 20 caused the largest decrease in surface tension although this reduction was relatively small, being approximately 5 mN/m.

The minimal effect that the addition of plasticizers has on the surface tension of 9 %w/w HPMC E5 solutions is perhaps not surprising since the surface tension of 2 %w/w solutions of these plasticizers is above 66 mN/m in each case.

Table 4.3 The effect of various formulation additives on the surface tension of 9%w/w HPMC E5 solutions over a range of temperatures

Formulation additive	Additive concentration (%w/w)	Temperature (°C)	Surface tension (mN/m)
PEG 200	3	20	45.6
PEG 200	3	30	45.0
PEG 200	3	40	44.9
PEG 400	3	20	45.6
PEG 400	3	30	45.2
PEG 400	3	40	44.7
PEG 1500	3	20	45.6
PEG 1500	3	30	44.9
PEG 1500	3	40	44.8
Glycerol	3	20	45.7
Glycerol	3	30	45.5
Glycerol	3	40	45.0
Propylene glycol	3	20	45.7
Propylene glycol	3	30	45.0
Propylene glycol	3	40	44.9
Opaspray	15	20	46.9
Opaspray	15	30	45.2
Opaspray	15	40	45.0
Polysorbate 20	0.5	20	42.1
Polysorbate 20	0.5	40	40.8
Polysorbate 20	1.0	20	41.2
Polysorbate 20	1.0	40	40.3
Sodium lauryl sulphate	0.5	20	41.3
Sodium lauryl sulphate	0.5	40	40.5
Sodium lauryl sulphate	1.0	20	39.9
Sodium lauryl sulphate	1.0	40	39.4

If the addition of a surfactant to HPMC E5 solutions was required, it may be preferable to use polysorbate 20 rather than sodium lauryl sulphate since the latter may cause significant increases in solution viscosity (see section 4.2.4, Fig. 4.7).

4.2.4   Viscosity

The rheological properties of a polymer solution depend mainly on the following parameters:

1. polymer size and shape;
2. polymer–polymer and polymer–dispersion medium molecular interactions;
3. polymer concentration;
4. solution or suspension temperature;
5. viscosity of the solvent or dispersion medium.

It is beneficial to assess how these factors influence the rheological profiles of film-coating polymer formulations in order to gain an understanding of how formulations may behave during the film-coating process.

Commercial grades of coating polymers are not monodisperse, but are known to contain polymer molecules covering a wide range of degrees of polymerization and hence chain lengths (Rowe, 1980; Tufnell *et al.*, 1983; Davies, 1985). Molecular weight fractions between 10^3 and 10^6 Da (Rowe, 1980) and 10^2 and 10^6 Da (Davies, 1985) have been found to exist for HPMC.

The molecular weight distribution of a polymer can be described by characteristic molecular weight averages. These include number-average molecular weights, M_N, and weight-average molecular weights, M_W where:

$$M_N = \frac{\sum n_i M_i}{\sum n_i} \tag{4.3}$$

$$M_W = \frac{\sum n_i M_i^2}{\sum n_i M_i} \tag{4.4}$$

and there are n_i molecules of molecular weight M_i.

Examination of these equations indicates that the value of M_N is particularly influenced by the presence of small amounts of low molecular weight fractions of the polymer and M_W by small amounts of high molecular weight fractions. It can also be calculated that, always, $M_W \geq M_N$.

The degree of polydispersity of a polymer can be defined by the polydispersity index (Q) where

$$Q = \frac{M_W}{M_N} \tag{4.5}$$

If the polymer is monosize, then $M_W = M_N$ and $Q = 1$.

The average molecular weight and molecular weight distribution of polymers are important factors in the coating process since they will influence not only solution viscosity, but also the mechanical properties of the final film coat (Rowe, 1976, see also Chapter 12).

Several authors have attempted to characterize the molecular weight of HPMC (Rowe, 1980; Tufnell *et al.*, 1983; Davies, 1985). Absolute methods of analysis, such as light scattering, which allow molecular weights to be determined directly from experimental data, have been found to be unsuitable for HPMC (Tufnell *et al.*, 1983; Davies, 1985). The technique that has been used successfully is gel permeation chromatography (GPC) which allows the determination of M_N, M_W and the degree of polydispersity (Q) for polymers having a wide range of molecular weights. GPC, however, suffers from the disadvantage that since no monodisperse fractionated samples of HPMC are available, the gel bed has to be calibrated with other standards, such as dextrans. The molecular weight values derived for HPMC must therefore be expressed as values equivalent to the standard molecule used. Since the hydrodynamic volume of an HPMC molecule may be different to that of the standard molecule and will vary depending on the solvent used, the molar mass expressed as an equivalent to a standard molecule is likely to be different to the absolute molecular weight. In practice, different GPC systems have been shown to produce different molecular weight values for the same HPMC sample (Davies, 1985).

The rheological properties of HPMC solutions

Dilute aqueous solutions of HPMC E5 consist of randomly orientated and randomly extended coils of hydrated molecules of a wide range of sizes, with their configuration and degree of solvation changing continuously due to random bombardment by solvent molecules. Each molecule will tend to act as a single entity with little or no intra- or intermolecular interactions (Davies, 1985). This would explain why dilute aqueous solutions of HPMC grades with low nominal viscosities exhibit Newtonian behaviour.

Polymer concentration

HPMC solution viscosity was found (Twitchell, 1990) to vary more than any other solution property for a range of coating formulations. Data for two commercial batches of HPMC E5 are shown in Table 4.4 as an indication of the interbatch variation that is typical of most polymeric coating materals. The concentration of HPMC in solution has a profound effect on solution viscosity, with this effect increasing with increasing concentration. For example, a doubling in concentration from 6 to 12 %w/w causes a greater than ten-fold increase in viscosity. The data in Table 4.4 are shown graphically in Figure 4.3.

Fig. 4.3 illustrates how the viscosity of HPMC solutions increases markedly with HPMC concentration. Note particularly how the gradient of the viscosity–concentration plot becomes extremely steep after solution concentrations above 10 %w/w. It is tempting when preparing a coating solution to have the concentration of dissolved polymer as high as possible (i.e. a 'high solids loading') in order to reduce the application time and the amount of solvent that needs to be evaporated. This is particularly so in the case of water, due to its high latent heat of vaporization.

Table 4.4   The effect of HPMC E5 concentration on aqueous solution
viscosity at 20°C for two batches of polymer

HPMC E5 concentration (%w/w)	Viscosity (mPa s)	
	Batch 1	Batch 2
2	4.6	4.8
4	14.0	—
6	37.5	44.9
9	136.9	166.0
10	227.7	—
12	437.0	519.5
15	1287.3*	1417.1*

* These solutions are non-Newtonian. The figures quoted are apparent Newtonian viscosities calculated using a power-law equation.

However, these solutions will be very viscous. The consequences of using high viscosity polymer solutions are discussed fully in Chapter 13.

Many attempts have been made by scientists to linearize such viscosity–concentration data. Pickard (1979), Delporte (1980) and Prater (1982), in attempting to determine a relationship between viscosity and HPMC E5 solution concentration, found that plots of log viscosity *versus* solution concentration were not linear. Philippoff (1936), however, had demonstrated for methylcellulose that if the eighth root of viscosity was plotted against concentration (%w/v) a straight line resulted. This latter relationship was also found by Aulton *et al.* (1986) to be applicable for HPMC E5. The result of a Philippoff plot for aqueous HPMC E5 solutions is shown in Fig. 4.4.

It is apparent from Fig. 4.3 that there is a very large increase in viscosity as increased concentrations of HPMC E5 are dissolved in water, a 12 %w/w solution, for example, being around 500 times more viscous than water alone. One contributing factor to this is the large hydrodynamic volume of the randomly coiled polymer chains and their associated hydrogen-bonded water molecules. These large flow units increase the resistance to flow and thus viscosity. The work of Davies (1985) suggests additionally that a significant amount of water is located within the random coil of the polymer. With HPMC E5 molecules this is thought to be non-draining, the water being mechanically trapped within the polymer coil and dragged along with the macromolecule during flow. This further increases resistance to flow and also decreases the amount of remaining free solvent.

As explained previously, commercial grades of HPMC are polydisperse in nature, consisting of a wide range of molecular weight fractions. Of these, the larger molecular weight fractions contribute to the viscosity to an extent which is disproportionate to their concentration on a weight basis. Thus a HPMC molecule with a degree of polymerization of 200 will produce a viscosity far higher than if the 200 individual units were present. This occurs since the cooperative nature of the flow of the 200 unit

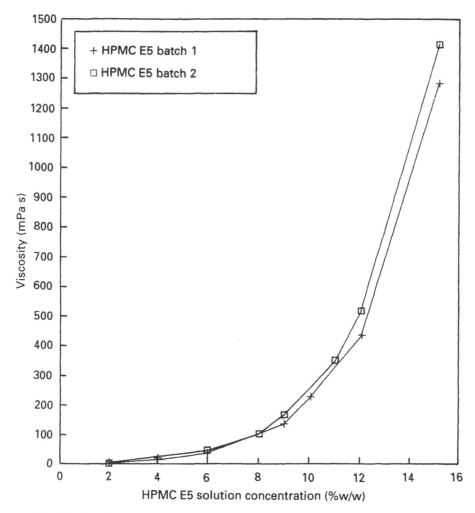

Fig. 4.3   Viscosity *versus* concentration curves for aqueous solutions of HPMC E5 at 20°C. Two sets of data are shown, corresponding to the two batches of HPMC E5 referred to in Table 4.4.

chain and its accompanying water molecules, which move together with the polymer, results in a very large flow unit. The work of Davies (1985) appears to support this although the data from Rowe (1980) show there to be no correlation between the viscosity at 2 %w/v and the value of the weight-average molecular weight.

For higher polymer concentrations where pseudoplastic flow is exhibited, the polymer chains, when under conditions of increasing shear, become progressively untangled and the hydrogen bonds may be broken, resulting in a reduction in the dimensions of the polymer and the release of any entrapped solvent, resulting in turn in a reduction in the disturbance to flow and therefore a reduction in viscosity.

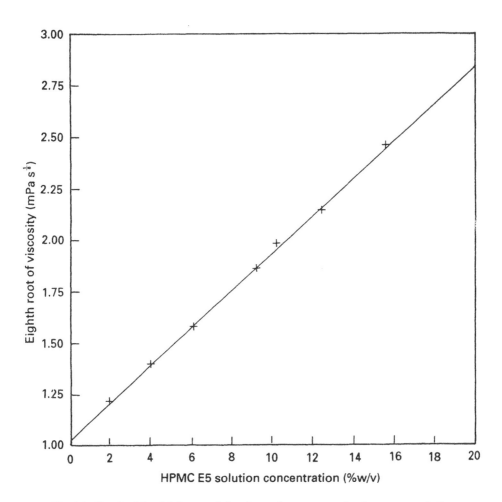

Fig. 4.4   Graph of the eighth root of viscosity against concentration for aqueous solutions
of HPMC E5 at 20°C.

During the film-coating process it is likely that film coat formulations will
encounter a wide range of shear rates. These range from the low values in the tubing
delivering solutions to the spray gun, to values of around 300 to 20 000 s⁻¹ as they
pass through the liquid spray nozzle (values calculated from equations in Henderson
et al., 1961) and to highly variable shear rates produced by the high-velocity atomizing air at the droplet production stage. Once impinged on the substrate, the shear
rate encountered will be dependent on the atomization conditions and the tumbling
action of tablets occurring in a coating pan or multiparticulates moving vigorously
in a fluidized bed. Newtonian solutions are likely to exhibit the same rheological
behaviour at all stages of the coating process irrespective of the shear rate encountered. At temperatures below approximately 45–50°C, dilute HPMC E5 solutions

behave as Newtonian liquids. It is probable, however, that coating solutions or suspensions which exhibit non-Newtonian behaviour may vary in viscosity at various stages during the coating process and when different coating conditions and coating equipment are used.

Fig. 4.3 showed that at the higher HPMC E5 concentrations small changes in concentration result in relatively large increases in viscosity. For example, the viscosity of an 11 %w/w solution is 350 mPa s whereas a 12% w/w solution has a viscosity of 520 mPa s. This concept may be of importance in relation to any evaporation that occurs from atomized droplets before they impinge on the substrate surface. If, for example, 20 % of the water is lost from the droplets during their passage to a tablet bed in a perforated pan coater, as suggested by Yoakam and Campbell (1984), then solutions initially of 6 %w/w and having a viscosity of 45 mPa s would hit the tablet with a concentration of 7.4 %w/w and a viscosity of approximately 80 mPa s. Similarly, droplets from 9 and 12 %w/w solutions may increase in viscosity from 166 to 360 mPa s and from 520 to 1265 mPa s, respectively. In the case of a 12 %w/w solution this is likely to be accompanied by a change in the rheological nature of the solution from Newtonian to pseudoplastic. Large differences may therefore potentially exist between the viscosity of the droplets and that of the bulk solution, with this effect becoming considerably greater as the initial solution concentration increases. The extent to which these changes in viscosity may occur during the coating process will be dependent on a number of factors, such as the temperature and humidity of the drying air, droplet size and the time taken to reach the tablet or multiparticulate surface.

The viscosity of most aqueous solutions is reduced by elevating their temperature. This is also true for HPMC, as is shown in Fig. 4.5.

As might be expected, a rise in temperature decreases solution viscosity, but one must be aware that HPMC solutions undergo thermal gelation at temperatures just above 50°C. The phenomenon of thermal gelation of HPMC solutions is discussed below.

The reduction in viscosity with increasing solution temperature is more pronounced at lower temperatures and higher solution concentrations. For the example data given, a temperature increase from 10 to 20°C results in a viscosity decrease of 17 mPa s for a 6 %w/w solution, 66 mPa s for a 9 %w/w solution and 216 mPa s for 12 %w/w solution. A temperature increase from 20 to 30°C, however, results in falls of only 10, 35 and 115 mPa s respectively.

Thermal gelation

Aqueous HPMC solutions exhibit the property of thermal gelation—that is, if a solution is heated above a certain temperature, a gel network is formed.

The thermal gelation temperature of HPMC E5 is often taken as the temperature at which the trend of decreasing viscosity with increasing temperature is reversed (Prater, 1982). This definition will generate, however, markedly different values of the gelation temperature depending on the shear rate at which the apparent viscosity is measured. Twitchell (1990) took the thermal gelation temperature as that

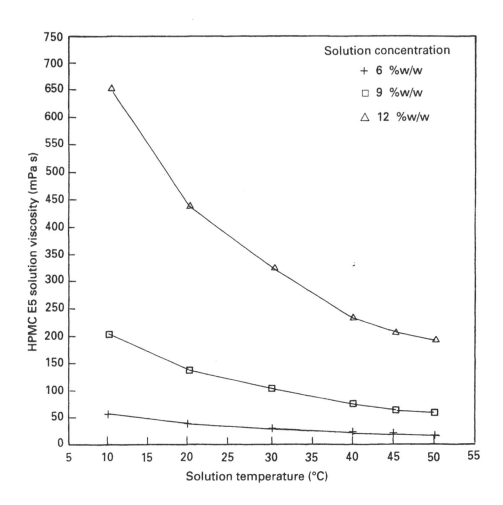

Fig. 4.5 The effect of solution temperature on the viscosity of aqueous HPMC E5 solutions of different concentrations.

temperature at which thixotropic behaviour was noted, since this is indicative of the formation of a gel structure and its breakdown on the application of shear forces.

If the temperature of dilute HPMC E5 solutions is raised above 50°C, there is a change in the shape of the rheological profile. Deviation from linearity occurs and there is evidence of pseudoplasticity.

Plots of the logarithm of viscosity *versus* the reciprocal of absolute temperature for 6, 9 and 12 %w/w aqueous solutions of HPMC E5 appear to be linear up to a temperature of approximately 45°C. At temperatures above 45°C deviation from linearity is observed. These findings are probably associated with the changing of rheological behaviour as the solution temperature approaches 50°C. Around this temperature, the extent of the desolvation of the polymer is such that polymer–water bonds are replaced by polymer–polymer bonds, resulting in associations between polymer chains and a restriction in the flow of the continuous phase. When the solution is sheared increasingly, the chains become more linearly orientated and any structure formed may be broken, resulting in a decrease in apparent viscosity.

At temperatures above about 52°C, thermal gelation occurs at most HPMC solution concentrations. This is due to the formation of a structured gel network in which the solvent is entrapped between chains of hydrogen-bonded polymer. For the many HPMC E5 solutions studied, Twitchell (1990) found no detectable differences in the thermal gelation temperature, this being 52 ± 1°C in each case.

Heating the HPMC E5 solutions to temperatures above approximately 60°C results in precipitation of the polymer and a decrease in viscosity. HPMC solutions which undergo thermal gelation will revert to their original rheological behaviour on cooling to 20°C.

A temperature rise from 20 to 40°C results in an approximate halving of the viscosities of the three concentrations studied (Fig. 4.5). It has been suggested that this behaviour could be exploited during the film coating process, since if HPMC E5 solutions were heated prior to use, then a greater solids loading could be achieved for a particular viscosity value, leaving atomization unchanged and the coating process time reduced (Hogan, 1982). Care must be taken, however, in controlling the temperature in industrial coating or employing temperature as a means of viscosity control for HPMC coating solutions, since heating HPMC solutions above their thermal gelation temperature will result in a semi-solid, unsprayable solution. Secondly, an excessive drying air temperature in a coater *may* result in atomized droplets gelling before they hit the substrate surface (however, this is unlikely, as a result of evaporative cooling).

It is important also to be aware that the gelation temperatures of the HPMC solutions used in aqueous film coating may be affected by the addition of commonly used formulation additives, so that factors leading to the phenomenon occurring in practice can be avoided. Reduction of the gelation temperature, to 37°C or below for example, has been associated with the reduction in release rate from coated tablets (Schwartz & Alvino, 1976).

In order to avoid changes in rheological behaviour and the problems associated with thermal gelation when using aqueous film coating, it is important that HPMC E5 solutions are not subjected to temperatures over approximately 45°C at any point in the coating process. Similarly, it should be remembered that the viscosity of a coating solution may vary considerably at different points in the coating process if it is subjected to fluctuating temperatures (Fig. 4.5). These temperature changes may occur in the coating solution holding vessel, during passage to the spray gun, at the spray gun itself, during passage to the tablet or multiparticulate surface, or at those surfaces.

Effect of plasticizer addition
The effect of including various commonly used plasticizers on the viscosity of aqueous HPMC E5 solutions at 20°C is illustrated in Fig. 4.6. The HPMC E5

concentration is constant at 9 %w/w for each test solution and the plasticizer concentration ranges from 0 to 5 %w/w. Generally, their addition at these levels raises solution viscosity, but causes no deviation from the original Newtonian behaviour of the solution.

The addition of the three different grades of polyethylene glycol (PEG) appeared to cause a linear increase in viscosity with increasing concentration, the increase being greater as the average molecular weight of PEG increased. The non-polymeric plasticizers, propylene glycol and glycerol, gave non-linear increases in viscosity with increasing concentration and gave rise to smaller increases in viscosity than the PEGs over the concentration range studied.

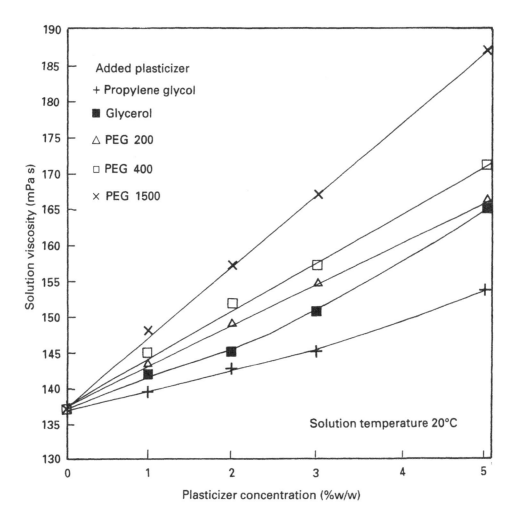

Fig. 4.6   The effect of plasticizer addition on the viscosity of an aqueous 9 %w/w HPMC E5 solution at 20°C.

In practice these plasticizers would be unlikely to be added to a 9 %w/w HPMC E5 solution at concentrations above 3 %w/w in the coating solution due to incompatibility encountered once the film coat has formed. Typical solution concentrations that would be used in practice lie between 1 and 2 %w/w. At these levels the viscosity increases caused by the plasticizers studied would range from approximately 4 to 20 mPa s, representing an approximate increase of between 3.5 and 15%.

The relationship between solution viscosity and solution temperature for 9 %w/w HPMC E5 solutions containing 2 %w/w of various plasticizers is similar to that observed when no plasticizers were present. The onset of pseudoplastic and thixotropic behaviour occurs at temperatures of approximately 50 and 52°C respectively, irrespective of the plasticizer present, and thus these changes occur at similar temperatures to those seen with the original additive-free HPMC E5 solution.

It has been shown by Okhamafe & York (1983) that the addition of PEG 400 and PEG 1000 at low concentrations (0.05 to 0.5 %w/v) to aqueous solutions of HPMC resulted in a decrease in the value of intrinsic viscosity. They attributed this decrease to an interaction between PEG and water. It was postulated that PEG removed the water molecules associated with HPMC, thereby reducing its molecular dimensions. If this was the case, however, it would be expected that PEG 400, being more hydrophilic than PEG 1000, would give rise to a greater reduction in intrinsic viscosity. The reverse was observed, however, by Okhamafe & York (1983). A minimum was observed in the intrinsic viscosity values at a PEG 1000 concentration of 50 %w/w and PEG 400 concentration of 60 %w/w, these concentrations being relative to the amount of HPMC E5. It was postulated that above these concentrations some of the PEG was interacting with the HPMC, leading to an increase in the molecular dimensions and thus to a viscosity increase, although it should be noted that PEG would not be used at these concentrations in coating formulations owing to compatibility problems in the dried film.

The effect of the addition of a plasticizer on the viscosity of HPMC E5 solutions is likely to be influenced by several factors. First, almost all plasticizers, when added to water, will cause an increase in viscosity. A second factor that may influence viscosity arises from the fact that all the plasticizers used are poor solvents for HPMC E5 compared with water—HPMC E5, for example, being virtually insoluble in glycerol at all temperatures. Their addition may therefore render the solvent system less favourable to the formation of a random, opened, coiled structure and thus cause a reduction in the hydrodynamic volume of the polymer. A consequence of the altered polymer dimensions would be a reduction in the values of intrinsic and actual viscosity and could explain the observations of Okhamafe & York (1983) with regard to the reduced intrinsic viscosity values observed when plasticizers were added.

Further contributing factors are the possibilities that either the plasticizers are interacting with the polymer itself or, more likely, with the water sheath surrounding the polymer, thereby altering the polymer dimensions. These interactions may either increase the dimensions of the polymer unit owing to association with the plasticizer, or decrease its dimensions by competing for and removing the attached water molecules. The latter effect would be more liable to occur with glycerol and propylene glycol since they are more hydrophilic than the PEGs.

In practice, it is probable that a combination of these factors influences solution viscosity, with the relative magnitude of each being different for each plasticizer.

Colouring agents, opacifiers, fillers and surfactants
The effect of including various other additives on the viscosity of 9 %w/w HPMC E5 solutions is shown in Fig. 4.7. It can be seen that all the additives studied caused an increase in the viscosity of HPMC E5 solutions, although the extent of the increase varies depending on the additive used and may differ at different shear rates if the additive imparts pseudoplastic behaviour.

It is recommended that for HPMC-based systems, a suitable maximum pigment-to-polymer ratio in the film coat is 1:2. This corresponds to 4.5 %w/w of solids being incorporated into a 9 %w/w HPMC E5 solution. At this concentration it can be seen that viscosity increases of up to approximately 80% may be encountered.

All the additives shown in Fig. 4.7 caused an increase in viscosity at concentrations likely to be used in practice. The inclusion of non-soluble components also caused a change in rheological behaviour from Newtonian to pseudoplastic, this arising from disturbances to the flow pattern and orientation of asymmetric particles as the shear rate increased. The extent of this change was dependent on the material used and generally was found to increase with increasing additive concentration. Formulations including these additives may therefore exhibit differing viscosities at different stages in the coating process.

Of the insoluble additives studied, the greatest increase in apparent Newtonian viscosity was caused by the brilliant blue HT aluminium lake followed by titanium dioxide and talc, with viscosity increases of over 80% (from 137 to 251 mPa s) being possible in the practical situation. The differences in the viscosity enhancing effect of the non-soluble additives will be dependent on complex relationships between factors such as the particle size, shape and density, particle–particle interaction and degree of agglomeration. Chopra & Tawashi (1985), for example, showed that as the mean volume diameter of talc was decreased from 39 to 16 μm, so the ability to enhance viscosity markedly increased. Substances such as talc, which have a flake-like structure, would (all other factors being equal) be expected to cause a greater deviation from Newtonian behaviour than titanium dioxide, for example, which is more rounded. Increasing the density of the solid may be expected to reduce the degree of viscosity enhancement due to a reduction in the surface area available for disturbance of the flow patterns.

Since there is likely to be considerable variation in the physical properties of most of these additives, depending on their source, it follows that the viscosity changes caused by their addition are also likely to vary.

Addition of the colorant dispersion Opaspray (which contains 30 %w/w solids) to a solution of HPMC E5 also imparts pseudoplastic behaviour, this being due to the presence of the insoluble solids, titanium dioxide and aluminium lake, included in its formulation. At the recommended concentration of 15 %w/w with a 9 %w/w

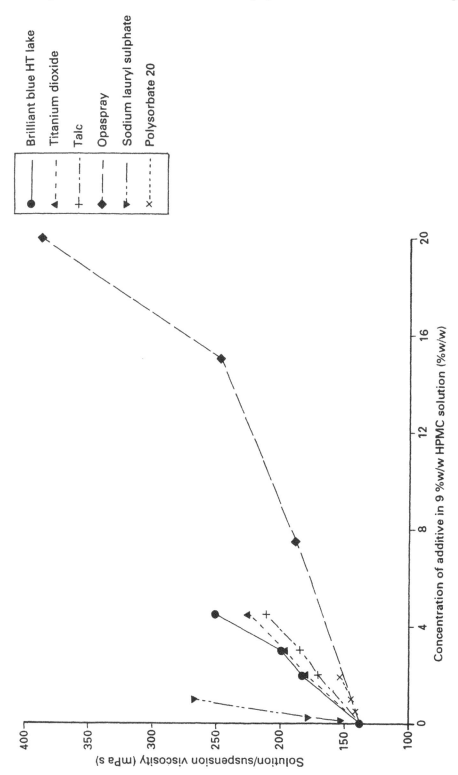

Fig. 4.7   Influence of the presence of some inclusions on the viscosity of 9 %w/w aqueous HPMC solutions.

HPMC E5 solution (giving a film pigment-to-polymer ratio of 1:2) Opaspray causes a viscosity increase of 109 mPa s (+80%). A further increase in Opaspray concentration to 20 %w/w more than doubles the viscosity increase to 250 mPa s.

The addition of insoluble solids dispersed in the formulation causes a change in the rheological profile with pseudoplastic behaviour being exhibited instead of Newtonian behaviour. However, viscosity values quoted are those of the apparent Newtonian viscosity. These are the viscosities that the formulations are calculated to possess at a shear rate of 1 per second. Viscosity values at any other shear rate can be calculated from a power-law equation by utilizing the calculated values of the apparent Newtonian viscosity and the index of non-Newtonian behaviour.

Rheograms also indicate that once the shear rate exceeds approximately 600 per second, there is generally a linear increase in shear stress with increases in shear rate, this being indicative of the existence of a Newtonian region at these shear rates.

The index of non-Newtonian behaviour for these formulations is generally close to 1, indicating that the deviation from Newtonian behaviour is not large. Over the concentration ranges studied, the value for the index of non-Newtonian behaviour did not appear to be related to the concentration of insoluble additive used.

The inclusion of the surface-active agents sodium lauryl sulphate (SLS) and polysorbate 20 at the concentrations detailed in Fig. 4.7 did not cause the 9 %w/w HPMC E5 solution to deviate from Newtonian behaviour. However, there was a large difference in their effect on solution viscosity, with SLS causing almost a doubling of viscosity from 137 to 268 mPa s when included at a concentration of 1 %w/w and polysorbate 20 having only a small effect at concentrations up to 2 %w/w. The inclusion of SLS at a concentration of 1 %w/w was found to cause a similar relative increase in the viscosity of a 12 %w/w solution of HPMC E5 from 437 to 821 mPa s. This, coupled with the fact that a 1 %w/w solution of SLS was found to possess a viscosity of 1.86 mPa s, suggests that the increases seen in the viscosity of the HPMC solutions is in effect due to an increase in the viscosity of the solvent rather than SLS interacting with the HPMC E5 molecules or their associated water sheath. In the absence of any difference in the effect of these surface active agents on the surface tension of HPMC solutions, it would seem sensible to use polysorbate 20 instead of SLS, since this may reduce any potential problems arising from increased viscosity values.

The effect of additives on gelation temperature
Care must be taken to ensure that any additives included in the coating formulation do not adversely reduce the gelation temperature. It has been shown by Levy & Schwarz (1958) that glycerol can cause a reduction in the gelation temperature of methylcellulose, whereas propylene glycol and PEG 400 can cause an increase. Prater (1982) found the inclusion of propylene glycol at a concentration of 20 %w/w to have a minimal effect on the gelation temperature of 5 %w/v solutions of HPMC E5. Twitchell (1990) studied the effect of the inclusion of five plasticizers at a solution concentration of 2 %w/w (the maximum at which they are likely to be used practically) in a 9 %w/w HPMC E5 solution and found them to have no detectable influence on the gelation temperature.

The thermal gelation temperature of the formulations which included Opaspray was found to occur at approximately 52°C, this being no different from the additive-free HPMC E5 solution.

Other polymers
Similar trends to those described above have been observed for other polymer solutions—for example, aqueous methylcellulose and alcoholic ethylcellulose solutions by Banker & Peck (1981) who also showed the lack of high viscosity for high concentrations of ethylcellulose pseudolatex dispersions.

4.2.5 Conclusions on solution properties
From the results presented and discussed in section 4.2 of this chapter it is apparent that the physical properties of HPMC E5-based solutions used in aqueous film coating may vary markedly and therefore potentially influence the coating process at a number of stages.

The main variable factor potentially influencing the atomization stage would appear to be the rheological properties of the solutions. The changes in surface tension and density values which may be encountered in practice seem unlikely to exert any significant effects. Variation in the rheological properties may arise from a variety of causes, including solution concentration and temperature, material batch variation, inappropriate storage conditions and whether plasticizing or colouring agents are present. In addition, some formulations may exhibit pseudoplastic behaviour which may give rise to variable values of viscosity at the point of atomization and at the substrate surface, these being dependent on the shear conditions encountered. Thus, any viscometer which provides for a variable rate of shear can be useful in evaluating effects of polymer concentration and effects of plasticizers and pigments on the viscosity of a polymer solution.

It has been demonstrated that the surface tension of the droplets produced on atomizing film-coating solutions may vary depending on the rheological properties of the solution from which they were produced, their droplet size (see Section 5.2.2), the concentration of HPMC E5 present and the time taken to travel to the substrate surface. Differences in droplet size, surface tension and viscosity may, in addition, influence the degree of evaporation and coalescence that occurs before the droplets impinge on the substrate which, in turn, may further influence the rheological properties.

Once impinged on the surface, the variations in droplet viscosity and surface tension may affect the ability of the droplets to adhere, wet, spread, coalesce and penetrate. This, in turn, may lead to differences in the occurrence of film coat defects, the adhesion to the tablet or multiparticulate core and the gloss and roughness of the coat. The extent to which the physical properties of the film-coating solutions affect the various stages of the coating process becomes clearer after examination of the actual droplet sizes produced during film coating (see section 4.4) and the properties of film coats produced in a practical situation (Chapters 12 and 13).

4.3   DROPLET SIZE MEASUREMENT

4.3.1   Methods of droplet size measurement

An understanding of the solution properties discussed above (section 4.2) is important since these properties can influence strongly the size and distribution of droplets produced during spraying which, in turn, will influence the fate of the droplet at the tablet or multiparticulate surface and the quality of the resulting film coat. Before we can discuss the interaction between droplets and surface we must be able to quantify the distribution of droplet sizes within the spray.

Droplet size analysis

The ideal droplet sizing technique should:

1. not interfere with the spray pattern and break-up process;
2. analyse large representative samples;
3. permit rapid sampling and counting;
4. have good size discrimination over the entire range of droplets being measured;
5. tolerate variations in the liquid and ambient gas properties;
6. permit determinations of both the spatial and temporal droplet size distribution.

Since it is very difficult to fulfil satisfactorily all of these criteria, the capabilities and limitations of a given technique must be recognized. Reviews of droplet measurement techniques have been presented by Jones (1977), Chigier (1982) and Lefebvre (1989). Of the numerous methods available for determining the droplet size distribution of an atomized spray, the following have been found to be the most useful:

- Captive methods.
- Photographic methods.
- Laser-light scattering methods.

Captive methods

Captive techniques commonly employed include impingement of the droplets onto either glass slides or plates coated with a powder or high-viscosity oil, or onto smoked paper. The diameter of the droplets is then measured individually using a microscope with an eyepiece graticule. Much of the earlier research into the atomization process relied on these captive methods for measuring droplet sizes. These techniques may, however, interfere with the spray pattern. They are also time consuming and tedious to perform since at least 1000 droplets should be counted in order to achieve a sufficiently accurate size distribution. There is also a common human error in that many of the smaller droplets are not counted, thus resulting in inaccuracies due to the collection of unrepresentative data. There may be additional problems associated with evaporation and/or coalescence.

Photographic methods

Photographic techniques utilizing double flash/double image photographs are capable of measuring both droplet size and droplet velocity. Cole *et al.* (1980), using such a technique, reported that droplets as small as 5 μm could be detected. Useful information on liquid jet disintegration mechanisms and droplet formation processes may also be gained. This method, however, also suffers from some major drawbacks. It is difficult to measure very small droplets accurately; there is a limited amount of information which can be gained from each photograph; and accurate analysis is both tedious and time consuming.

Laser-light scattering methods
Both the above methods are unsatisfactory for routine or extensive testing. Fortunately, a far superior method is available. Major advances in the measurement of droplet sizes have occurred in recent years with the advent of sophisticated optical systems. Many instruments are commercially available, based on forward light scattering, diffraction, laser doppler velocimetry and holography. Such techniques are invariably very quick, non-intrusive and permit coupling to a microprocessor for data analysis.

Chigier (1982), in a review of the sizing techniques available, concluded that the Fraunhofer diffraction particle sizer (e.g. Malvern Instruments Ltd) was the simplest of the methods to use and reported that it had been extensively adopted in laboratories testing overall spray characteristics; its use has also been reported by Lefebvre (1989). It provides accurate, repeatable, representative and reliable results in a wide range of environments and is now widely used, although it does not give information on individual droplets.

The Malvern droplet and particle size analyser
The Malvern analyser, a schematic representation of which is shown in Fig. 4.8, is based on the theory of Fraunhofer diffraction. A small, safe laser transmitter produces a parallel beam of monochromatic light (He/Ne, λ = 632.8 nm) through which is passed the spray to be analysed. When the light falls on the droplets a diffraction pattern is formed whereby some of the light is diffracted by an amount dependent on the size of the droplet. The diffraction angle is largest for small droplets (for example, 11° for droplets of 1 μm diameter) and decreases as the droplet size increases. A Fourier transform lens is used to focus the light pattern onto a multi-element photodetector in order to measure the diffracted light energy distribution. Undiffracted light is brought to focus at a hole in the centre of the detector and the diffracted light is focused concentrically around the central axis. The radius of the concentric rings is therefore a function of the focal length of the lens and the size of the droplet which diffracted the light, the light from larger droplets being focused a smaller distance from the centre. The diffraction pattern generated by the droplets is independent of the position of the droplet in the beam, hence measurements can be made with droplets moving at any speed. Since the spray is not monosize, a series of concentric rings of different radii corresponding to droplets of different sizes are generated. The photodetector consists of 30 concentric, semicircular, light-sensitive ring detectors, with a hole in the centre. Behind the hole is a photodiode which is used for alignment and measuring the intensity in the centre of the pattern. Each pair of detectors corresponds to droplets of a particular

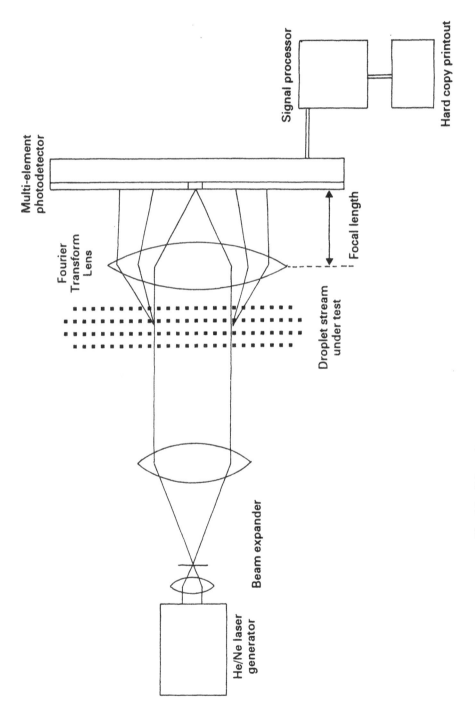

Fig. 4.8.   Schematic representation of the Malvern droplet size analyser.

diameter range (thus giving fifteen size bands), the size range being dependent on the focal length of the lens used. Lenses with focal lengths of 63, 100 and 300 mm correspond to total droplet measuring size ranges of 1.2–118 μm, 1.9–188 μm and 5.8–584 μm respectively. The signal from the multi-element detector is amplified, digitized and processed by a microcomputer.

The data can either be presented as a best fit to a chosen mathematical function (such as normal, log normal and Rosin–Rammler) or analysed independently (model-independent mode) using the Malvern algorithm. Results can be stored on disc and a hard copy produced. Results detailed include the percentage by weight in each different size band and the cumulative weight percentages above and below the size bands.

4.3.2   Characteristic droplet size distributions and representative mean diameters

Droplet size distributions
An accurate knowledge of the distribution of droplet sizes within a spray is a prerequisite for the understanding of how the many factors involved in film coating affect both the atomization process and the resultant film coat. To describe fully the spray produced from a stated set of atomization conditions, it is necessary to give the number, weight or volume of droplets of a particular size or in a particular size band. In studies where a large variety of different atomization conditions are investigated, describing the droplet sizes in this way yields a large amount of data and it is difficult to assess the relative importance of the variables involved. Consequently, droplet distributions are often characterized by a single value representing a 'mean diameter' as described below.

An alternative approach to representing the size distribution of the sprays is to determine if the data can be expressed by well-defined mathematical functions, as shown by Rosin & Rammler (1933), Mugele & Evans (1951), Fraser & Eisenklam (1956) and Kumar & Prasad (1971). These functions include normal, log–normal, Rosin–Rammler and upper–limit log–normal distributions. They are empirical in nature, and because of the complex liquid break-up mechanisms associated with most sprays, have no theoretical basis. The selection of the function to describe a system is only dependent on its ability to fit the actual data. The advantage of characterizing sprays in this way is that the entire distribution can be represented by two or three parameters, these usually describing a 'mean' diameter and an indication of the dispersity of sizes.

Characteristic mean diameters
The majority of workers investigating the atomization process have characterized the droplet distribution in terms of characteristic mean droplet diameters, and have presented equations to show the effect of process variables on these diameters. Although they have no fundamental meaning, unless it is known that the droplets fall in a defined distribution function, characteristic droplet diameters serve as a useful simple method of comparing large quantities of data. When expressing an

average diameter, a given polysize system is replaced by either an equivalent mono-size system which has the same number of droplets and one other property (such as length, surface or mass) in common, or by a system where the polysize and mono-size systems do not have the same number but have other properties in common, such as specific surface.

It is necessary therefore to define these characteristic droplet diameters. Those commonly used are described below.

Mean length diameter. The mean length diameter (D_L), also known as the *arith-metic mean diameter*, is defined as the diameter of a monosize system having the same number and total length as the polysize system. Thus,

$$D_L = \frac{\sum (x.\Delta n)}{N} \qquad (4.6)$$

where Δn is the number of droplets of diameter x, and N is the total number of droplets.

Volume mean diameter. The volume mean diameter (D_{VM}) is defined as the diam-eter of a monosize system which has the same number and total volume as the poly-size system. Thus, with symbols as defined in equation (4.6),

$$D_{VM} = \left[\frac{\sum (x^3.\Delta n)}{N} \right]^{1/3} \qquad (4.7)$$

Surface mean diameter. The surface mean diameter (D_{SM}), also referred to as the *Sauter mean diameter*, is the diameter of a monosize system having the same specific surface as the polysize system. Thus, again with symbols as defined in equation (4.6),

$$D_{SM} = \frac{\sum (x^3.\Delta n)}{N} \bigg/ \frac{\sum (x^2.\Delta n)}{N} \qquad (4.8)$$

Mean evaporative diameter. The mean evaporative diameter (D_{ME}) is the diam-eter of a monosize system which has the same specific evaporation rate as a given polysize spray and can be calculated by symbols (as defined in equation (4.6)),

$$D_{ME} = \left[\frac{\sum (x^3.\Delta n)}{N} \bigg/ \frac{\sum (x.\Delta n)}{N} \right]^{0.5} \qquad (4.9)$$

Mass median diameter. The mass median diameter (D_{MM}) is the diameter above or below which lies 50% of the total mass. It can be read from a cumulative weight percentage undersize or oversize graph.

Other diameters determined by the percentage of the total mass which lies below their size include $D_{0.1}$ (10% below), $D_{0.9}$ (90% below), and the Rosin–Rammler diam-eter (63.2% below, as long as the data fit a Rosin–Rammler distribution).

Values for a range of calculated characteristic mean diameters for the same HPMC spray are shown in Table 4.5. Note the wide range of values listed. The data emphasize that we must decide carefully which d_{mean} is calculated since this can make a significant difference to the figure quoted. Similarly, as in all size analysis

Table 4.5 Characteristic calculated mean droplet diameters for a typical aqueous HPMC E5 spray (Twitchell, 1990)

Descriptive name	Characteristic mean diameter (μm)
Mean length diameter (D_L)	3.7
Volume mean diameter (D_{VM})	6.4
Surface mean diameter (D_{SM})	14.3
Mean evaporative diameter (D_{EM})	9.3
Mass median diameter (D_{MM})	24.1
$D_{0.1}$	6.7
$D_{0.9}$	64.9

techniques, the method of measurement and correct full description of the type of mean size calculated should always be quoted.

Of the droplet diameters listed in Table 4.5, the most commonly quoted are the volume mean diameter, surface mean diameter and mass mean diameter. In the case of the above example, the values of the mean length diameter and volume mean diameter are lower since they are affected disproportionately by a large number of very small droplets (below 10 μm). In addition, the accuracy of the smaller mean droplet diameters is likely to be lower since the ability of early Malverns to determine droplet sizes is reduced at diameters of approximately 10 μm and below (Weiner, 1982; Naining & Hongjian, 1986).

It can be concluded from the above discussion that each of the methods of expressing the data has its advantages and disadvantages. It is most convenient to express data in the form of characteristic droplet diameters. These can be supplemented where necessary by the use of graphical representations of the complete distribution.

4.4 THE INFLUENCE OF FORMULATION AND ATOMIZATION CONDITIONS ON SPRAY DROPLET SIZE AND SIZE DISTRIBUTION

4.4.1 Introduction

General introduction to atomization
Atomization is the process whereby a liquid is broken up into a spray of droplets. It is employed in a wide range of industrial processes including paint application, air-conditioning humidification, fuel ignition, spray drying, fluidized-bed granulation and film coating. In film coating the utilization of atomization techniques enables the coating polymer to be efficiently applied to a granule, pellet, bead or tablet core surface. Atomized droplets hitting the substrate during film coating should be in such a state that they spread evenly over the surface and form a

smooth continuous film of even thickness. The atomization stage of the coating process therefore encompasses all factors which influence the state at which the droplets arrive at the substrate surface and their behaviour once there. Inadequate control of the atomization process can result in film coat defects such as picking, sticking and excessive roughness.

Although much research has been carried out in recent years into various aspects of the film-coating process, characterization of the atomization stage and its influence on the final film properties has been largely ignored. Satisfactory film coats have been achieved in the pharmaceutical industry using atomization techniques arising from a combination of trial-and-error and previous experience. It can be argued, however, that if the development scientist and the process operator have knowledge of how the coating formulation, spray-gun type and operating parameters influence the atomization process and the resulting film properties, a more rational approach could be adopted to predict the conditions likely to produce a satisfactory end-product.

Methods of achieving atomization

Many different methods of atomizing solutions are available. They all tend to produce a distribution of droplet sizes and all, except those using ultrasonic energy, tend to be relatively inefficient; the energy required to produce the increase in surface area is typically less than 1% of the total energy consumption (Masters, 1976).

Ultrasonic atomization

Ultrasonic atomizers form droplets by subjecting the fluid to intense high-frequency vibrations. They have not tended to be used for tablet, granule or multiparticulate film coating to date, since those available either have difficulty in coping with the flow rates required for either organic or aqueous film coating, produce droplets which do not possess sufficient momentum or have nozzles which are easily fouled.

Hydraulic (airless) atomization

In a hydraulic atomizer, droplets are produced by forcing a liquid under high pressure through a small orifice. The form of the resulting liquid can be varied by changing the pressure used, by altering the direction of flow into the orifice or by the use of different nozzles. Flat or conical spray patterns may be produced. Hydraulic atomization is the system of choice when organic solvents are used to dissolve the film-forming polymer, since premature droplet drying is inhibited as air is not used to produce and shape the spray. The high pressures needed to produce adequate atomization of viscous coating solutions demand that the flow rates produced are relatively high even with very small orifice diameters. This is acceptable with highly volatile organic solvents, but when water is used, as is the preferred practice in pharmaceutical coating, the ability of the coating equipment to evaporate the solvent satisfactorily may be overcome and the product overwetted, resulting in poor-quality coatings.

Pneumatic atomization

This is the method of choice for aqueous pharmaceutical film coating. The energy for atomization is derived from a high-speed airstream which impinges on a jet of the solution to be atomized. In order to produce droplets this airstream has to both accelerate the liquid above a critical speed whereby it becomes unstable, and provide energy to overcome the viscous and surface tension forces resisting droplet formation. Since air has a low density, a comparatively large volume moving at high speed is required to impart a portion of its energy to heavy viscous materials such as film-coating solutions. Each part of the solution that leaves the spray gun must be accompanied by a high volume proportion (relative to liquid) of fast-flowing air. The droplets so produced move with and are propelled by the expanding stream of atomizing air towards the product surface. The correct balance between atomizing air and fluid flow is essential for correct droplet formation. Details of pneumatic guns are given in Chapter 8.

Factors affecting the size distributions of droplets produced by pneumatic atomization

Previous studies into the atomization process have encompassed a wide range of substances, spray-guns and atomization conditions. The results of such work have often been found to apply only for the particular set of conditions used and difficulty has been encountered when trying to extrapolate results of one study to those of another. Since the atomization process is complex with many interacting variables, prediction of the size of droplets produced on a purely theoretical basis have proved unsatisfactory to date. The conditions encountered in aqueous pharmaceutical film coating are also quite unlike most of those in other atomization applications.

However, a survey of work in other fields yields the following general conclusions about the factors most likely to influence the atomization process during aqueous film coating:

1. The size of droplets produced during atomization will depend on the design of the atomizer, the properties of the liquid and the conditions under which atomization takes place.
2. Larger droplets are usually produced from liquids of increasing viscosity, surface tension and density.
3. The method of imparting the energy from the high-velocity and high-pressure air to the liquid is an important influencing factor.
4. The relative velocity of the atomizing air to that of the liquid being atomized, and thus the shear rate produced, is a major determinant of the final droplet size.
5. An increasing air/liquid mass ratio up to a value of around 4:1 will tend to produce smaller droplets, but a further increase in the ratio is unlikely to result in any additional reduction in droplet size.
6. The liquid flow rate may influence atomization in other ways in addition to its effect on the air/liquid mass ratio.

7. Heating the liquid to be atomized will reduce its viscosity and may result in a reduction in atomized droplet size.
8. There may be axial and radial differences in droplet sizes within the spray, depending on the atomizer used and the extent of coalescence and evaporation.

Spherical droplets produced during pneumatic atomization will not be monosize; they will exist in a range of diameters. In order to characterize fully the spray and to assess the influence of the atomization stage on the properties of the resulting film coat, it is necessary to analyse the droplet size distributions produced under defined atomization conditions. The data obtained can then be examined to determine whether the droplet sizes fit mathematically defined distribution patterns and characteristic mean droplet diameters can be calculated. This has been discussed in section 4.3.2.

The factors influencing the size distribution of film-coating droplets can be subdivided broadly into two categories: formulation factors and process factors.

Formulation factors
The formulation factors which influence the formation of droplets in a binary nozzle (i.e. one in which the liquid is atomized with high-pressure air) are numerous. Of the properties mentioned in previous studies, the following are likely to have the greatest effect on film coat formulations (see section 4.2): density, surface tension and viscosity.

These properties of solutions have been investigated in some detail for aqueous hydroxypropyl methylcellulose (HPMC E5 (Methocel E5, Colorcon Ltd) solutions and were discussed in section 4.2. Density was found to change little over concentration ranges used in practice. HPMC is itself surface active and reduces the surface tension of water; this reduction occurs at very low concentrations and little further change occurs over the concentration range of HPMC solutions used in practice.

Polymer solution viscosity has been found to be by far the most important variable. The concentration of HPMC solutions and the inclusion of additives has a profound effect on solution viscosity and thus, possibly, droplet size.

Process factors
The following processing parameters may have an influence on the atomization process and the size of the droplets when they contact the substrate:

1. atomizing air pressure
2. coating liquid flow rate (spray rate)
3. distance from the spray gun to the tablet, granule or pellet bed
4. spray-gun design
5. spray shape
6. radial distance from the spray centre
7. liquid nozzle diameter
8. atomizing air mass flow rate and velocity
9. heating of the coating solutions.

4.4.2 Concentration of polymer in solution (viscosity effects)

The effect of formulation viscosity on the atomization of film-coating solutions
Changes in solution concentration produce a marked effect on the distribution of droplet sizes from a given spray gun.

The relationship between HPMC E5 concentration and solution viscosity has been detailed in section 4.2.4. Three concentrations have been atomized in a study by Twitchell (1990): 6, 9 and 12 %w/w HPMC in water. These solutions have viscosities of 45, 166 and 520 mPa s, respectively, at 20°C. The data presented below are from that study.

Size distribution
The influence of viscosity on the distribution of droplet sizes can be seen in Figs 4.9 and 4.10 which show the size distribution of droplets produced by a Schlick model 930/7-1 spray gun using an atomization air pressure of 414 kPa and spray rate of 50 g/min.

First, note the bimodal nature of the distribution. This is probably caused by the pulsation of the peristaltic pump used in the experiment. This is significant because such pumps are commonly used in industrial coating.

Lower concentrations (and therefore lower viscosities) yield a larger number of smaller droplets (less than 25 μm diameter), whereas a higher polymer concentration shows a shift to larger droplets. This latter effect can be attributed to the greater energy necessary to overcome the increased viscous forces resisting formation of new surface during atomization.

When a solution with a concentration of 6 %w/w HPMC is atomized under these conditions, all the droplets were found to be below 65 μm and over 75% by weight below 25 μm. With 9 %w/w solution, 99.7% by weight of droplets were found to be below 113 μm and with the 12 %w/w solution all droplets were below 160 μm. The respective values for amounts below 25 μm were 52 and 40%.

The cumulative distribution of sizes is shown in Fig. 4.10. As expected, changes in solution concentration produce a marked effect on the cumulative size distribution of droplet sizes produced using a given set of conditions.

Mean size
Fig. 4.11 shows how the different solution concentrations, and thus viscosities, influence the droplet mass median diameter (D_{MM}) produced by the Schlick model 930/7-1 spray-gun at different atomizing air pressures.

Increases in HPMC E5 solution concentration increased the average size of the atomized droplets at each of the air pressures studied. The increase in droplet size is thought to have arisen mainly from the increased energy required to overcome the viscous forces resisting liquid acceleration and droplet formation. The tendency for more viscous liquids to exhibit reduced evaporation and resist coalescence may also have been contributing factors.

The relationship between viscosity and mean droplet size takes the form of a linear plot of the logarithm of the mean droplet size against the logarithm of

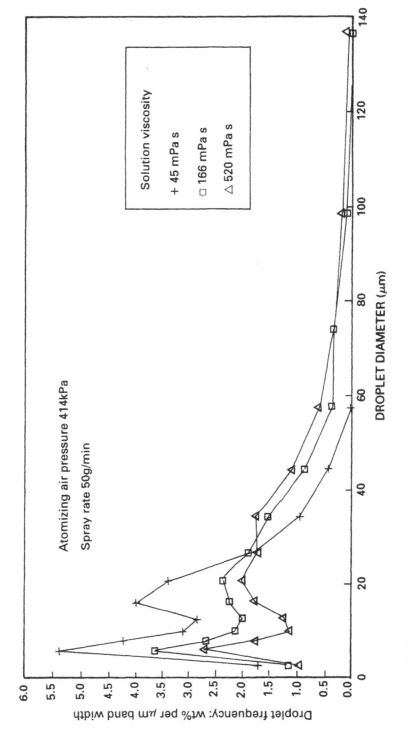

Fig. 4.9　The effect of HPMC E5 solution viscosity on droplet size/weight frequency distributions produced by a Schlick model 930/7-1 spray gun: 180 mm from the gun, flat spray shape, measured at centre of spray.

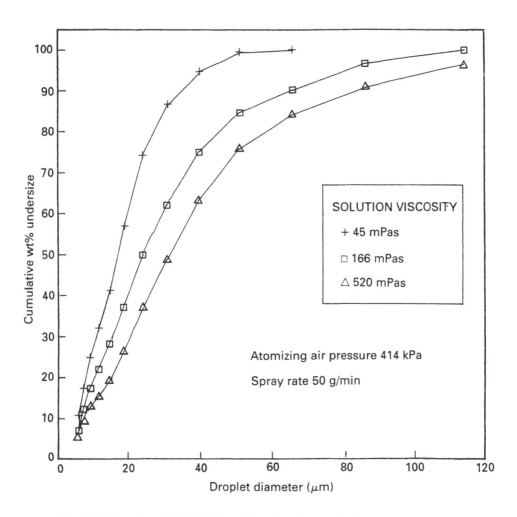

Fig. 4.10 The effect of HPMC E5 solution viscosity on the droplet cumulative wt%
undersize curves for a Schlick model 930/7-1 spray-gun (data from Fig. 4.9).

solution viscosity. This linearity indicates that the relationship between the mean
atomized droplet diameter and viscosity can be described in the form $D \propto \mu^n$.

The effect of heating film-coating solutions prior to atomization

Heating film-coating solutions has been shown to cause a reduction in their viscosity (see section 4.2.4). It may be considered, therefore, that the heating of formulations prior to atomization may be used as a method of reducing the atomized
droplet size. Twitchell (1990), with solutions atomized by a Schlick spray-gun, has
shown that heating the coating solutions up to temperatures of 37°C before they
enter the spray-gun has a minimal effect on the resultant atomized droplet size.

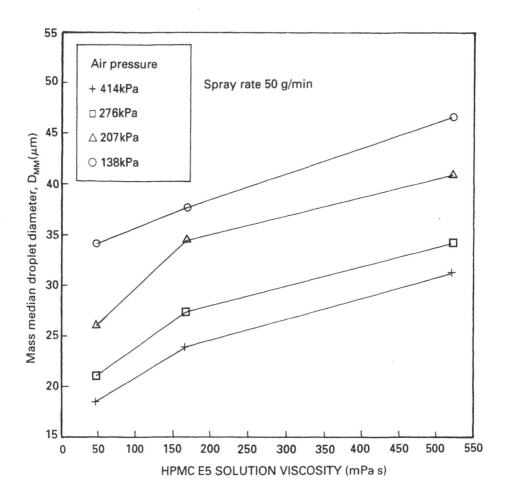

Fig. 4.11　The effect of HPMC E5 solution viscosity on the mass median diameter of droplets from a Schlick model 930/7-1 spray-gun: 180 mm from the gun, flat spray shape, measured at centre of spray, 50 g/min.

Similar findings were reported by Shæffer and Wørts (1977) for the pneumatic atomization of fluidized-bed granulation solutions.

There are two factors which may explain these results. First, the reduction in droplet size arising from the lower solution viscosities is likely to be relatively small. The second possible explanation is that, at the point of droplet detachment, the viscosity has returned to its original (unheated) value. Since the coating solution travels relatively slowly through the liquid nozzle of the spray-gun in comparison with the cool atomizing air in the surrounding chamber of the gun, a type of heat exchanger system exists within the gun which will cool the solution before it leaves the liquid nozzle. As the solution leaves the liquid nozzle in the form of a small diameter cylindrical jet, it is immediately surrounded by a large volume of high-velocity expanding cool air. This again may provide a sufficiently good heat transfer system to cool the liquid before it is accelerated and broken up into droplets.

It would thus appear that attempts to reduce the spray droplet size by heating the coating solutions would prove unsuccessful.

4.4.3 Atomizing air pressure

The effect of atomizing air pressure on the atomization of film-coating solutions

Mean size
Fig. 4.12 shows the influence of atomizing air pressure on the mean droplet sizes produced by the Schlick model 930/7-1 spray-gun when atomizing a 9 %w/w aqueous HPMC E5 solution fed to the gun at various spray rates. The droplet sizes were measured in the centre of a flat spray at a distance of 180 mm from the spray-gun.

There is a progressive change to finer droplets as the air pressure is increased, this being observed at all the spray rates investigated. The effect of increasing atomizing air pressure is most noticeable at pressures below 276 kPa (40 lb/in²), and the quality of the atomized spray is shown to deteriorate rapidly as the atomizing air pressure falls to 69 kPa (10 lb/in²). At atomizing air pressures between 276 and 414 kPa there appears to be only a relatively small reduction in droplet size with increasing air pressure.

Size distribution
The influence of the atomizing air pressure on the droplet size distribution can be seen in Fig. 4.13. This figure represents the distributions measured at the centre of the spray 180 mm from a Schlick model 930/7-1 spray-gun, when 9 %w/w HPMC E5 solution was sprayed at a rate of 50 g/min.

The cumulative percentage undersize curves for the same data are shown in Fig. 4.14.

Increasing the atomizing air pressure produced an increase in the weight of droplets in the smallest size bands and a reduction or elimination in the weight in the largest size bands, with a consequent reduction in the range of droplet diameters encountered. At an air pressure of 414 kPa (60 lb/in²) for example, only 10% by weight of droplets greater than 65 μm were encountered, whereas at 69 kPa (10 lb/in²) there was 56% by weight. It can also be observed that, when using the atomization conditions stated, there is a change in the frequency distribution pattern. A much more even weight distribution is apparent as the atomizing air pressure decreases with an accompanying absence of the large weight frequency of droplets below 10 μm.

Although there was a tendency for only small changes in the characteristic mean diameters to occur as the atomizing air pressures increased above 276 kPa (40 lb/in²), the reduction in the droplet size range and increase in the weight frequency in the smallest size bands were still apparent.

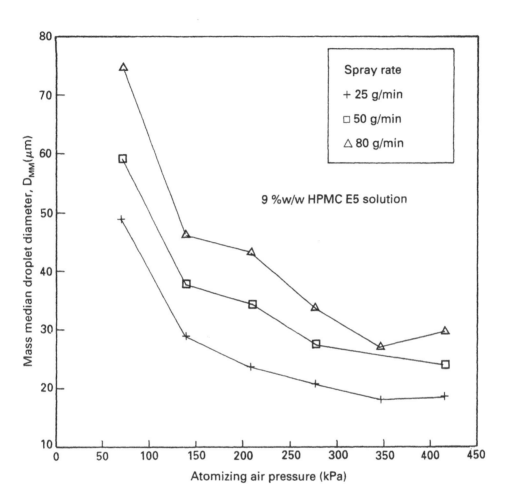

Fig. 4.12   The effect of atomizing air pressure on the mass median diameter of droplets
produced by a Schlick model 930/7-1 spray-gun at a range of spray rates.

4.4.4   Liquid flow rate (spray rate)

The effect of spray rate on the atomization of film-coating solutions

Liquid flow rate through the gun has been shown to also influence droplet size. The
effect of the spray rate on the size distribution of droplets produced during the
atomization of aqueous film-coating solutions was examined by Twitchell (1990) at
different atomization air pressures, with different spray guns and with different
solution viscosities. Spray rates between 25 and 80 g/min were investigated. In each
case droplets were measured at the centre of a flat spray at a distance of 180 mm
from the spray-gun.

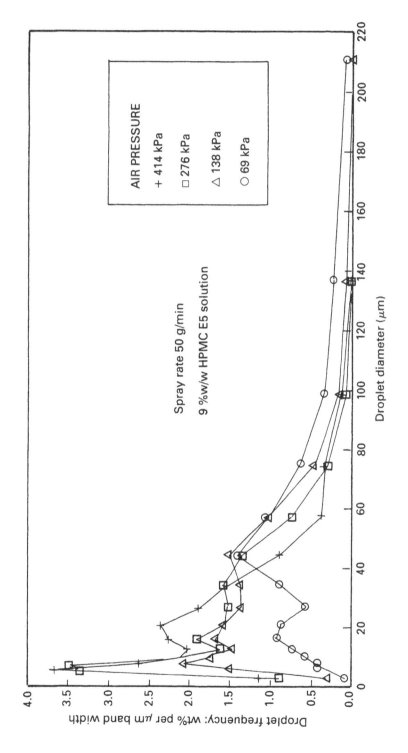

Fig. 4.13 The effect of atomizing air pressure on the droplet size wt% frequency distributions produced by a Schlick model 930/7-1 spray gun.

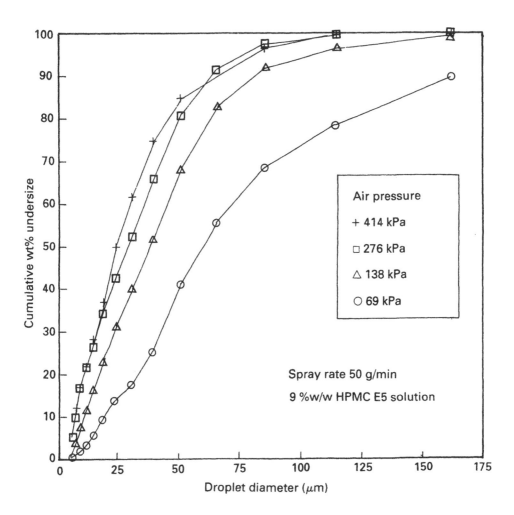

Fig. 4.14   The effect of atomizing air pressure on the droplet cumulative wt% undersize curves for a Schlick model 930/7-1 spray-gun.

The influence of spray rate on the droplet mass median diameter produced by the Schlick gun at different atomizing air pressures is illustrated for a 9 %w/w HPMC E5 solution in Fig. 4.15.

An increase in liquid flow rate between 25 and 80 g/min increases mean droplet size. This effect can be attributed to the reduction in the mass ratio of atomizing air to film-coating liquid which results in a reduction in the energy available per unit mass of liquid during droplet formation.

Figs 4.16 and 4.17 emphasize that these effects and trends are also observed at other solution concentrations.

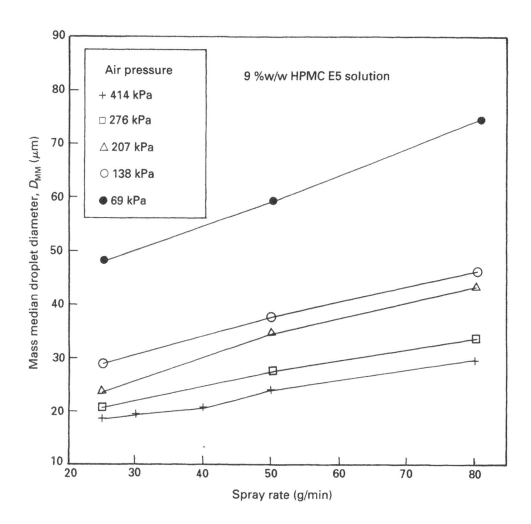

Fig. 4.15 The effect of spray rate on the mass median diameter of droplets produced by
a Schlick model 930/7-1 spray-gun (9 %w/w HPMC E5 aqueous solution).

In general it can be seen that the increase in droplet size with increasing spray
rate becomes more pronounced as the air pressure falls and as the solution concentration, and hence viscosity, increases.

It can be concluded, therefore, that during the film-coating process an increase in
liquid flow rate will give rise to larger droplets, the extent of which will be dependent on solution viscosity and the atomizing air pressure.

It is shown in section 4.4.3 that, at a fixed liquid mass flow rate (spray rate), an
increase in the atomizing air pressure (with the corresponding increase in air mass
flow rate) has only a small effect on droplet size providing that the air/liquid mass
ratio is above a critical value (which occurs at 276 kPa for examples given). Data in

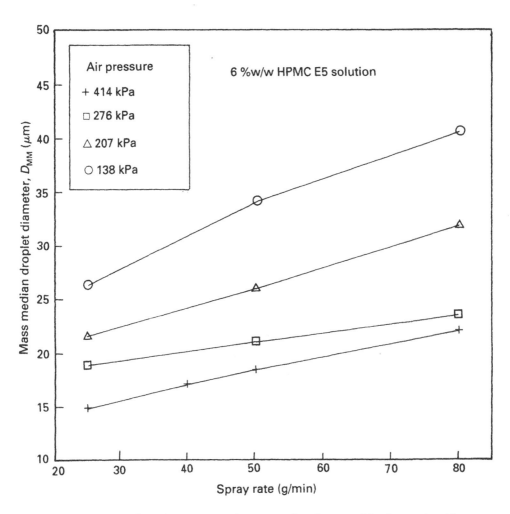

Fig. 4.16   The effect of spray rate on the mass median diameter of droplets produced by a Schlick model 930/7-1 spray-gun (6% w/w HPMC E5 aqueous solution).

the above figures, however, demonstrate that at a fixed air pressure, increases in spray rate cause an increase in droplet size, this occurring despite a air/liquid critical ratio being exceeded. This indicates that spray rate influences the droplet size independently of the other atomization parameters, a finding also reported by Kim and Marshall (1971). This independent effect of the spray rate will act in addition to its influence on the air/liquid mass flow ratio, the latter effect tending to become important at low atomizing air pressures.

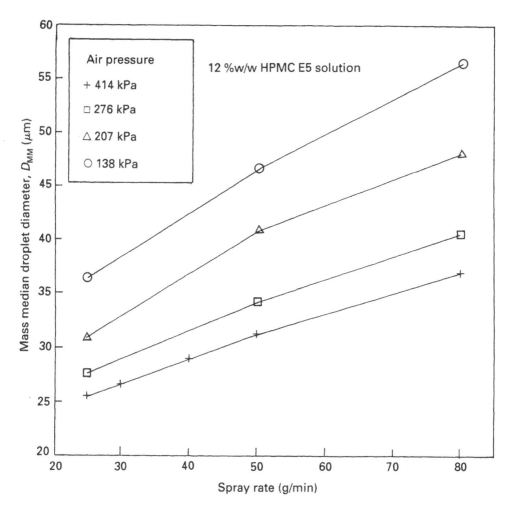

Fig. 4.17   The effect of spray rate on the mass median diameter of droplets produced by
a Schlick model 930/7-1 spray-gun (12 %w/w HPMC E5 solution).

4.4.5   Distance from spray gun

The effect of distance from the spray gun on the droplet diameters of atomized film-coating solutions

Spray guns used in a Model 10 (24 in., 600 mm diameter) Accela–Cota are usually positioned between approximately 150 and 300 mm from the tablet bed, depending on gun design. The maximum distance is restricted by space constraints within the Accela–Cota, this being especially true with the bulky Binks Bullows and Walther Pilot spray-guns. A gun-to-bed distance of 300 mm is commonly encountered in the larger model Accela Cotas (48 in., 1200 mm and 60 in., 1500 mm) used for production scale film coating. Fig. 4.18 shows the variation in mass median diameters with increasing distance from the spray-gun.

Surprisingly, the droplet size increases with increasing distance from the gun. It may have been expected that evaporation of the droplets would have caused the opposite effect. It can be seen that there is an approximate doubling of the mass median droplet diameters from 24 to 45 μm for the 9 %w/w solution and from 31 to 59 μm for the 12 %w/w solution. The reason for this observation can be elucidated from the droplet size distributions shown in Fig. 4.19. As measurements of the droplets within the spray are taken at increasing distance from the point of

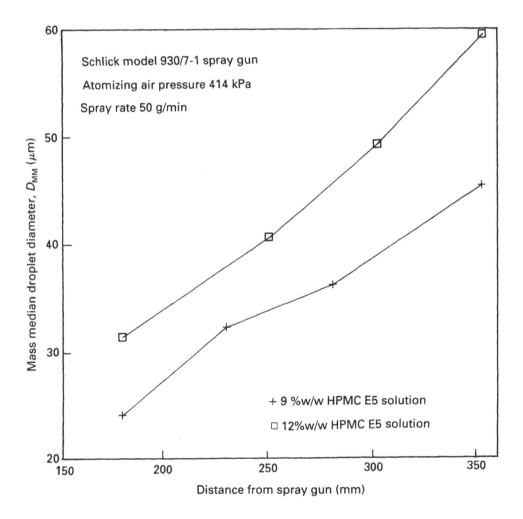

Fig. 4.18   The effect of distance from the spray gun on the measured mass median droplet diameter for both 9 and 12 %w/w HPMC E5 solutions fed to a Schlick model 930/7-1 spray gun set to produce a flat spray.

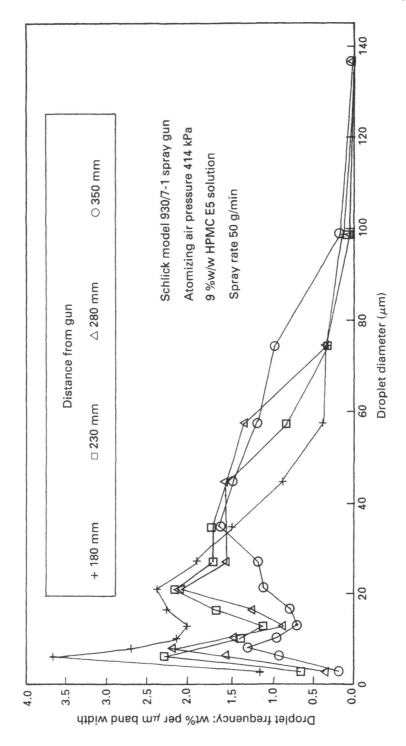

Fig. 4.19   The effect of distance from the spray gun on droplet size/weight frequency distribution.

atomization at the spray-gun, there is a reduction in the number of very fine droplets and an increase in the numbers of larger droplets. There is, in addition, an increase in the range of droplet sizes encountered at the furthest two distances from the spray-gun, droplets being encountered in the size range 160–260 μm. This suggests collision and coalescence as the mechanism.

Changes in droplet size which occur between leaving the spray gun and hitting the product surface potentially may arise from two sources: evaporation of volatile components from the droplets (Arai et al., 1982; Yoakam & Campbell, 1984; Meyer & Chigier, 1985; Tambour et al., 1985) or droplet coalescence (Wigg, 1964; Meyer & Chigier, 1985; Tambour et al., 1985).

Increasing mean droplet diameter at the centre of the spray with increasing distance from the atomizer has been reported also by Wigg (1964), Prasad (1982), Arai et al. (1982) and Meyer & Chigier (1985). An increase in distance from 180 to 350 mm was found to give rise to an approximate doubling of the calculated mean droplet diameters for HPMC E5 solutions (Fig. 4.18). There are two possible explanations for these results. It may be that droplets coalesce on their way to the bed, which would reduce the number of the smaller droplets, increase the number of the larger droplets and increase the range of droplet sizes encountered. Alternatively, although evaporation would be expected to reduce the mean droplet size, evaporation may result in the smaller droplets effectively disappearing from the measuring range, thereby increasing the relative proportion of the larger droplet sizes and giving artificially high values for the droplet diameters (Arai et al., 1982).

Droplet size data suggest that, at the centre of the flat spray where the droplets were measured, little evaporation takes place. The predominant cause of the increase in measured droplet sizes with increasing distance from the spray-gun is therefore likely to be due to droplet coalescence effects.

Although droplet size measurements indicate that at the centre of the spray the predominant effect that is occurring is coalescence, it is not suggested that evaporation does not take place. Indeed, the occurrence of spray drying during aqueous film coating demonstrates that evaporation can occur. It is likely that evaporation will be most prevalent where the spray density is lowest—that is, at the edges of the spray. This arises from reduced local relative humidity levels and is potentiated by the increased distances that need to be travelled and the associated increased time for evaporation to occur. An increased spray surface area arising from the production of smaller droplets will also increase the evaporation potential.

Droplet coalescence is likely to arise from the different momentum and velocities exhibited by droplets of differing sizes. The larger droplets are likely to be travelling at a greater speed (Meyer & Chigier, 1985) and thus may collide with the smaller droplets, resulting in coalescence. This will be aided by the natural turbulence created in the spray by the atomizing air, which tends to potentiate the speed and directional differences. Since the average droplet speed drops rapidly after leaving the spray gun, the time taken to travel a unit distance will increase as the distance from the gun increases. This, coupled with the greater differential between droplet velocities at increasing distances, may tend to increase the amount of coalescence that occurs. Spray density (number of droplets per unit volume) will, however, reduce as the distance from the spray gun increases, this occurring as a consequence of the natural expansion of the spray. This reduction in spray density would reduce the tendency for coalescence to occur, although its influence in this study (where measurements were taken at the centre of the spray) would appear to have been small relative to the increase in size arising from droplet velocity effects.

A further factor which might be expected to influence evaporation is the temperature of the coating solution, with higher temperatures increasing the driving force for evaporation. Information in section 4.4.2 indicates that even if solutions are heated prior to entering the spray-gun, cooling effects within the gun may cool the coating solution close to that of the compressed air temperature. Evaporative cooling effects during droplet-travel to the substrate bed will also influence the temperature of the droplets at the point of contact with the substrate.

Since the droplets contain dissolved polymer, it may be that a 'crust' is formed on the droplet surface after a small amount of evaporation has taken place. This 'crust' may then serve to maintain the diameter of the evaporating droplet despite further solvent loss. If this was occurring, even considerable evaporation may only result in small decreases in the measured droplet size. This effect would be potentiated with HPMC E5 solutions due to the surface active nature of the polymer.

4.4.6 Spray–gun design

The effect of the spray–gun design on the atomization process
The type of spray gun used to atomize film-coating solutions has also been shown to have an effect on the distribution of droplet sizes. Binks-Bullows, Schlick, Walther Pilot and Spraying Systems guns have been investigated (Aulton *et al.*, 1986). The details of these guns and their associated air caps and liquid caps are shown in Table 4.6. Further details of the design, structure, adjustment and use of spray-guns for film coating can be found in Chapter 8.

Figs 4.20 and 4.21, which are plots of mean droplet size against atomizing air pressure and spray rate, respectively, for five different gun combinations, show this effect.

It can be noted that the overall trends (i.e. droplet size decreasing with increasing atomizing air pressure and decreasing spray rate) are not altered by changing the spray-gun. However, there are differences in the mean sizes of the droplets produced, despite otherwise identical atomization conditions.

The differences in spray characteristics and the consequent effects on the properties of film coats (see Chapter 13) could have arisen potentially from differences in:

1. the spray dimensions and the distribution of droplets throughout the spray;
2. the liquid nozzle internal diameter;
3. the area of the annulus between the liquid nozzle and the air cap and thus the volume flow rate, mass flow rate and velocity of the atomizing air in the annulus;
4. the total volume of air accompanying the spray to the point of analysis.

Table 4.6   Details of spray gun types, air caps and liquid caps used by Twitchell (1990) in the generation of the data presented in this chapter and in Chapter 13

Spray gun make	Model	Air cap designation	Liquid nozzle designation	Liquid nozzle diameter (mm)	Annulus area (mm^2)
Schlick	930/7-1	Standard	Standard	0.8	2.30
Schlick	931/7-1	Standard	Standard	1.2	2.30
Schlick	932/7-1	Standard	Standard	1.8	2.30
Walther Pilot	WA/WX	0.5–1.0	Standard	1.0	2.16
Binks Bullows	540	63PB	66	1.8	3.13
Spraying Systems	$^1/_4$J Series	62240–60°	2850	0.71	0.68
		67228–45°	2850	0.71	1.01
		67228–45°	2050	0.51	1.01

A potentially important factor which has been shown to vary between different spray guns and at different air pressures is the air consumption—the total volume of cool air which accompanies the spray after it has been produced. This comprises a combination of the atomizing and spray-shaping air after they have expanded on leaving the air cap of the spray gun. Although shown not to be a determinant of the atomized droplet size (this being dependent on the annulus air velocity and mass flow rate), the total volume of air may influence the behaviour of the droplets on the way to and on arrival at the substrate surface. The momentum of the droplets after leaving the spray gun will be obtained from the kinetic energy of the atomizing spray and shaping air, and will thus be a function of the total air mass flow rate and velocity. The momentum of the air and droplets at the point of reaching the bed will therefore be dependent on both the air velocity on leaving the annulus and the side-port holes, the air density and total air volume. Increases in atomizing air pressure (which increase air consumption) and the use of spray guns with higher air consumption values will both increase the momentum of the droplets and may therefore influence the penetration and spreading behaviour of droplets on the substrate surface (see Chapters 5 and 13).

Changes in air consumption may also have a small influence on the total volume and temperature of the air passing through the coating pan. This, in turn, may influence the tablet-bed or fluidized-bed temperature, rate and extent of evaporation from the droplets on the way to the bed and the drying characteristics of the droplets on the product surface. The likely extent of these effects may be calculated if the drying air volume flow rate and temperature and the spray gun air consumption and air temperature are known.

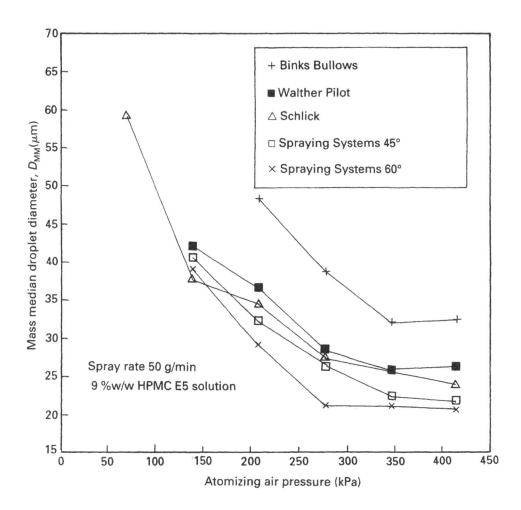

Fig. 4.20   The effect of atomizing air pressure on the mass median diameter of droplets produced by different spray guns. Droplets were measured at the centre of a spray at a distance of 180 mm from the gun.

4.4.7   Spray shape

The effect of spray shape on the droplet sizes of atomized film-coating solutions
The droplet size results presented so far in this chapter have all been calculated from distributions measured in the centre of a flat spray shape of the type commonly employed in aqueous film coating. Many spray guns, including Schlick, Walther Pilot and Binks Bullows, are however capable of producing a variety of spray shapes ranging from a narrow angle solid cone (of approximately 10° exit angle) to a wide angle flat spray (Fig. 4.22) by increasing the volume of air allowed to enter the side-port holes.

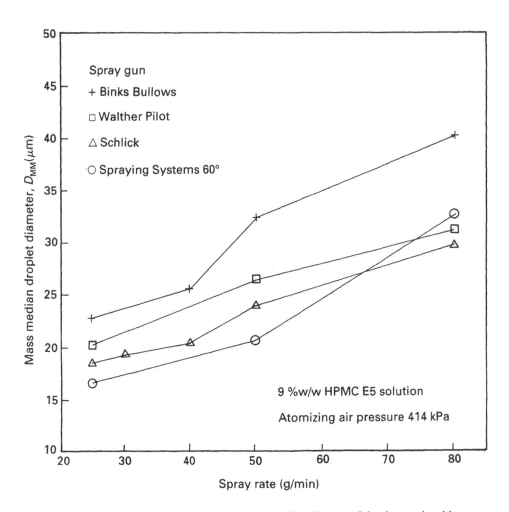

Fig. 4.21   The effect of spray rate on the mass median diameter of droplets produced by different spray guns.

The flat spray was that which would commonly be used during film coating; a solid cone is achieved when no air was allowed to enter the side-ports of the air cap; and an elliptical spray is obtained when approximately half the air needed to produce the flat spray is allowed to enter the side-ports.

Droplet sizes from the centre of sprays of different shapes produced under otherwise identical conditions by the Schlick model 930/7-1 and Walther Pilot spray guns have been measured by Twitchell (1990). The results of this study indicate that with the Walther Pilot gun there is minimal difference in the droplet sizes produced by the flat and cone-shaped sprays. Analysis of sprays produced by the Schlick gun, however, indicates that droplets measured from the cone-shaped spray are larger

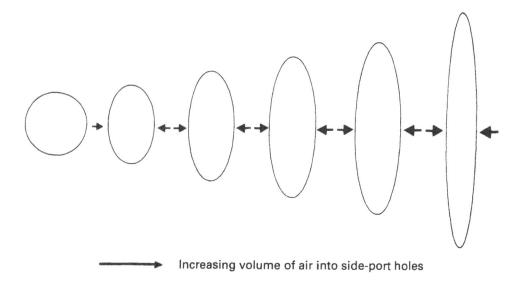

Increasing volume of air into side-port holes

Fig. 4.22 Evolution of a spray pattern from a cone to a flat spray.

than from the flat spray. It would appear, therefore, that different droplet sizes may exist in different shaped sprays. The differences in sizes were, in general, more apparent both in absolute and percentage terms as the average mean droplet size increased. There appeared to be no significant differences between droplet sizes determined for the elliptical and flat spray shapes of the Schlick gun.

When the Walther Pilot gun is set to produce a flat spray, the spray contains a dense region of droplets in the spray centre. The Schlick gun, although also producing a more dense central region, does so to a lesser extent than the Walther Pilot gun and consequently produces a more evenly distributed spray. The cone-shaped sprays produced by both guns cover a similar area (approximately one-third of that of the flat sprays) and have a similar droplet density. Thus, when the spray is changed from a flat shape to a cone, there is a greater increase in droplet density in the centre of sprays produced by the Schlick gun than the Walther Pilot gun and, consequently, a greater likelihood of the droplet size increasing due to increased frequency of coalescence. The reduction in total atomizing air volume which accompanies the change to the cone-shaped spray is thought unlikely to be a contributing factor, since this reduction is greater with the Walther Pilot gun than with the Schlick gun.

Spray density, as well as changing with liquid flow rate, may also differ at different areas within the spray. The extent to which this occurs will depend on the type of spray gun (especially the design of the air cap) and the relative proportions of atomizing and spray-shaping air. An increased density of droplets in the centre, and thus the increased coalescence taking place in this zone, is thought to contribute to the larger droplet sizes encountered in the centre of the sprays produced by the Walther Pilot gun compared with the Schlick gun.

4.4.8   Liquid nozzle diameter

The effect of liquid nozzle diameter on the atomization of film-coating solutions
Pneumatic spray guns are often available with a choice of liquid nozzle diameters.
It is therefore necessary to ascertain whether the droplet size produced by the spray
guns is dependent on the liquid nozzle diameter and, if so, how the liquid nozzle
influences droplet production. Liquid nozzle diameter differences could potentially
alter the speed that the liquid exits from the nozzle and thus both its speed relative
to the atomizing air and the shear forces it encounters.

This has been investigated by Twitchell (1990) who atomized a 9 %w/w HPMC E5
solution with both Schlick and Spraying Systems spray guns, using identical conditions except for changes in the inner diameter of the liquid nozzle. Schlick model
930/7-1, 931/7-1 and 932/7-1 spray-guns with corresponding liquid nozzle diameters
of 0.8, 1.2 and 1.8 mm and Spraying Systems $^1/_4$J series guns with 2850 (nozzle diameter 0.71 mm) and 2050 (nozzle diameter 0.51 mm) liquid nozzles were used.

Increasing the nozzle diameters reduces the average liquid nozzle exit velocity
and thus potentiates the velocity difference and reduces the shear forces exerted on
the liquid. Liquid exit velocities have been calculated (Twitchell, 1990) to range
from an average 0.17 m/s at a spray rate of 25 g/min through a 1.8 mm nozzle, to
6.8 m/s when spraying at 80 g/min through a 0.5 mm nozzle. The atomizing air
velocity as it exits the air annulus was calculated to be greater than 130 m/s, and
thus the relative difference in velocities will be little affected by changes in liquid
nozzle diameter.

The results of this study indicate that over the range of liquid nozzle diameters
studied, which covers the majority of the range available for the spray-guns used in
aqueous film coating, the liquid nozzle diameter has no influence on the mean
droplet sizes produced upon atomization. Examination of the distribution of droplet
sizes also failed to show any detectable differences.

4.4.9   Atomizing air velocity and mass flow rate

*The effect of spray-gun air cap annulus, atomizing air velocity and mass flow rates
on atomization*
It has been shown that differences exist between droplet sizes produced by different
spray guns under otherwise identical conditions. Since the energy used to atomize
the droplets is derived from the kinetic energy of the atomizing air, differences in
this energy may potentially influence droplet production. Differences arise from
variance in gun design, particularly in the geometry of the annulus around the liquid
nozzle, which may in turn lead to differences in the atomizing air velocity and
mass/volume flow rates and therefore the energy available for atomization.
Variation in the liquid nozzle diameter itself has been shown to have no effect on
the droplet size (section 4.4.8).

The results of Twitchell (1990) show the air mass flow rate (calculated from
air density and volumetric flow rate) to increase with the area of the annulus,
irrespective of the air pressure used. The Binks Bullows gun was found to exhibit

the largest air mass flow rates but the lowest air exit velocities. Both values for the Walther Pilot gun are slightly higher than the Schlick gun, although, with the latter, air velocity is shown to vary less with changes in atomizing air pressure. The Spraying Systems guns both have considerably lower annulus atomizing air mass flow rates than the other three guns. The Spraying Systems 60° gun exhibits the highest air exit velocity values. The air velocity values for the Spraying Systems 45° gun are similar to those of the Schlick and Walther Pilot guns. Although the air exit velocity values all increase with increasing atomizing air pressure, the increase is relatively small compared with the corresponding increase in air mass flow rate.

This information, and the relationships described in sections 4.4.6 and 4.4.7, suggest that at the higher atomizing air pressures the most important factor in determining the size of droplets is not the atomizing air mass flow rate, but the velocity of the air as it exits the air cap. Since with the Schlick gun the air velocity is virtually the same across the range of air pressures, the rise in droplet size with decreasing air pressure must be due to the reduction in air mass flow rate, with its accompanying reduction in the air/liquid mass ratio.

The comparatively low annular mass flow rates exhibited by the two Spraying System guns means that the critical air/liquid mass ratio is reached at a lower atomizing air pressure than for the other spray guns examined. This would account for the shape of the curves in Fig. 4.20 where the increase in mean droplet size with decreasing air pressure is greater for the two Spraying Systems guns.

The resultant droplet size is therefore likely to be dependent on a complex relationship between the air velocity and the mass flow rate. Also, as explained previously, the air mass flow rate is an important factor in governing the behaviour of droplets once they impinge on the substrate surface.

4.5 CONCLUSIONS

It is apparent from examination of the influence of atomization conditions on the droplet size distributions and characteristic mean droplet sizes that many factors will influence the size and momentum of the droplets impinging on a surface of the granules, pellets or tablets during aqueous film coating. These factors include the atomizing air pressure, spray rate, solution viscosity, spray gun type, distance from the spray gun, spray shape and the velocity and mass flow rate of the atomizing air. These influencing factors in general cannot be considered or altered in isolation since the effect of one variable is dependent to a varying extent on one or more of the other variables.

Formulation and process variables will not only exert a considerable influence on the atomized droplet size, but also on the droplet momentum, spray density and the degree of evaporation and coalescence that occurs during travel to the product. Increasing coating solution concentration (and thus increasing viscosity) will increase the atomized droplet size, although over the viscosity range used in practice this effect is likely to be relatively small. Heating the solutions prior to atomization appears to have little effect on droplet size. Liquid flow rate influences the droplet size independently of the other atomization parameters. During their passage to the substrate surface, the droplets in the centre of the spray are likely to increase in size since droplet coalescence effects predominate over solvent evaporation effects.

The effect of the atomization stage of the aqueous film-coating process on resultant film coat properties is discussed in Chapter 13.

REFERENCES

Arai, M., Kishi, T. & Hiroyasu, H. (1982) *ICLASS Proceedings*, 11–4.

Aulton, M.E., Twitchell, A.M. & Hogan, J.E. (1986). *Proc. 4th Int. Conf. Pharm. Tech., APGI, Paris, France* V, 133–140.

Banker, G.S. & Peck, G.E. (1981) *Pharm. Technol.* **5(4)**, 55.

Banks, M. (1981) Studies on the fluidised bed granulation process. Ph.D. Thesis, De Montfort University, Leicester.

Bikerman, J.J. (1970) In *Physical surfaces* (ed. Bikerman, J.J.), Academic Press, London.

Chigier, N. (1982) *ICLASS Proceedings*, 29–47.

Chopra, S.K. & Tawashi, R. (1985) *J. Pharm. Sci.* **74(7)**, 746–749.

Cole, G.C., Neale, P.J. & Wilde, J.S. (1980) *J. Pharm. Pharmacol.* **32** Suppl., 92P.

Davies, M.C. (1985) Ph.D. Thesis, University of London.

Delporte, J.P. (1980) *J. Pharm. Belg.* **35(6)**, 417–426.

Fair, J.R. (1974) In *Chemical engineers' handbook*, 5th edn, 18.58–18.67.

Fraser, R.P. & Eisenklam, E.P. (1956) *Trans. Inst. Chem. Eng.* **34**, 294–307.

Henderson, N.L., Meer, P.M. & Kostenbauder, H.B. (1961) *J. Pharm. Sci.* **50**, 788–791.

Hogan, J.E. (1982) *Int. J. Pharm. Tech. Prod. Mfr* **3(1)**, 17–20.

Jones, A.R. (1977) *Prog. Energy Combust. Sci.* **3**, 225–234.

Kim, K.Y. & Marshall, W.R. (1971) *AIChE Journal* **17**, 575-584.

Kumar, R. & Prasad, K.S.L. (1971) *Ind. Eng. Chem. Des. Develop.* **10**, 357–365.

Lefebvre, A.H. (1989) In *Atomization and sprays* (ed. Lefebvre, A.H.), Hemisphere Publishing Corporation, New York.

Levy, G. & Schwarz, T.W. (1958) *J. Amer. Pharmaceut. Assoc.* **47**, 44–46.

Masters, K. (1976) In *Spray drying.* (ed. Masters, K.), George Goodwin, London.

Meyer, P.L. & Chigier, N. (1985) *ICLASS Proceedings*, IVB(b)/1.

Mugele, R.A. & Evans, H.D. (1951) *Ind. Eng. Chem.* **43**, 1317–1324.

Naining, W. & Hongjian, Z. (1986) *Partic. Sci. Technol.* **4**, 403–408.

Nukiyama, S. & Tanasawa, Y. (1939) *Trans. Soc. Mech. Eng. (Japan)* **5**, 68–75.

Okhamafe, A.O. & York, P. (1983) *Proc. 3rd APGI, Int. Conf. Pharm. Tech., Paris, France* III, 136–144.

Philippoff, P. (1936) *Cellulose Chem.* **17**, 57–77.

Pickard, J.F. (1979). Ph.D. Thesis, CNAA.

Prasad, K.S.L. (1982) *ICLASS Proceedings*, 4–3.

Prater, D.A. (1982) Ph.D. Thesis, University of Bath.

Rosin, P. & Rammler, E. (1933) *J. Inst. Fuel* **7**, 29–36.

Rowe, R.C. (1976) *Pharm. Acta Helv.* **51**(11), 330–334.

Rowe, R.C. (1980) *J. Pharm. Pharmacol.* **32**, 116-119.

Schæfer, T. & Wørts, O. (1977) *Arch. Pharm. Chemi. Sci. Ed.* **5**, 178–193.

Schwartz, J.B. & Alvino, T.P. (1976) *J. Pharm. Sci.* **65**(4), 572–575.

Tambour, Y., Greenburg, J.B. & Albagli, D. (1985) *ICLASS Proceedings*, VIA/2.

Tufnell, K.J., May, G. & Meakin, B.J. (1983) *Proc. 3rd Int. Conf. Pharm. Tech., Paris, France, APGI*, **V**, 111–118.

Twitchell, A.M. (1990) Studies on the role of atomisation in aqueous tablet film coating, Ph.D. Thesis, De Montfort University, Leicester.

Weiner, B.B. (1982) In *Particle sizing* (ed. Chigier, N.), Wiley, New York.

Wigg, L.D. (1964) *J. Inst. Fuel* **37**, 500-505.

Yoakam, D.A. & Campbell, R.J. (1984) *Pharm. Tech.* **8**(1), 38-44.

5

Surface effects in film coating

Michael E. Aulton

SUMMARY

This chapter will explain the significance of the stages of impingement, wetting, spreading and penetration of atomized droplets at the surface of tablet or multi-particulate cores. It will explain some of the fundamental aspects of solid–liquid interfaces which are important to the process of film coating. This chapter will emphasize the importance of controlling the 'wetting power' of the spray and the 'wettability' of the substrate, and will explain how this can be achieved by changes in formulation and process parameters.

Both surface tension and contact angle are important properties in influencing the wetting of a substrate surface (whether this be tablets, granules or spheronized pellets) by the coating formulation. These properties have been evaluated in coating polymer systems because of their possible relationship with wetting, spreading and subsequent adhesion. These aspects are discussed in detail in this chapter.

The chapter also contains a discussion on the adhesion properties of the final dried film coats and some data are presented to illustrate the factors influencing the magnitude of these adhesive forces.

5.1 INTRODUCTION

In our deliberations on the process of film coating of pharmaceutical solid dosage forms, one cannot escape a consideration of surface aspects relating to the wetting of granule, pellet or tablet cores by the coating solution and the subsequent adhesion of the dried films.

This chapter will consider some fundamental aspects of these stages and explain the mechanisms involved in the spreading and wetting of droplets once they hit the substrate. While it is not always necessary to have a firm grasp of these concepts to produce a satisfactory film coat in practice, an awareness and understanding of some of these theories will help to produce much more efficient and elegant films.

Film coatings are invariably applied in the pharmaceutical industry by spraying a coating solution or suspension onto the surface of a bed of moving tablet cores or onto fluidized multiparticulates. Hot air is blown through the bed to evaporate the solvent in order to leave a continuous polymer film around the cores. Droplet generation, droplet travel from the gun to the bed, impingement, spreading and coalescence of the droplets at the surface, and subsequent gelation and drying of the film, are all important factors which need to be understood and, where possible, controlled.

This chapter will concentrate on those processes which occur at the interface between the droplets of coating liquid and the surface of the substrate cores. It will consider the importance of solution and core properties and process conditions, although the latter will be explained in more detail in other chapters.

Once the sprayed droplets of film-coating solution hit the surface of the substrate core, they will (hopefully) adhere to the surface and then wet and spread over the underlying surface. They should then form a strongly adhered, coherent dried film coat.

Control over the collision of the droplets with the substrate is primarily a function of apparatus design, and the positioning and settings of the spray-guns. The velocity of the droplets as they hit the cores ensures that they have a momentum. This momentum will provide some of the energy required for spreading. Since momentum is the product of mass and velocity, its value is obviously a function of the size, speed and direction of the droplets at the point of contact. This aspect is also discussed more fully in Chapter 13 in the context of the effects that droplet size, gun-to-bed distance and other processing variables have on the quality of the resulting coat.

5.2 WETTING

5.2.1 Wetting theory
First, let us consider briefly the relevant theory relating to wetting.

True wetting is defined as *the replacement of a solid–air (or more correctly solid–vapour) interface with a solid–liquid interface*, i.e. in simple terms, a 'dry' surface becomes 'wet'. During this process individual gas and vapour molecules must be removed from the surface of the solid and replaced by solvent molecules. The relative affinity of these molecules will dictate whether this process is spontaneous or not. It should be appreciated that this process is influenced by the two properties of *wetting power* and *wettability*.

In the context of film coating, 'wetting power' can be defined as *the ability of the atomized droplets to wet the substrate* and 'wettability' can be defined as *the ability of the substrate to be wetted by the atomized droplets*.

An appreciation of this subdivision of wetting helps us to appreciate that in practice it is possible to manipulate the interfacial process by adjustment of either (or indeed both) the properties of the droplets, or those of the tablet or multiparticulate cores.

5.2.2   Surface tension

Introduction
The following discussion attempts to introduce the reader to the concepts of interfacial tensions within the context of film coating. It is not intended to be a full explanation of the science of the subject. The reader is referred to standard physical chemistry texts for a fuller, more fundamental explanation of these principles.

All interfaces between various states of matter will have an excess surface free energy. This arises as a result of the unsatisfied molecular or atomic bonds present at a surface of the material, since these particular molecules or atoms are not completely surrounded by other like molecules or atoms.

We are all familiar with the concept of liquid surface tension, but from the above description you can appreciate that *all* surfaces will have this excess free energy (or *surface tension*). In the context of film coating, we have to consider the following interfaces.

Liquid–vapour (LV) interface
This will exist between the droplet of coating solution and its surrounding environment. This is often referred to as the liquid–air interface but this is not strictly correct since the air directly at the interface will be saturated with solvent vapour from the droplet. Note also that the same basic principles apply whether or not the liquid in question is water (as in aqueous film coating) or an organic solvent (as used in organic film coating).

The symbol for the liquid–vapour interfacial free energy (or surface tension) is γ_{LV}. Its typical SI units are mN/m.

Solid–vapour (SV) interface
This is the 'dry' solid surface. The word 'dry' is quoted since the surface will not be free of solvent molecules. There will be an equilibrium between solvent molecules present in the air and those adhered to the solid surface. Thus, again, solid–vapour interface is a more accurate description than solid–air. The corresponding symbol and unit are γ_{SV} and mN/m, respectively.

Solid–liquid (SL) interface
This is the wetted solid. There will still be a residual surface free energy between the two phases because they are different materials. The magnitude of the SL interfacial free energy is influenced by the properties of *both* the phases. This is an important point to grasp because it indicates that the process of wetting (i.e. the generation of a SL interface) can be influenced by changes to either the spray or the solid, as was discussed earlier when the terms 'wetting power' and 'wettability' were introduced.

The corresponding symbol and unit for SL interfacial free energy are γ_{SL} and mN/m, respectively.

Measurement of liquid surface tension

The measurement of SL and SV interfacial free energy is extremely difficult to perform and is beyond the scope, not only of this book, but also of most companies involved in film coating. The measurement of LV interfacial free energy (or liquid surface tension as it is commonly called) is relatively easy, however. Furthermore, it is possible to obtain an insight into the γ_{SL} and γ_{SV} values by measurement of the *contact angle* of a sessile drop of liquid on a horizontal solid surface. This is explained later in section 5.2.3.

There are two simple and commonly used techniques for determining γ_{SV}. These are referred to as the Du Nuoy tensiometer and Wilhelmy plate techniques. The Du Nuoy technique consists of measuring the force (often using a torsion balance) needed to pull a horizontal metal ring free from the surface of a liquid. In the Wilhelmy technique the horizontal ring is replaced by a vertical plate. In both techniques surface tension can be calculated since the experiments measure the downward force on the ring or plate resulting from the excess surface free energy in the surface of the liquid.

For further details of these techniques, the reader is referred to textbooks on physical chemistry.

Surface activity of HPMC solutions

The surface activity of HPMC solutions was discussed in Chapter 4 (section 4.2.3). Data were presented which showed that the addition of HPMC greatly reduced water surface tension at low concentrations, but over those concentrations likely to be used in practice there is little further change in equilibrium liquid surface tension.

Surface ageing

HPMC E5 solutions at concentrations of approximately 5×10^{-3} %w/w or less were found to take a considerable time to reach their equilibrium surface tension values. This time-dependent reduction in surface tension of aqueous HPMC E5 solutions has been studied by Twitchell (1990) and is illustrated in Fig. 5.1 for solution concentrations in the order of 10^{-4} %w/w and Fig. 5.2 for more dilute solutions in the order of 10^{-5} %w/w.

It can be seen that the time taken for the equilibrium surface tension to be reached decreases as the concentration increases. For concentrations below 5×10^{-4} %w/w, time periods in excess of 30 minutes were required under the conditions of test. At least 900 minutes was required before the 2×10^{-5} %w/w solution attained equilibrium. This phenomenon of time-dependent surface tension is known as *surface ageing*. This has also been reported for high molecular weight hydroxypropyl cellulose samples at aqueous solution concentrations of 2×10^{-5} %w/w and below (Zografi, 1985).

Surface ageing occurs since, when a fresh liquid surface is formed (such as in atomization), it will be relatively free of actively adsorbed HPMC molecules. This is

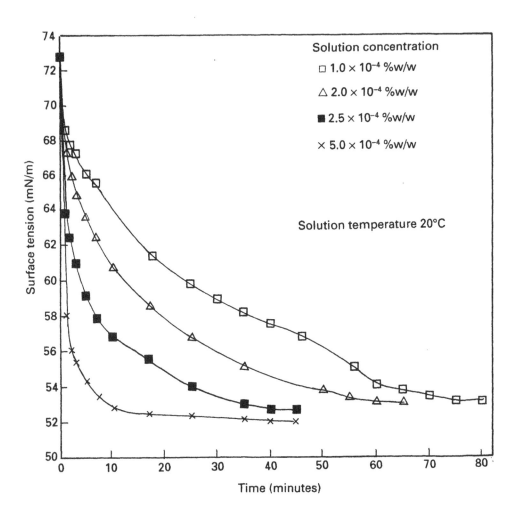

Fig. 5.1 The relationship between surface tension and time for aqueous HPMC E5 solutions of various concentrations.

not, however, the equilibrium state. There will be a gradual diffusion of solute molecules from the bulk of the solution to the droplet surface and orientation of the molecules once at the surface until an equilibrium situation is achieved. The wide distribution of molecular weight fractions in HPMC E5 (Rowe, 1980a; Davies, 1985) is likely to contribute to the time-dependent nature of the surface tension, with the larger molecules diffusing less rapidly and being more sterically hindered. The attainment of the equilibrium surface tension will correspond to that of equilibrium adsorption, this being a dynamic state with molecules continuously leaving and entering the surface layer at the same rate. The time-dependent non-equilibrium surface tension is referred to as the *dynamic surface tension.*

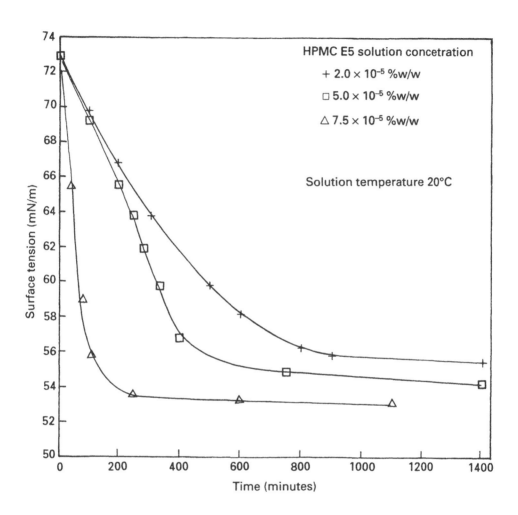

Fig. 5.2 The relationship between surface tension and time for aqueous HPMC E5 solutions of various concentrations.

Non-ionic surface active agents, into which category HPMC E5 can be classified, tend to exhibit marked surface activity at considerably lower concentrations than ionic ones with identical hydrophobic groups. If the surfactants form micelles, this leads to a subsequent tendency for lower values of the critical micelle concentration. The attainment of equilibrium surface tension values at concentrations below the critical micelle concentration has been found to be considerably slower with non-ionic surfactants, and for a specific surfactant to be slower for lower concentrations (Lange, 1971; Wan & Lee, 1974). At concentrations below the point of inflection in the surface tension/concentration curve (see Fig. 4.2 for HPMC), it can be considered that the surface can accommodate all the HPMC molecules in the solution, and thus before the equilibrium surface tension is reached these molecules must make their way to the surface. As the solution concentration increases, the molecules which are required to reach the surface have, on average, a shorter distance to travel and thus equilibrium is attained more quickly. HPMC E5 solutions with a concentration greater than approximately 5×10^{-3} %w/w attain equilibrium surface tension values sufficiently quickly such that no time-dependent reduction in surface tension can be detected.

Surface tensions of atomized droplets
The above discussion implied that the surface tension of atomized droplets may not be as expected. Twitchell *et al.* (1987) took this argument one stage further. Surface tension data measured on the surface of bulk liquid at equilibruim could give a misleading result. As Table 4.2 showed, the surface tension under such conditions changes little over a wide range of concentrations that are likely to be used in practice, with an abrupt rise in surface tension only being significant at concentrations below 2×10^{-5} %w/w HPMC.

However, there are two factors which are very different in film-coating atomization compared to the experimental situation. First, there is the sudden generation of a very large area of fresh surface (i.e. LV interface). A typical film-coating spray could have between 15 and 60 m^2 of surface for each 100 ml of liquid sprayed! So, even at high bulk solution concentrations, are there going to be enough molecules to saturate the liquid surface to enable its surface tension to fall to bulk equilibrium values? Additionally, even if there are enough molecules in the bulk, will they have enough time to migrate to the surface of the droplet before the droplets collide with their target substrate?

Twitchell *et al.* (1987) used the Gibbs absorption equation to calculate the number of molecules that would be needed to saturate the large surface area of a spray, and concluded that, with droplets up to about 140 μm mean diameter, there would be insufficient molecules, even with an aqueous HPMC E5 solution with a bulk concentration of 9 %w/w, to saturate the fresh liquid surface generated during atomization.

The smaller the droplet, the larger the fresh surface area generated, thus the lower will be the degree of surface saturation and therefore the higher the surface tension. Twitchell *et al.* (1987) estimated that the surface tension of a 100 μm droplet of 9 %w/w HPMC E5 would be 61 mN/m; for a 50 μm droplet this would be 67 mN/m and a 25 μm diameter droplet would have a surface tension of 70 mN/m. They also calculated that above a mean droplet size of 143 μm there would be sufficient HPMC molecules to theoretically saturate the surface (as long as time was not a factor). It can be seen from the data in section 4.4 that the figures for droplet sizes quoted above are realistic for typical film-coating sprays.

It will be appreciated that as the HPMC molecules migrate to the surface of the droplets, the concentration of HPMC remaining in the bulk of the droplet will be very low. This fact introduces another potential detrimental phenomenon, in that with dilute solutions there is a considerable time required for equilibrium surface tensions to be set up (as discussed above in the section on surface ageing).

The above observations lead to the conclusion that the surface tension of droplets hitting a tablet surface may be considerably greater than that predicted from measuring the bulk surface tension, this effect being more pronounced with smaller droplets and less concentrated solutions and possibly will be potentiated by the time taken for HPMC molecules to migrate to the freshly produced droplet surface. Wetting, penetration and spreading of film-coating solutions on tablet or multiparticulate surfaces may therefore not follow expected trends. Factors such as solvent evaporation during travel to the tablet, polymer polydispersity and the inclusion of formulation additives may also influence this phenomenon.

5.2.3 Contact angle

Introduction
When a droplet is in static (non-dynamic, equilibrium) contact with a flat surface, a number of things could happen. At the two extremes, the droplet could either sit as a discrete droplet with just a single point of contact (no wetting) or it could spread out completely to cover the whole surface (full wetting). In practice, film-coating droplets usually form a discrete entity somewhere in between these extremes (see Fig. 5.3). The angle of a tangent drawn from a point at the contact between solid–liquid–vapour at the edge of the drop is known as the *contact angle*.

If the value of the contact angle (θ) is equal to 0° then the surface is completed wetted. As the degree of wetting decreases the contact angle increases. At 180° no wetting occurs. From this it can be concluded that any factors which influence the surface tension of the formulation and/or the interfacial tension will influence the degree of wetting. Surface-active agents, for instance, may decrease both γ_{LV} and γ_{SL}, the latter arising from their adsorption at the solid–liquid interface.

The degree of spreading of a droplet is determined by Young's equation:

$$\frac{\gamma_{SV} - \gamma_{SL}}{\gamma_{LV}} = \cos \theta \tag{5.1}$$

where γ_{SV} is the solid–vapour interfacial tension, γ_{SL} is the solid–liquid interfacial tension and γ_{LV} is the liquid–vapour interfacial tension. The principle of Young's equation can be better understood by examining the sketches in Figs 5.4 and 5.5.

At the periphery of the droplet there exists an equilibrium between the surface forces associated with the three surfaces at that point, i.e. the solid–vapour interface force in the plane of the solid surface in one direction is balanced by the sum of the resolved forces associated with the solid–liquid and liquid–vapour interfaces in the opposite direction. Therefore, at equilibrium

$$\gamma_{SV} = \gamma_{SL} + \gamma_{LV}.\cos \theta \tag{5.2}$$

Rearranging equation (5.2) gives

$$\gamma_{LV}.\cos \theta = \gamma_{SV} - \gamma_{SL} \tag{5.3}$$

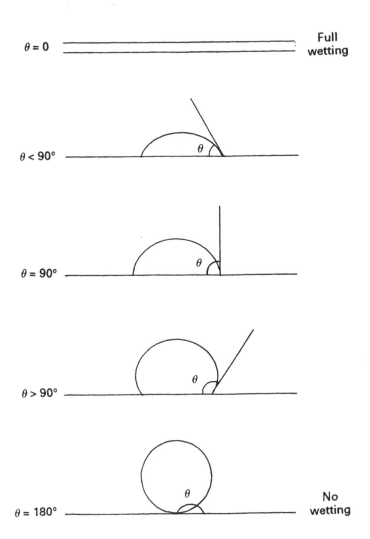

Fig. 5.3   Illustration of droplet contact angles θ ranging between 0 and 180°.

then

$$\cos \theta = \frac{\gamma_{SV} - \gamma_{SL}}{\gamma_{LV}} \tag{5.4}$$

Thus we have Young's equation (equation (5.1)).

Determination of the contact angle made by a liquid, solution or suspension of film-coating formulation on a surface has often been undertaken to assess the wettability of powders or tablet compositions and the wetting characteristics of

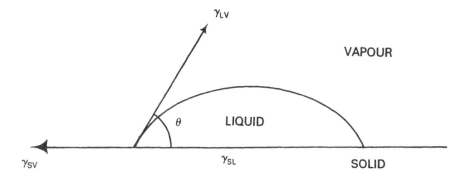

Fig. 5.4   Diagram of a droplet in equilibrium with a solid substrate, showing the balance of forces between γ_{SV}, γ_{LV} and γ_{SL}.

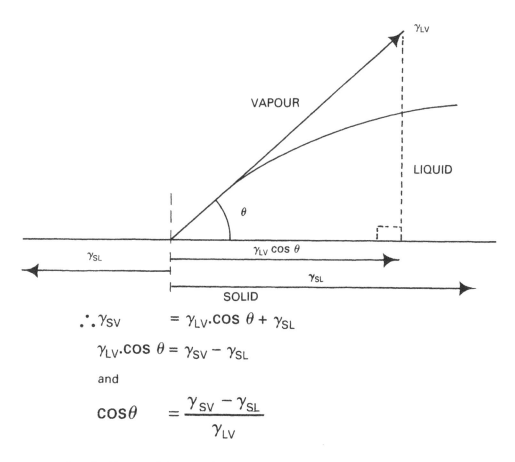

$$\therefore \gamma_{SV} = \gamma_{LV}.\cos\theta + \gamma_{SL}$$

$$\gamma_{LV}.\cos\theta = \gamma_{SV} - \gamma_{SL}$$

and

$$\cos\theta = \frac{\gamma_{SV} - \gamma_{SL}}{\gamma_{LV}}$$

Fig. 5.5   Close-up of the edge of a liquid droplet on a solid surface and the explanation of Young's equation.

of test liquids (Harder *et al.*, 1970; Zografi & Tam, 1976; Lerk *et al.*, 1976; Fell & Efentakis, 1979; Buckton & Newton, 1986; Odidi *et al.*, 1991). In addition, surface characteristics and surface energy values have been elucidated from contact angle measurements (Harder *et al.*, 1970; Zografi & Tam, 1976; Liao & Zatz, 1979; Costa & Baszkin, 1985; Davies, 1985), as has the relationship between the contact angle and adhesion of coating formulations to different substrates (Wood & Harder, 1970; Harder *et al.*, 1970; Nadkarni *et al.*, 1975). Alkan & Groves (1982) used contact angle measurement as an aid to calculating the penetration behaviour of an organic film-coating solution.

The tablet surface free energy and polarity and interactions with the coating solution components have been shown by Costa & Baszkin (1985) to influence the contact angle, spreading and penetration at the tablet surface. They showed that the contact angles made by a series of polyols on tablets of various formulations were dependent on the tablet surface free energy, and that the constituents played a part in modifying this surface energy. The authors also showed the tablet core constituents to influence tablet pore size and, consequently, penetration rates into the tablet.

Thus, as far as aqueous film coating is concerned, measurement of contact angles may provide useful information on film adhesion, droplet spreading and penetration tendencies, and also interactions between the constituents of the coating formulation and those of the tablet substrate.

Measurement of contact angle

Various methods have been used to assess contact angles. These include direct measurement using, for example, a telemicroscope or photographic technique; indirect measurement such as the h–e method, which involves measuring the maximum droplet height on a surface (Kossen & Heertjes, 1965; and see Fig. 5.6) and by measurement of liquid penetration. A review of the methods available has been made by Stamm *et al.* (1984) and a comparison of the h–e method and a direct measurement technique reported by Fell & Efentakis (1979). Contact angle determination methods have been reviewed critically by Buckton (1990).

The relationship between the maximum height of a sessile drop on a horizontal surface and contact angle was first derived by Padday (1951) as

$$\cos \theta = \frac{1 - \rho_L g h^2}{2 \gamma_{LV}} \tag{5.5}$$

In equation (5.5), ρ_L and γ_{LV} are the density and equilibruim liquid surface tension of the coating solution and h is the measured height of the drop. This equation was later amended by Kossen & Heertjes (1965) to allow for the volume porosity of the compact (ε_v). They derived two equations.

For $\cos \theta < 90°$:

$$\cos \theta = 1 - \sqrt{\frac{\rho_L g h^2}{2 \gamma_{LV}} \cdot \frac{2}{3(1 - \varepsilon_v)}} \tag{5.6}$$

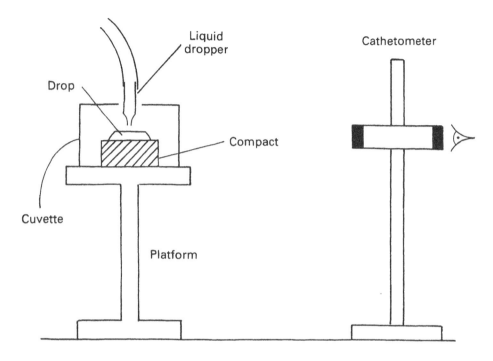

Fig. 5.6 Determination of contact angle by the maximum droplet height technique of Kossen & Heertjes (1965).

For $\cos \theta > 90°$:

$$\cos \theta = -1 + \sqrt{\frac{(2 - \rho_L g h^2)}{2\gamma_{LV}} \cdot \frac{2}{3(1 - \varepsilon_v)}} \qquad (5.7)$$

One further complication with contact angle determinations that is relevant to its measurement in the context of a coating droplet on a tablet surface is the effect of surface roughness. This can be understood by examining Fig. 5.7. Close examination will show that the actual true contact angle (θ_t) at the point of contact is the same in each case, but the measured (apparent) contact angles (θ_m) are very different.

Contact angles in film coating

Most work performed on the wetting of pharmaceutical materials utilizing contact angle measurement has concentrated on measuring the angles of drops which have been placed carefully on a flat substrate surface. In addition, the substrates have tended to be specially prepared, for example, either by using a high compaction pressure to minimize liquid penetration and reduce surface roughness or by using test solutions saturated with the components of the compacts in order to avoid any dissolution of the substrate. Although these techniques may give information of a

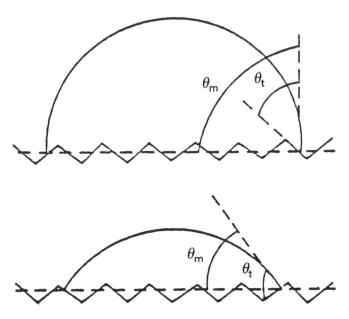

Fig. 5.7 The effect of surface roughness on the apparent contact angle.

fundamental nature, they do not reflect what may happen when film-coating solutions are applied in practice. Little information is available at present regarding the influence of droplet momentum on the contact angle formed, the role of changes in film-coating formulations, or the contact angles formed on coated tablets.

The contact angles formed by droplets on a substrate during aqueous film coating may potentially influence the roughness and appearance of the coated product. The contact angle will also reflect the degree of liquid penetration into the substrate and, consequently, coat adhesion. Young's equation (equation (5.1)) equates the forces acting on a drop of liquid on a solid surface. This equation implies that the contact angle is dependent upon the surface tension of the liquid, the solid–liquid interfacial tension and the surface tension of the solid. Low contact angles are favoured by high solid and low liquid surface tensions and a low solid–liquid interfacial tension.

Table 5.1 shows the data of Twitchell *et al.* (1993) for some contact angle measurements of droplets of HPMC E5 solutions approximately 1 s after being placed gently on uncoated and coated compacted tablet cores. These results also indicate that the contact angles formed by HPMC-based formulations on coated tablets can be different from those formed on uncoated tablets. Droplets placed gently on the surface of coated tablets showed greater initial contact angles than those on uncoated tablets, this being particularly apparent with the low-viscosity solutions. Droplet viscosity appeared to have minimal influence on the contact angles formed by droplets placed gently on coated tablet surfaces. These latter two findings are due to a reduction in droplet penetration into the coated tablet surface compared with the uncoated tablet surface. The potential for very rough coated

Table 5.1 Contact angle of droplets of aqueous HPMC E5 solutions on uncoated and coated tablet cores

Coating formulation	Concen-tration (%w/w)	Viscosity (mPa s)	Uncoated tablets	Coated tablets $R_a = 1.75~\mu$m	Coated tablets $R_a = 2.60~\mu$m	Coated tablets $R_a = >5.0~\mu$m
HPMC E5	6	45	39	98	96	102
HPMC E5	9	166	62	99	98	106
HPMC E5	11	350	72			
HPMC E5	12	520	73	105	106	108
HPMC E5	15	1417*	82			
HPMC E5 + PEG 400	9 1	171	57	102	103	111
Opadry-OY	11	161*	63	98	97	107

*Formulations exhibited pseudoplastic behaviour. Viscosity values quoted are the apparent Newtonian viscosity values (Twitchell, 1990). All other formulations exhibited Newtonian behaviour.

surfaces to increase the observed contact angle of droplets placed gently on the surface is also demonstrated in Table 5.1. This is likely to have arisen from a tendency for the rougher surface to resist movement across the surface, thereby reducing the advancement of the droplet.

If we assume that (i) HPMC coating formulations of the type used in practice exhibit minimal differences in their surface tension (section 4.2.3), (ii) the uncoated tablets are the same and (iii) the solid–liquid interfacial tensions are the same, it might be expected from theoretical considerations that the contact angles which the droplets make on the tablets during a coating process would be of the same order, irrespective of the coating conditions. This indeed may be the case if (i) the substrate has zero porosity, (ii) the droplets have time to reach equilibrium on the substrate, (iii) the droplets are saturated with components of the substrate so that dissolution does not occur and (iv) no other external forces are acting on the spreading process. In practical situations, however, the above conditions do not exist and there is therefore the potential for the droplet contact angles to be dependent upon the application conditions.

The latter point (iv) is discussed further in section 5.4 in which the concept and usefulness of determining dynamic contact angles is discussed in the context of droplet spreading on the substrate surface.

5.2.4. Types of wetting

The process of wetting, as defined in section 5.2.1 above, can be subdivided into three distinct types: *adhesional*, *immersional* and *spreading* wetting. Each of these control the fate of the droplet of coating solution after initial impact.

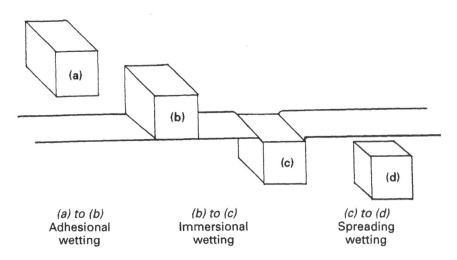

(a) to (b)
Adhesional
wetting

(b) to (c)
Immersional
wetting

(c) to (d)
Spreading
wetting

Fig. 5.8   Schematic diagram of adhesional, immersional and spreading wetting.

A pictorial theoretical representation of these types of wetting is shown in Fig.
5.8. It depicts the gradual immersion of a cube from air into liquid. It helps to illustrate the changes (either gains or losses) in the surface areas of various interfaces
that occur as this sequence proceeds. It is the differences in the disappearance or
appearance of the various interfaces that define the differences between the various
types of wetting.

In the transition from stage (a) to stage (b) in Fig. 5.8, i.e. to the point at which
the cube just touches the surface of the liquid, there is a loss in area of both the
solid–vapour and liquid–vapour interfaces and a corresponding gain in a wetted
solid–liquid interface. This is adhesional wetting.

As the cube becomes immersed in the liquid (stage (b) to stage (c) in Fig. 5.8)
there is loss of solid–vapour (i.e. 'dry') interface and a corresponding gain in
solid–liquid (i.e. wetted) interface. Note, however, that there is no change in the area
of the liquid–vapour interface, i.e. there is neither loss nor gain of the liquid–vapour
interface during this process of immersional wetting.

Spreading wetting occurs between stages (c) to (d) in Fig. 5.8, i.e. as the liquid
spreads over the top surface of the cube. In this case there is again loss of
solid–vapour and gain of solid–liquid interfaces but this time there is an increase in
the area of liquid–vapour interface.

The common thread in all types of wetting described above is that 'dry'
solid–vapour interface is replaced by 'wetted' solid–liquid interface. The differences
in the fate of the liquid–vapour interface defines which type of wetting is occurring.
These differences are summarised below.

- *In all cases*   solid–vapour interface disappears
                          solid–liquid interface forms
- *Adhesional wetting*   liquid–vapour interface disappears

- *Immersional wetting* no change in liquid–vapour interface
- *Spreading wetting*   liquid–vapour interface forms.

So much for 'textbook' explanations, but what does this mean in the context of the film coating of tablets or multiparticulates? In the following set of diagrams, these concepts have been converted into visualizations of situations that arise during actual film coating.

Adhesional wetting

Fig. 5.9, which is a diagrammatic representation of adhesional wetting, shows a droplet of coating formulation approaching and hitting the surface of a tablet core or multiparticulate pellet. The resulting collision will result in a loss of

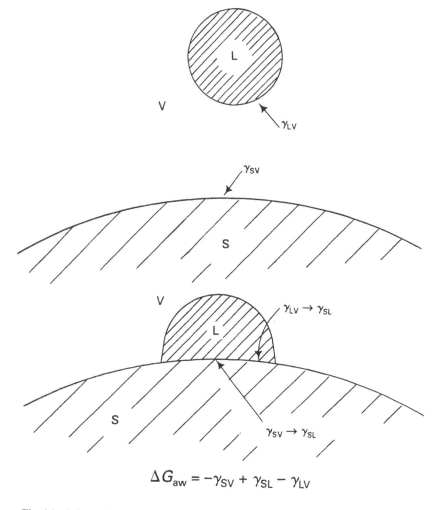

$$\Delta G_{aw} = -\gamma_{SV} + \gamma_{SL} - \gamma_{LV}$$

Fig. 5.9 Schematic representation of adhesional wetting in the context of film coating—
1: Droplet collision.

liquid–vapour interface (the original surface of the drop), loss in solid–vapour interface (the 'dry' surface of the core) and gain of a solid–liquid interface (i.e. the now
wetted area of surface on the core).

The corresponding changes in the surface free energies occurring during this
process are also shown in the diagram. Thus, the overall change in surface free
energy during adhesional wetting (ΔG_{aw}) is the summation of all these changes.

This type of wetting is obviously *essential* for all film-coating processes.

A second example of adhesional wetting is shown in Fig. 5.10, which depicts a
substrate particle (the lower diagram) on which is an adhered droplet of coating
formulation that has not fully dried. A second core approaches at the point of
contact where the wet drop is situated. Adhesional wetting will occur with the same
changes in surface and interfacial energies as described above in Fig. 5.9.

This second example of adhesional wetting will be detrimental since, if the
droplet meniscus dries while the two cores remain in contact and the two cores are
separated during the tumbling action of the coater or fluidized bed, the film will be
ripped away from one core, leaving a partially or uncoated area, and the other core
will have an irregular, extra-thickness coating at one point. The resulting defect is
known as 'picking'.

Immersional wetting
A depiction of immersional wetting is shown in Fig. 5.11. Remember that in immersional wetting there is no change in the area of liquid–vapour interface. An example
of this is the penetration of the coating solution or suspension into a pore in the
substrate core. Strictly, this pore should be parallel to ensure no change in the
liquid–vapour interface area, but the principle holds for most tablet or pellet pores.

The corresponding changes in the individual and overall surface energies are
shown in the diagram.

This type of wetting should be actively encouraged during film coating since it
markedly increases the subsequent adhesion of the dried film. This results not only
from an increase in interfacial contact area as the coating formulation penetrates
into the pores, but also as a consequence of the film drying within the pores,
providing 'roots' to strongly attach the dried polymer coat.

Spreading wetting
Fig. 5.12 is a representation of spreading wetting in the context of film coating.

This diagram shows a droplet spreading out on the surface of a tablet or pellet
after it has collided with the surface (i.e. subsequent to the initial adhesional wetting
described in Fig. 5.9). Again there is a loss of 'dry' solid–vapour interface and a
corresponding increase in the area of solid–liquid interface beneath the newly
spreaded area. This scenario also fits in with the requirement to increase the
liquid–vapour interfacial area during spreading wetting.

As with the other types of wetting, it is important to encourage spreading
wetting. This will lead to a greater area of coverage by each droplet and will also
yield a smoother, dried coat. This latter aspect is discussed further in Chapter 13.

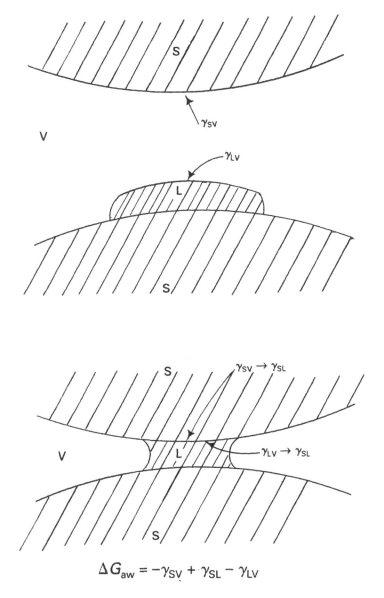

$$\Delta G_{aw} = -\gamma_{SV} + \gamma_{SL} - \gamma_{LV}$$

Fig. 5.10   Schematic representation of adhesional wetting in the context of film coating—
2: Tablet or pellet sticking.

The determination of work of wetting from measurements of contact angle and liquid surface tension

It is now possible to calculate the changes in surface free energy occurring during each type of wetting. The great significance of this is that if the result of the calculation gives a negative value for the change in free energy, it means that the wetting will be spontaneous. This is obviously the desired situation. Furthermore, the more

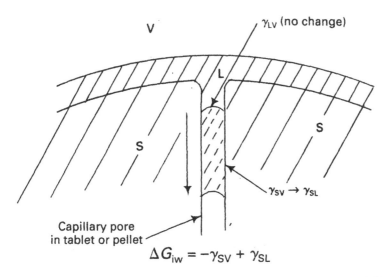

$$\Delta G_{iw} = -\gamma_{SV} + \gamma_{SL}$$

Fig. 5.11   Schematic representation of immersional wetting in the context of film coating.

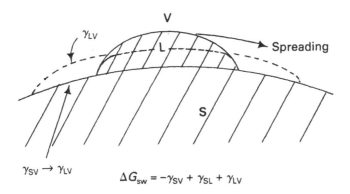

$$\Delta G_{sw} = -\gamma_{SV} + \gamma_{SL} + \gamma_{LV}$$

Fig. 5.12   Schematic representation of spreading wetting in the context of film coating.

negative is the value of the free energy change, the greater will be the ease and degree of wetting, penetration and spreading. On the other hand, if the free energy change is positive, wetting will not be spontaneous. Thus it will either not happen at all or energy will have to be provided in order for spreading to occur (which will be discussed later). It should also be mentioned here that surface free energy change (ΔG) is often referred to as the work of wetting (W). These two terms are interchangeable and the concept of spontaneity is true for both a negative free energy charge and negative work.

However, for the moment there is a potential problem in obtaining the data necessary to calculate the energy changes associated with adhesional, immersional and spreading wetting. Values for γ_{SL}, γ_{SV} and γ_{LV} must be known (see the equations in Figs 5.9 to 5.12). While it is relatively easy to measure γ_{LV} (as described in section 5.2.2), γ_{SL} and γ_{SV} are not easily measurable in practice.

However, we can make use of Young's equation (equation (5.1), section 5.2.3). A rearrangement of this equation introduced earlier (equation (5.4)), and reproduced here,

$$\cos\theta = \frac{\gamma_{SV} - \gamma_{SL}}{\gamma_{LV}} \tag{5.4}$$

gives

$$\gamma_{SV} - \gamma_{SL} = \gamma_{LV}.\cos\theta \tag{5.8}$$

Thus our two unknowns can be replaced by the more easily measured term $\gamma_{LV}.\cos\theta$.

Thus, from determinations of equilibrium liquid surface tension and contact angle it is possible to calculate the changes in free energy (ΔG) (or work of wetting, W) for each type of wetting. These calculations are followed through here using adhesional wetting as an example to yield simple and usable formulae for ΔG_{aw} and W_{aw}.

$$\Delta G_{aw} = -\gamma_{SV} + \gamma_{SL} - \gamma_{LV}$$

$$\cos\theta = \frac{\gamma_{SV} - \gamma_{SL}}{\gamma_{LV}}$$

Therefore

$$\gamma_{SV} - \gamma_{SL} = \gamma_{LV}\cos\theta$$

Therefore

$$\Delta G_{aw} = -(\gamma_{LV}\cos\theta) - \gamma_{LV}$$

Therefore, since $\Delta G_{aw} = -\gamma_{LV}\cos\theta - \gamma_{LV}$,

$$\Delta G_{aw} = -\gamma_{LV}(\cos\theta + 1)$$

and

$$W_{aw} = -\gamma_{LV}(\cos\theta + 1)$$

Note also that the negative of the value of W_{aw} is equal to the work of adhesion, i.e. the work required to restore initial conditions, in this case $+\gamma_{LV}(\cos\theta + 1)$.

A summary of the changes in free energy and work of wetting for the three types of wetting is shown below.

Adhesional wetting

$$\Delta G_{aw} = W_{aw} = -\gamma_{SV} + \gamma_{SL} - \gamma_{LV} = -\gamma_{LV}(\cos\theta + 1) \tag{5.9}$$

Immersional wetting

$$\Delta G_{iw} = W_{iw} = -\gamma_{SV} + \gamma_{SL} = -\gamma_{LV}(\cos\theta) \tag{5.10}$$

Spreading wetting

$$\Delta G_{sw} = W_{sw} = -\gamma_{SV} + \gamma_{SL} + \gamma_{LV} = -\gamma_{LV}(\cos\theta - 1) \tag{5.11}$$

The similarity of the three equations will be noticed. In each case there is a loss of SV and a gain in SL interfacial energy. The equations differ only as a result of the differing fate of the liquid–vapour interface during each of the three types of wetting (see section 5.2.4).

Insufficient data are available to follow such calculations through for film-coating systems. However, in an analogous experiment, Banks (1981) made some useful determinations in the context of fluidized-bed granulation. He measured the equilibrium contact angles of aqueous PVP solutions by the maximum drop height technique on compacts compressed from powder mixes of different ratios of lactose (hydrophilic, $\theta < 30°$) and salicylic acid (hydrophobic, θ greater than $90°$). Calculations based on his data are shown in Table 5.2.

Examination of the data in Table 5.2 shows that the work of adhesion is always negative, irrespective of contact angle. Thus, adhesional wetting will *always* be spontaneous. This is a mixed blessing as the two sketches of adhesional wetting (Figs 5.9 and 5.10) indicated. On the one hand, adhesional wetting is essential in order for the droplet to adhere to the surface of the substrate. However, the defect known as picking may also result from adhesional wetting. This defect can be reduced, however, by careful manipulation of process conditions (see Chapters 13 and 15). As would be expected, the work of adhesional wetting is more negative for more hydrophilic systems.

Thus, improving either the wetting power of the spray or the wettability of the core (by the use of surfactants, for example) will improve adhesional wetting. Either (or both) will improve the interfacial contact between the droplet and core.

The column in Table 5.2 that lists the work of immersional wetting shows that it is negative (and therefore spontaneous) when the contact angle is less than $90°$ but positive when above $90°$. The significance of the positive value of work has been explained above and should be avoided if immersional wetting is to occur. As

Table 5.2 Calculated values for the free energy changes associated with the three types of wetting using substrates of compacts prepared from various ratios of salicylic acid and lactose wetted with a 5% aqueous PVP solution

Salicylic acid (%)	Lactose (%)	Contact angle ($\theta°$)	Work of wetting (mN/m)		
			Adhesional $-\gamma_{LV}(\cos\theta + 1)$	Immersional $-\gamma_{LV}(\cos\theta)$	Spreading $-\gamma_{LV}(\cos\theta - 1)$
0	100	26.7	−96.2	−45.4	+ 5.4
20	80	41.4	−88.9	−38.1	+12.7
40	60	58.0	−77.7	−26.9	+23.9
50	50	64.8	−72.5	−21.7	+29.1
60	40	71.6	−66.8	−16.0	+34.8
80	20	76.5	−62.7	−11.8	+39.0
100	0	92.9	−44.2	+ 6.6	+57.4

explained in section 5.2.4, it is advantageous to encourage immersional wetting in film coating.

The column of work of spreading wetting shows that this is always positive. This is very significant since it means that the spreading of film-coating droplets over a tablet core will never be spontaneous. Spreading, therefore, requires energy to be provided before it can proceed. In film coating this energy must come from the momentum of the droplets as they hit the tablets. The effect of droplet momentum on the measured contact angle of film-coating droplets is discussed later in this chapter (section 5.4) and the role of droplet momentum in contributing towards the production of a smooth film coat is discussed in Chapter 13.

5.3 PENETRATION

Introduction

During the initial stages of the aqueous film-coating process, the droplets will impinge onto an uncoated surface and simultaneously penetrate into and spread onto the tablet or multiparticulate surface. The degree of penetration will be governed by the degree of interaction between the ingredients and pore structure of the substrate and by the ingredients and physical properties of the coating formulation (Alkan & Groves, 1982). The degree of spreading (see section 5.4) will be dependent mainly on the droplet properties and the interaction between the components of the tablet and those of the droplet.

Pharmaceutical tablets, granules and pellets contain numerous pores into which the applied film-coating solutions may penetrate. Penetration time (t) has been demonstrated to follow closely equation (5.9), which was developed by Alkan & Groves (1982) from the earlier work of Washburn (1921)

$$\frac{1}{t} = \frac{1}{4}\left[\frac{2\pi}{3V_v}\right]^{\frac{2}{3}} \times \left[\frac{\cos\theta.\gamma_{LV}}{\mu}\right] \times \left[\varepsilon^{\frac{2}{3}}.D\right] \qquad (5.12)$$

where D is the mean pore diameter, V_v is the void volume of the penetrated space, ε is the porosity of the powder bed, θ is the solid–liquid contact angle and μ and γ_{LV} are the viscosity and surface tension of the solution, respectively.

The final volume of liquid which can penetrate into the bed will be the same as the void volume, and the rate of penetration of a film-coating solution will be dependent on its viscosity, liquid surface tension and interaction with the solid surface. The validity of this equation was confirmed by following the depth of penetration of an organic film-coating solution based on HPMC into a tablet with respect to time (Alkan and Groves, 1982).

The penetration behaviour of aqueous film-coating solutions

The penetration behaviour of film-coating solutions into the substrates used in coating should yield information to explain more fully the role of coating formulation in governing the film properties and the incidence of film coat defects.

The concept of different rates of penetration into tablet surfaces by solutions of different viscosities was utilized by Fisher & Rowe (1976) to explain the variation in film adhesion between formulations of different grades of HPMC. The authors postulated that the increased rate and depth of penetration of solutions prepared from lower molecular weight grades of HPMC resulted in an increase in the effective area of coating-to-tablet contact, and therefore higher adhesion.

Penetration times for aqueous HPMC E5 solutions into tablet cores have been investigated by Twitchell (1990). Some of his data are shown in Table 5.3.

It can be seen that over the range of solution concentrations likely to be used practically (6–12 %w/w), there is the potential for an eighteen-fold difference in penetration rate. The test tablets used in this study consisted of microcrystalline cellulose, pregelatinized starch and stearic acid. The former two components can both be used as tablet disintegrants and allow water to penetrate quickly into the tablet surface, resulting in the disruption of tablet bonds and rapid tablet disintegration. This, coupled with the relatively high porosity of the test tablets, would facilitate the formation of low aqueous coating solution contact angles. Counteracting those factors which aid penetration are droplet viscous forces. The wide range of penetration times listed in Table 5.3 demonstrates the potential importance of HPMC solution concentration/viscosity in governing the degree of atomized droplet penetration into a substrate. The extremely slow penetration rates found for the higher solution concentrations (despite the favourable substrate properties described above) suggests that problems associated with poor adhesion, e.g. intagliation bridging, may occur with these solutions, especially if applied to low-porosity or hydrophobic substrates.

The penetration behaviour of the coating solution may influence film properties and the incidence of film defects.

5.4   SPREADING

Dynamics of contact angle and spreading in the context of film coating
Young's equation (equation (5.1), section 5.2.3) relies strictly on surface forces to

Table 5.3   Penetration into tablets of 9 %w/w aqueous HPMC E5 solutions

HPMC E5 solution concentration (%w/w)	Solution viscosity (mPa s)	Penetration time ± s.d. ($n = 10$) (s)
0	1	0.9 ± 0.1
6	45	52 ± 5
9	166	379 ± 54
11	350	468 ± 68
12	520	939 ± 89
15	1287	1374 ± 115

determine the tendency of the droplet to wet and will give *equilibrium* contact angles for drops placed carefully on the surface. During aqueous film coating, however, there is a very short time period between the droplet hitting the surface and a film being produced. There may therefore be insufficient time for equilibrium values of γ_{SL} and γ_{LV} to be reached (as discussed in section 5.2.2). In addition equilibrium contact angles may not be achieved if spreading is slow due to a high droplet viscosity. The potential for the latter effect to occur was illustrated by Zografi (1985) who showed, for a series of polydimethylsiloxanes on metal surfaces, that the time taken for the equilibrium contact angle to be reached increased markedly as the liquid viscosity increased.

Droplets contacting tablet surfaces do not do so gently, but impinge with a relatively high velocity, the kinetic energy being derived from the atomizing air. Data gathered from studies under equilibrium conditions may therefore not be applicable to droplets spreading during the actual coating process. Zografi (1985) reported that droplets forced to move across a surface at high velocities exhibited larger dynamic contact angles. He concluded that forced spreading may therefore induce ordinarily good wetting systems to have less wetting power during a process like film coating.

The contact angles of droplets of HPMC solution allowed to fall from various distances onto uncoated 15 mm flat–faced, circular tablets have been reported by Twitchell *et al.* (1993). Some of their data can be seen in Table 5.4.

It is apparent from these results that the contact angle is dependent on both the viscosity of the formulation and the momentum possessed by the droplet. When the droplets are carefully placed on the tablet surface (i.e. 0 mm column in Table 5.4), increasing the HPMC E5 concentration from 6 to 15 %w/w, with the resultant viscosity increase from 45 to 1417 mPa s, gave rise to an increase in the contact angle. The inclusion of PEG 400 in the HPMC E5 formulation appeared to have a minimal effect on the contact angle formed. Opadry formulations with viscosity values similar to HPMC E5 solutions gave comparable contact angles. This indicates that when droplets are placed on a tablet surface, it is solution viscosity rather than the presence of additives in the formulation which has the major influence on the contact angle formed.

Droplets that were allowed to fall from a height of either 100 or 200 mm were shown (with the exception of the 15 %w/w HPMC E5 solution) to produce smaller contact angles than droplets placed on the surface. Again, the contact angle formed by the droplets was dependent primarily on the viscosity of the formulation. The 12 %w/w HPMC E5 solution showed only a small reduction in contact angle (6°) when allowed to fall from 200 mm and the 15 %w/w solution showed no change at all.

Only a small amount of energy will need to be imparted to droplets atomized from low HPMC E5 solution concentrations (6 %w/w and below) in order for them to spread well. The fact that these concentrations are applied to produce smooth, high-gloss coats (Reiland & Eber, 1986) suggests that sufficient energy to spread the droplets is imparted during typical coating processes. With higher HPMC E5 solution concentrations, however, it was demonstrated that the contact angle was dependent on the kinetic energy and viscosity of the droplets. The data indicated

Table 5.4   The influence of droplet formulation and momentum on the
contact angle formed on uncoated tablets.

Coating formulation type	Component concentration (%w/w)	Viscosity (mPa s)	Contact angle (°)		
			Distance of droplet fall (mm)		
			0	100	200
HPMC E5	6	45	39		29
HPMC E5	9	166	62	50	46
HPMC E5	11	350	72		58
HPMC E5	12	520	73	71	67
HPMC E5	15	1417*	82		82
HPMC E5 with PEG 400	9 1	171	57		45
Opadry-OY	7	51*	42	33	27
Opadry-OY	11	161*	63		48
Opadry-OY	16	514*	70		65

*Formulations exhibited pseudoplastic behaviour. Viscosity values quoted are the apparent Newtonian viscosity values (Twitchell, 1990). All other formulations exhibited Newtonian behaviour.

that considerably greater amounts of energy need to be imparted to highly viscous droplets in order to force them to spread on a tablet surface after contact. The extent of spreading will therefore be dependent on the droplet viscosity and the atomization conditions. The reader will also recall that spreading is not a spontaneous process (see section 5.2.4).

Data are presented in Table 5.5 for the contact angle of droplets either placed or dropped onto *coated* tablets (Twitchell *et al.*, 1993).

When the droplets were given kinetic energy during the contact angle measurements, droplet viscosity was found to be important in determining the resulting contact angle formed on coated tablets, and differences in contact angles formed on the coated and uncoated tablets became much smaller.

The roughness of the coated tablet surfaces were found by Twitchell *et al.* (1993) in most cases not to influence significantly droplet contact angles, when the droplets were given kinetic energy. The resistance to droplet advancement presumably being overcome by the momentum of the droplet. Only very rough tablets ($R_a > 5$ μm) showed significantly higher contact angles. This general finding may not necessarily occur, however, during practical film coating, since the droplets hitting the tablet are much smaller and their size relative to the undulations in the surface is also much smaller.

On coated tablets, therefore, the spreading behaviour and contact angle formed by atomized coating solution droplets are likely to be dependent mainly on droplet

Table 5.5 The influence of droplet formulation and momentum on the contact angle formed on coated tablets with an arithmetic mean roughness of 2.6 μm. (Twitchell *et al.*, 1993)

Coating formulation type	Component concentration (%w/w)	Viscosity (mPa s)	Contact angle (°) Distance of droplet fall (mm)			
			0	50	100	200
HPMC E5	6	45	96	52	36	34
HPMC E5	9	166	98	69	55	47
HPMC E5	12	520	106	99	93	80
HPMC E5	15	1417*	109	—	—	98
HPMC E5 with PEG 400	9 1	171	103	—	—	49
Opadry-OY	11	161*	97	—	—	50

*Formulations exhibited pseudoplastic behaviour. Viscosity values quoted are the apparent Newtonian viscosity values (Twitchell, 1990). All other formulations exhibited Newtonian behaviour.

viscosity and kinetic energy. If, however, the droplets are so viscous that the kinetic energy gained from the atomizing air causes minimal forced spreading on the surface, or the substrate is sufficiently hydrophobic, surface tension and interfacial tension forces may play a more dominant role.

It should be noted that the determination of contact angles can only give an indication of the likely effects in practice and serve to offer explanations for subsequent coat properties. In the practical situation, the time taken for droplet penetration and spreading to occur is very small (<1 s) and if the droplet is evaporating its viscosity will be changing continually. The droplets will also impinge on the tablets or multiparticulates at various collision angles, with the momentum of the substrate itself making a major contribution to the forced spreading process. The results of Twitchell *et al.* (1993) demonstrate, however, that formulation viscosity and droplet kinetic energy are likely to play important roles in governing the degree of penetration and spreading on uncoated tablets, and the spreading behaviour on partially coated and fully coated tablets.

The manner in which coating variables influence the surface roughness of the coats has also been reported by Twitchell *et al.* (1993) and is discussed in detail in Chapter 13. The degree to which this will influence the contact angle of the droplets hitting partially coated cores is as yet unclear.

A practical consequence of poor spreading properties of film-coating solutions is manifest in a film defect known as 'orange peel', where the surface is rough and has the characteristic appearance of an orange or lemon skin (see Chapter 13).

5.5 ADHESION

5.5.1 Introduction

A major factor in the choice of coating formulations and processes is the need to have strong adhesion of the polymer film to the product surface. Surprisingly, few studies measuring the adhesion of such coatings to well-defined solid surfaces have been defined; Johnson & Zografi (1986) list some relevant early publications. Experimental work has been somewhat inconclusive in demonstrating any quantitative relationship between the surface energetics of the coating solution and substrate and the resulting adhesive strength. One reason for this is the difficulty in accounting for the effect of bulk film properties on the adhesion measurement.

The adhesion of film coats to tablet substrates is of importance if coating defects such as bridging of the intagliations are to be avoided (Rowe, 1981). The extent of film adhesion will be dependent on the properties of the core and the coating formulation. In order to assure good adhesion, there should (after initial wetting) be both good intrinsic bonding between the chemical groups of the polymer and solid and a maximum true area of contact. The presence of gaps or air pockets between the polymer and solid will tend to weaken the adhesive strength.

The work of adhesion (W_A) between a solid and a liquid can be defined as the energy per unit area required to separate molecules bonding across the interface. It is described by the Young–Dupré equation:

$$W_A = \gamma_{LV} (\cos \theta + 1) \tag{5.13}$$

where γ_{LV} is the solution surface tension and θ the equilibrium contact angle formed when a drop is placed on the substrate surface. You can compare this with equation (5.9) to see that the work of adhesion is of the same magnitude, but opposite sign, to the work of adhesional wetting.

Thus, an increase in the coating solution surface tension or a decrease in the contact angle formed should, in principle, promote adhesion. Maximum attractive forces between a liquid and solid should occur when $\cos \theta = 1$, i.e. when the contact angle θ is zero. In this case, the forces of attraction between the liquid and solid are greater than the cohesive forces of the liquid and $W_A = 2\gamma_{LV}$.

The surface interactions responsible for adhesion have been explained above in the context of wetting theory. Rowe (1988) has developed a theoretical approach based on solubility parameters. He derives equations which will predict both the interaction parameter and ideal butt-test adhesive strength from solubility parameters readily available in the literature. This approach assumes that film/substrate adhesion is due entirely to the summation of the interactions of the intermolecular bonding forces in a perfectly bonded system. Trends predicted by these relationships were found to be comparable to data obtained in practice for the adhesive strength of films of a series of cellulose derivatives on microcrystalline and anhydrous lactose substrates.

Methods for determining adhesion of polymer film coats on tablet surfaces
The principle of the technique is simple. It is necessary to pull off the coat from the core in tension and measure the force needed in order to quantify adhesion. A force–displacement (or stress–strain) tensometer of the 'Instron-type' is satisfactory, although a special apparatus was built and used successfully by Fisher & Rowe (1976). The principle of polymer film adhesion testing is shown in Figure 5.13.

There are a number of considerations to be taken into account in order that the correct value is measured. One is to scrape away the film coat from the sides of the tablet so its presence does not interfere with the application of a pure tensile force to the film. Secondly, it should be appreciated that the actual force needed to pull off the coat is not the true adhesion force since the measured value is influenced by the true area of contact and internal stress within the film.

Rowe (1981) has shown with pharmaceutical systems that these residual stresses are related (among other factors) to film thickness and that such effects are reduced as film thickness is reduced. He proposed a model, shown in Fig. 5.14, where residual stresses, P, cause the theoretical adhesion, A, to be reduced by a factor, R (which is a reaction at the interface arising due to the non-flexibility of the substrate). Thus, the measured adhesion, F, is actually less than theoretical adhesion, A, which can be calculated from intermolecular forces. Thus $F = A - R$, and if R is greater than A then spontaneous failure will occur during storage and will become apparent as bridging of intagliations, for example.

Three factors can contribute to the value of the total internal stress within the film, P: the internal stresses (P_S) due to shrinkage of the film during solvent evaporation, the thermal stresses (P_T) due to differences between the thermal properties of

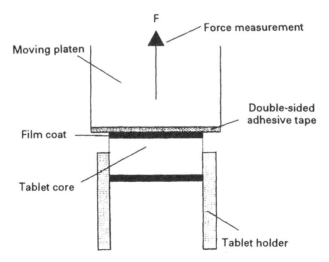

Fig. 5.13   Simple apparatus for the measurement of the apparent adhesion of a polymer
film coat on a tablet substrate.

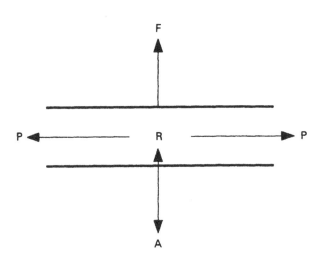

Fig. 5.14   True and apparent adhesion.

the coat and the core; and stresses (P_V) within the film as a result of volumetric changes if the core expands during or after coating. These factors are discussed more fully in Chapter 12.

5.5.2   Factors affecting adhesion

There are very many factors which influence the strength of adhesion between a polymer coat and a tablet or multiparticulate core. These are considered in turn below and representative data are provided.

Wetting (contact angle)

The theories of wetting discussed above (section 5.2.4) suggest that wetting is optimized with high values of both liquid surface tension and the cosine of the contact angle (i.e. contact angles well below 90° are preferred). Thus, an increase in initial wetting should increase the area of available contact between the film and the core. This was also discussed in section 5.2.4. The work of Harder *et al.* (1971) explains specifically some of the surface forces responsible for the adhesive process during the film coating of tablets.

Nadkarni *et al.* (1975) investigated the effect of solution surface tension and contact angle formed on various substrates when coating with poly(methyl vinyl ether/maleic anhydride) plasticized with glyceryl triacetate and dissolved in a variety of solvents. They found that, in accordance with the theory of the Young–Dupré equation, the film adhesion of sprayed coats was greatest with solution/substrate systems exhibiting the lowest contact angles and with solutions of the highest surface tension.

Solvent

Fung & Parrott (1980) showed how the solvent used in film coating can influence the adhesion of the final dried film. It is interesting to note that the lowest adhesion value was achieved with water, presumably as a result of the poorer wetting and higher viscosity with this solvent compared with the organic solvents studied. Similarly, Johnson & Zografi (1986) observed lower adhesion of HPC films cast or sprayed from aqueous rather than from ethanolic solutions.

Polymer type and molecular weight

The influence of polymer grade on the adhesion properties of film coats was reported by Fisher and Rowe (1976) & Rowe (1977b, 1978). Lower molecular weight grades were shown to lead to higher adhesion values. This is probably due to viscosity differences between the solutions, those containing low molecular weight grades being able to penetrate further into the pores of the tablet and thus enhance adhesion.

However, the situation is not always this clear. Experience and work on biconvex tablets (Rowe, 1977b) has shown that neither high nor low molecular weight grades of HPMC consistently produce a higher adhesion and thus no simple deduction can be made in the context of recommending a particular polymer grade for improving adhesion.

Solution concentration

Johnson & Zografi (1986) have measured the effect of the original concentration of solutions of HPC on the adhesive strength of films of varying thicknesses. The higher initial concentration of HPC appeared to produce stronger adhering films at equivalent film thicknesses, yet the authors had no clear explanation for this observation, since one may have predicted better penetration of the less viscous solution leading to greater adhesion of the dried film.

Plasticizer

Plasticizers are obviously important coating components. So how do their presence and concentration affect the adhesion of the coat? Fisher & Rowe (1976) reported that the inclusion of glycerol and propylene glycol at concentrations of up to 20 %w/w in HPMC films sprayed from organic solutions did not have a significant effect on the film/tablet adhesion properties. There is a slight reduction in adhesion but probably not enough to be significant in practice.

In contrast, Porter (1980) found a slight increase in adhesion with glycerol and propylene glycol but a slight decrease with PEG 400 and with low concentrations of PEG 4000. However he observed a marked increase in adhesion with the addition of very high concentrations of PEG 4000.

Opacifier

Film adhesion was shown by Fisher & Rowe (1976) to be reduced by 45% by the addition of 10 %w/w of titanium dioxide. Additional increases in titanium dioxide content to 50 %w/w were shown, however, to have little further effect.

This phenomenon was not found by Porter (1980) who, instead, showed both titanium dioxide and FD&C Yellow No.5 aluminium lake to have little effect on adhesion at concentrations of up to 40 %w/w. This discrepancy may have arisen either from the use of different solvent systems (Porter using an aqueous system and Rowe an organic one) or to differences in the equipment used to measure the adhesion.

Film thickness

Johnson & Zografi (1986) measured the adhesion of HPC to well-defined solid substrates as a function of dry film thickness. They used a well-controlled butt adhesion test, providing a constant slow rate of film detachment. This ensured that the viscoelastic contribution of the film to the adhesion measurement remained constant. They noticed that the method of film preparation, whether cast or sprayed, had no significant effect on the adhesion measurement. They observed that the adhesive strength of HPC films on a range of substrates decreased linearly with increasing film thickness. They suggested that extrapolating this line back to zero film thickness reflected the fundamental value for the work of adhesion between film and substrate.

Earlier, Rowe (1978) had found the relationship less well defined, particularly at film thicknesses greater than about 35 μm. Rowe (1981) had also suggested that extrapolation to zero film thickness might provide a better measure of intrinsic adhesion, or at least could normalize the contribution of film thickness when comparing different systems.

Core excipients

One of the most intriguing aspects of improving adhesion is the influence of core excipients. The tablet core constituents play an important role in achieving a successfully coated product. Rowe (1977b) examined the effect of some direct compression excipients and tablet lubricants on adhesion values of HPMC film coats and showed that tablet core excipients can have a marked effect on observed adhesion. This, however, should not be too surprising since it has been emphasized before in this chapter that wetting is an *inter*-facial phenomenon and thus is influenced by both the droplets and the substrate core.

Rowe (1977b) found adhesion to be influenced by the polarity of tablet surface. Tablets prepared from microcrystalline cellulose were shown to exhibit high adhesion values, this being attributed to the presence of hydroxyl groups at the surface which were able to form hydrogen bonds with the HPMC. Lactose and some other sugars showed intermediate values with the lowest value being observed with the addition of inorganic excipient dicalcium phosphate dihydrate.

The effect of tablet lubricants was found to be dependent on their non-polar hydrocarbon content (Rowe, 1977b). Of the lubricants studied, stearic acid was found to be preferable as far as adhesion was concerned, a factor accredited to the presence of the free polar carboxyl group. When this carboxyl group was combined with either calcium (calcium stearate) or magnesium (magnesium stearate) the measured adhesion was reduced. High concentrations of lubricants should be avoided—although this is well appreciated for other reasons, of course.

It appears from these data that adhesion problems might be overcome by the addition of some microcrystalline cellulose to the formulation of the core. The latter comment is further evidence of that commonly recommended, but not so commonly followed, advice that the core and coat should not be developed in isolation. It is not good practice to expect coating scientists to overcome poor core formulation.

Core porosity
The role of porosity in improving wetting has been discussed earlier in this chapter (sections 5.2.4 and 5.3). It could be predicted that there would be an improvement in adhesion with increasing substrate porosity as a result of increased adhesional and immersional wetting. Fisher & Rowe (1976) observed a general decrease in measured adhesion with increasing tablet compaction pressure and thus decreasing substrate porosity. Rowe (1978) found a linear increase in adhesion with increasing porosity for two grades of HPMC. The slope of this line was lower for the higher viscosity grade, reflecting the reduced rate of penetration of this solution into the substrate.

5.5.3 Consequences of poor adhesion
Strong adhesion is obviously desirable. The consequences of weak adhesion are visible and damaging film-coating defects, such as bridging of intagliations, etc. These are discussed fully in Chapter 13.

5.6 CONCLUSIONS

This chapter has shown the importance of a knowledge of what is happening at the interface between a tablet or multiparticulate core and a film-coating formulation—both as a liquid during its application and as a dried polymer film in the final state.

The wetting, spreading and adhesion stages of the film-coating process are all extremely important aspects to be controlled since they strongly determine the integrity, strength and performance of the film coat in practice. We have seen how the wetting properties of the droplets are a function of formulation and droplet size and that, in addition, the spreading stage is influenced by the momentum of the droplets hitting the substrate surface.

The link between good wetting and good adhesion cannot be overemphasized. In this chapter the influence of various factors on film adhesion has been described.

While it is not always necessary to have a firm grasp of these physicochemical concepts to produce a satisfactory film coat in practice, an awareness and understanding of some of the theories discussed in this chapter should assist in the development of more efficient and elegant film coats.

REFERENCES

Alkan, M.H. & Groves, M.J. (1982) *Pharm. Tech.* **6**, 56–67.

Banks, M. (1981) Studies on the fluidised bed granulation process. Ph.D. Thesis, De Montfort University, Leicester.

Buckton, G. (1990) *Powder Technol.* **61**, 237–249.

Buckton, G. & Newton, J.M. (1986) *Powder Tech.* **46**, 201–208.

Costa, M.D.L. & Baszkin, A. (1985) *J. Pharm. Pharmacol.* **37**, 455–460.

Davies, M.C. (1985) Ph.D. Thesis, University of London.

Fell, J.T. & Efentakis, E. (1979) *Int. J. Pharm.* **4**, 153–157.

Fisher, D.G. & Rowe, R.C. (1976) *J. Pharm. Pharmacol.* **28**, 886–889.

Fung, R.M. & Parrott, E.L. (1980) *J. Pharm. Sci.* **69(4)**, 439–441.

Harder, S.W., Zuck, D.A. & Wood, J.A. (1970) *J. Pharm. Sci.* **59(12)**, 1787–1792.

Harder, S.W., Zuck, D.A. & Wood, J.A. (1971) *Canadian J. Pharm. Sci.* **6(3)**, 63–70.

Johnson, B.A. & Zografi, G. (1986) *J. Pharm. Sci.* **75(6)**, 529–533.

Kossen, N.W.F. & Heertjes, P.M. (1965) *Chem. Eng. Sci.* **20**, 593–599.

Lange, H. (1971) In: *Non-Ionic Surfactants.* (ed. Schick, M.). Wiley Interscience, London.

Lerk, C.F., Schoonan, A.J.M. & Fell, J.T. (1976) *J. Pharm. Sci.* **65(6)**, 843.

Liao, W. & Zatz, J.L. (1979) *J. Pharm. Sci.* **68**, 488–494.

Nadkarni, P.D., Kildsig, D.O., Kramer, P.A. & Banker, G.S. (1975) *J. Pharm. Sci.* **64(9)**, 1554–1557.

Odidi, I.O., Newton, J.M. & Buckton, G. (1991) *Int. J. Pharmaceut.* **72**, 43–49.

Padday, J.F. (1951) *Proc. 2nd Int. Congr. Surface Activity*, Butterworths, London, **3**, 81–121.

Porter, S.C. (1980) *Pharm. Technol.* **4(3)**, 66–75.

Reiland, T. L. & Eber, A.C. (1986) *Drug Dev. Ind. Pharm.* **12(3)**, 231–245.

Rowe, R.C. (1976) *J. Pharm. Pharmacol.* **28**, 310–311.

Rowe, R.C. (1977a) *J. Pharm. Pharmacol.* **29**, 58–59.

Rowe, R.C. (1977b) *J. Pharm. Pharmacol.* **29**, 723–726.

Rowe, R.C. (1978) *J. Pharm. Pharmacol.* **30**, 343–346.

Rowe, R.C. (1980) *J. Pharm. Pharmacol.* **32**, 116–119.

Rowe, R.C. (1981) *J. Pharm. Pharmacol.* **33**, 610–612.

Rowe, R.C. (1988) *Int. J. Pharmaceut.* **41**, 219–222.

Stamm, A., Gissinger, D. & Boymond, C. (1984) *Drug Dev. Ind. Pharm.* **10**, 381–408.

Twitchell, A.M. (1990) Studies on the role of atomisation in aqueous tablet film coating, Ph.D. Thesis, De Montfort University Leicester.

Twitchell, A.M., Hogan, J.E. & Aulton, M.E. (1987) *J. Pharm. Pharmacol.* **39** Suppl., 128P.

Twitchell, A.M., Hogan, J.E. & Aulton M.E. (1993) *Proc. 12th Pharm. Tech. Conf., Solid Dosage Research Unit, Helsingør, Denmark*, March–April, **1**, 246–257.

Wan., L.S.C. & Lee, P.F.S. (1974) *J. Pharm. Sci.* **63**, 136–137.

Washburn, W.E. (1921) *Physiol. Rev.* **17**, 273.

Wood, J.A. & Harder, S.W. (1970) *Canadian J. Pharm. Sci.* **5(1)**, 18–23.
Zografi, G. (1985) Presented to the Institute of Applied Pharmaceutical Sciences, Center for Professional Advancement, Amsterdam.
Zografi, G. & Tam, S.S. (1976) *J. Pharm. Sci.* **65**, 1145–1149.

6

The development of film-coating processes

Graham C. Cole

SUMMARY

To develop a film-coating process requires a laboratory test rig that can be scaled-up to meet production requirements. All the process parameters need to be optimized. A scheme is discussed here that provides an integrated computer-controlled system designed for aqueous film coating in a side-vented pan. A comparison is made of energy requirements of a column-coating system and a coating pan.

All the major operational coating parameters can be measured and recorded under the overall control of a microcomputer. The monitored values are displayed on a computer screen at selected short intervals, e.g. 5 s, and, at selected longer intervals, e.g. 1 min, they can be printed as hard copy.

This chapter describes the selection of instruments to measure the appropriate parameters; how the coating process may be optimized using a laboratory side-vented pan; the loop closed to provide automatic control, and the process scaled-up to control successfully the coating of production size batches.

6.1 INTRODUCTION

To set up a suitable experimental rig required for the general development of all coating processes, instruments are required to measure and record data from the process parameters. First it is necessary to determine which parameters have a critical effect on the performance of the coating system to produce a tablet that is pharmaceutically acceptable.

The following process parameters are possibilities:

- Inlet air flow rate.
- Inlet air temperature.
- Inlet air humidity.
- Outlet air flow rate.
- Outlet air temperature.
- Outlet air humidity.
- Leakage air rate to the atmosphere through the casing.
- Spray concentration.
- Spray temperature.
- Spray flow rate.
- Quantity of attrition from cores (by filtration of the exhaust air).
- Quantity of spray not applied to tablets (by filtration of the exhaust air).
- Tablet-bed temperature.
- Power/torque to keep the drum turning.
- Rotational speed of the drum.
- Electrical power consumption of fans.
- Heat input to inlet air.
- Pressure drop, inlet–outlet airstream.
- Atomizing air pressure. (The atomizing air flow can be neglected as a calculation will show that it is less than 2% of the total air throughput.)

After conducting a number of preliminary experiments, a number of these parameters can be rejected as they do not critically affect the appearance and quality of the film-coated tablet. This list is then reduced to ten which, by installing the appropriate instruments, are used to record the raw data. These instruments are linked through an analogue-to-digital converter to a computer and printer and the values for each parameter recorded on a specifically numbered channel.

Channel
0   Coating spray rate.
1   Inlet air flow rate.
2   Inlet air temperature.
3   Outlet air flow rate.
4   Outlet air temperature.
5   Outlet air dew-point.
6   Fan rotational speed.
7   Coating drum drive torque.
8   Coating suspension temperature.
9   Tablet surface temperature.
10   Atomising air pressure.
15   10-volt reference source.

These are designated the critical parameters. Each can easily be scanned, measured and recorded. The next stage in the set-up of the test rig is the selection of a coating pan, coating accessories, instruments, computer and printer. An example is a model 10 Accelacota (Manesty Machines Ltd). However, any suitable manufacturer's coating pan could be used, depending on the objectives of the coating development programme.

6.2   DEVELOPMENT OF THE EXPERIMENTAL RIG

The coating pan
As an example, a model 10 Accelacota could be used. A unit is shown diagrammatically in Fig. 6.1.

The unit has a horizontal rotating cylindrical drum, the curved surface of which is uniformly perforated. The ends of the cylinder are conically dished, so that tablets in the drum are turned over and also mixed laterally. There are baffles to assist this stirring action. Hot drying air enters the drum through the perforations on the side remote from the tumbling tablet bed, and is drawn through the bed by a fan in the exhaust plenum. This plenum has a mouth that fits closely to the outside of the perforated curved surface of the drum.

The angles of the front and rear sides of the pan are 56° and 61° respectively, which was originally intended to ensure complete mixing of the tablets from the top of the bed to the bottom and from front to rear. However, it was found that this was insufficient to ensure homogeneous mixing and baffles were fitted. Generally, they are of the same shape but of different size for each model and can be easily removed or replaced with baffles of different design, depending on the physical

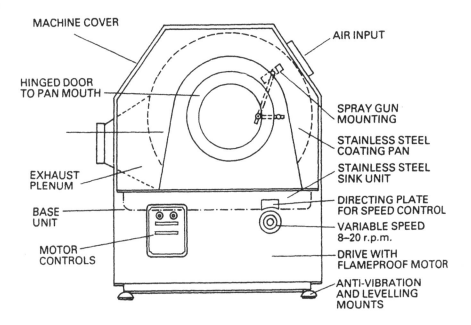

Fig. 6.1   Schematic diagram of Model 10 Accelacota.

characteristics of the tablet to be coated, e.g. friability, and the properties that the coat is designed to impart to the tablet, e.g. enteric coating. In this case the degree of mixing becomes a critical parameter.

A means is required of applying the coating suspension or solution and storing it during application to ensure that it remains homogeneous. Most manufacturers supply suitable units. A typical unit designed for the application of aqueous film-coating solutions and suspensions is shown in Fig. 6.2. The controls are mounted on the top face of the unit and comprise gauges for pump speed, fluid pressure, atomizing air pressure and on/off switches. Below each gauge is the regulator which controls the circuit to which the pressure gauge applies. The adjustment is effected by rotating the main control knob of each regulator while the adjustment is secured by the inner lockscrew. On the panel there are also two valves controlling the flow and return of coating solution.

The operation of the unit is briefly as follows: Compressed air is supplied to the air inlet manifold and from there to three different internal supplies. One supply passes through an air-pressure regulator to the liquid pump and the pressure of this air is shown on the pump air-pressure gauge. This pressure governs the pressure of the liquid. A second air supply passes through a regulator which controls the atomizing air-pressure gauge and the air is then supplied direct to the atomizing air connection on the spray bar in the coating pan. Also connected into this circuit is a

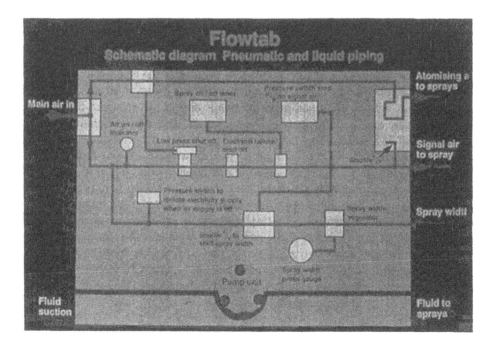

Fig. 6.2 Spray unit control unit.

pressure stop valve which controls the signal air to the spray bar. The signal air is used to provide an option for stopping and starting the spray. In some cases continuous spraying results in overwetting.

The third air supply taken from the air inlet manifold passes through an air-pressure regulator which feeds air to two air-controlled diaphragm type fluid-pressure regulators. Two regulators are necessary to supply the relatively large volumes of fluid used on the larger models of coating pans. This method of control has been employed so that there is no differential pressure between the outputs from the two regulators.

Coating fluid is picked up from the storage container by a peristaltic pump, and pumped at pressure to the fluid-pressure regulators where the supply pressure is controlled and maintained. This pressure is shown on the fluid-pressure gauge. The coating solution is then fed through a valve to the coating pan spray bar, spray nozzle and the excess is returned by means of a second pipe, through a second valve, to the solution container. In the case of low-viscosity liquids, the return control valve can be used to create a back pressure in the system to keep the flow rate constant.

The flow is controlled by:

1. the speed of the pump;
2. the internal diameter of the flexible silicone tube which provides a range of flow rates from 0.002 to over 8 g/s;
3. the nozzle setting.

This arrangement is versatile and easy to clean. No metal surfaces of the pumping system are in contact with the coating suspension during the spray operation, which reduces the risk of cross-contamination. It is possible to control the speed of the pump by linking it to a signal such as the temperature of the exhaust air, inlet air or tablet-bed temperature. One way of controlling the process is to use the exhaust temperature as a controlling parameter as this is an indirect measure of the tablet-bed temperature and is sensitive to process changes. By using a minimum exhaust temperature of 35°C and linking the spray rate directly to this temperature, the pump would automatically stop if the temperature fell below this level. For each degree rise in temperature above this level the speed of the pump increased, up to a maximum of 50 rev/min thus increasing the spray rate. This relationship is illustrated in Fig. 6.3. The relationship between these three variables is inserted as an instruction in the computer programme. By altering this instruction different spray rates can be obtained, depending on the size of the coating pan used and the spray rate required. It can also be demonstrated that a balance can be achieved between the inlet temperature, exhaust temperature and spray rate during the coating operation.

To do this a simplified programme must be written to provide automatic control of the coating process. For example:

Channel

0	Inlet drying air temperature	°C
1	Outlet drying temperature	°C

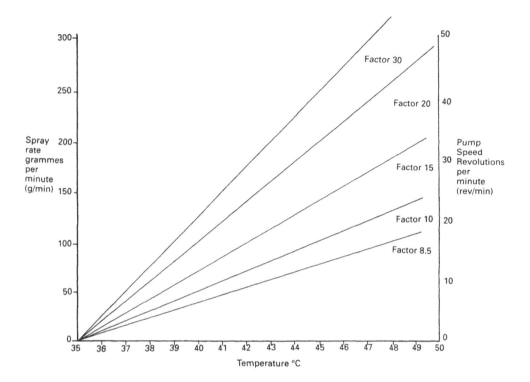

Fig. 6.3   Relationship between pump speed, temperature and spray rate.

2	Pump speed	rev/min
3	Coating suspension used	$kg \times 10^{-3}$
4	Atomizing air pressure	lb/in^2 or bar

The advantage of a computer-based system means that these parameters can be scanned and measured rapidly, say every 5 s, and displayed on the VDU. The results can then be recorded every minute, and every 5 min the spray flow rate can be calculated and recorded. An example of part of the type of a printout is shown in Fig. 6.4.

At the completion of the coating process and when a predetermined quantity of coating suspension has been applied, a 'batch completed' sign is flashed onto the VDU, the pump is automatically switched off and a summary of the processing parameters recorded on the printout.

This process and control programme is schematically represented in Fig. 6.5.

The spray bar fitted to larger coating pans consists of three chambers, one of which contains the coating fluid, one the atomizing air, and one the signal air. The spray guns are mounted directly on the chamber which contains the coating solution and separate pipe connections are made between the gun and the two air chambers.

INLET TEMP	OUTLET TEMP	PUMP SPEED	SUSP'N USED	ATM. PRESS.	FLOW RATE	ELAPSED TIME	
60	40	10	1399	30	34	40 MIN.	M
60	39	10	1442	30			M
60	39	10	1484	30			M
60	39	10	1526	30			M
60	39	10	1526	30			M
INLET TEMP	OUTLET TEMP	PUMP SPEED	SUSP'N USED	ATM. PRESS.	FLOW RATE	ELAPSED TIME	
60	39	10	1569	30	34	45 MIN.	M
60	39	10	1611	30			M
60	38	10	1654	30			M
59	39	10	1696	30			M
59	38	10	1738	30			M
INLET TEMP	OUTLET TEMP	PUMP SPEED	SUSP'N USED	ATM. PRESS.	FLOW RATE	ELAPSED TIME	
60	38	10	1738	30	34	50 MIN.	M
59	38	10	1781	30			M
59	38	10	1823	30			M
61	38	10	1866	30			M
61	38	10	1908	30			M
INLET TEMP	OUTLET TEMP	PUMP SPEED	SUSP'N USED	ATM. PRESS.	FLOW RATE	ELAPSED TIME	
61	38	10	1950	30	42	55 MIN.	M
60	38	10	1993	30			M
60	38	10	1993	30			M
60	38	10	2035	30			M
60	38	10	2078	30			M
INLET TEMP	OUTLET TEMP	PUMP SPEED	SUSP'N USED	ATM. PRESS.	FLOW RATE	ELAPSED TIME	
60	38	10	2120	30	34	60 MIN.	M
60	38	10	2120	30			M
60	38	10	2162	30			M
60	38	10	2205	30			M
60	38	10	2247	30			M
INLET TEMP	OUTLET TEMP	PUMP SPEED	SUSP'N USED	ATM. PRESS.	FLOW RATE	ELAPSED TIME	
60	38	10	2290	30	34	65 MIN.	M
59	39	10	2290	30			M
60	38	10	2374	30			M
60	39	10	2374	30			M
60	38	10	2417	30			M
INLET TEMP	OUTLET TEMP	PUMP SPEED	SUSP'N USED	ATM. PRESS.	FLOW RATE	ELAPSED TIME	
60	38	10	2459	30	34	70 MIN.	M

WEIGHT OF SUSPENSION USED = 2502 GRAMMES   ELAPSED TIME = 71 MINS

Susp'n used – Suspension used
ATM. Press – Atomizing pressure
Temp   – Temperature

Fig. 6.4   Recorded data

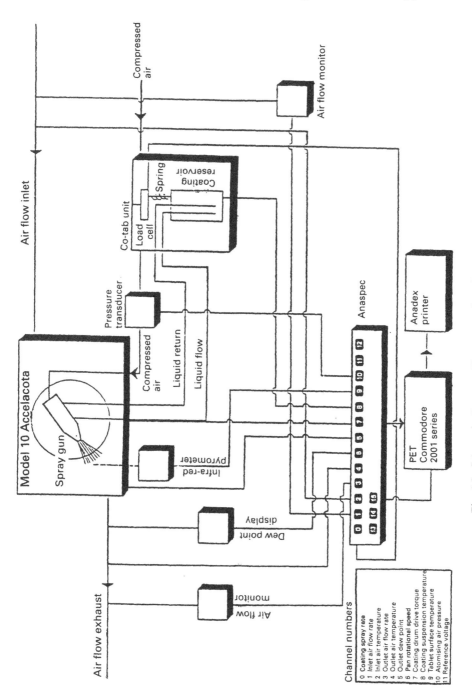

Fig. 6.5 Schematic diagram of instrumented coating pan.

Channel numbers

0 Coating spray rate
1 Inlet air flow rate
2 Inlet air temperature
3 Outlet air flow rate
4 Outlet air temperature
5 Outlet dew point
6 Pan rotational speed
7 Coating drum drive torque
8 Coating suspension temperature
9 Tablet surface temperature
10 Atomising air pressure
11 Reference voltage

The spray gun is an automatic unit with micro-adjuster for spraying. Connections are provided for the supply of coating solution, atomizing air, and signal air.

6.2.1 Instrumentation

The following are examples of instruments that can be used, giving a general approach to what should be done. Many scientists will have their own preference so the choice here should not be considered as cast in stone.

Dew-point hygrometer

This hygrometer is of the optical condensation type. In this instrument a surface is cooled by a thermoelectric or Peltier cooler until dew or frost begins to condense on a mirror. The condensate surface is maintained electronically in vapour pressure equilibrium with the surrounding gas, and surface condensation is detected by an optical or an electrical technique. The condensation surface, when maintained at the temperature at which the rate of condensate exactly equals the evaporation, is then the dew-point temperature. Such a sensor is a fundamental measuring device. The temperature of the surface when so controlled is typically measured with a platinum resistance thermometer, thermocouple or thermistor embedded in the mirror surface.

The main drawback of this type of hygrometer is its complexity and high cost when compared to most other humidity sensors. It is also subject to contamination by materials other than water condensing on the cooled surface.

Air flow measurement

The air flow is measured by two turbine flow meters, a Pitot tube and a differential pressure transmitter.

Because of the problems of obtaining reliable air flow measurements, two straight circular cross-sectional sections of duct should be built to incorporate the turbine flow meters: one for the inlet air and one for the exhaust duct air. The meters must be inserted at a position in the ducts to ensure fully developed air flow using the total flow rate calculated from the velocity distribution across the section.

This inlet air duct plus the meter assembly needs to be calibrated. The second turbine flow meter, mounted in the exhaust, can be calibrated against the first meter. Good correlation is obtained when the coating pan is completely sealed and no air leaks into the pan from the environs.

Pitot tubes determine local or point velocities by measuring the difference between impact pressure and static pressure. In use the Pitot is connected to a low-pressure transmitter which operates on a diaphragm capacitance principle. Two pressure cavities are separated by a taut metal diaphragm with an electrode supported close to it on either side producing two air di-electric capacitors. A pressure difference between the cavities deflects the diaphragm changing the capacitance of the circuit. The volume displacement for full-scale definition is typically 0.003 cm^3.

The capacitors on either side of the diaphragm form two tuned circuits with inductors in the circuit board. These tuned circuits are equally coupled to an R.F.

transitor oscillator which provides a stable signal. A change in the transducer alters the capacitance in each of the tuned circuits, unbalancing the voltages across them. A differential rectifier voltmeter across the tuned circuits provides a D.C. signal from the change in pressure in the transducer. This transmitter has an output of 0–10 V which is linear with respect to the air velocity.

The Pitot tube consists of an impact tube whose opening when positioned in the duct faces directly into the stream of air to measure the impact pressure. It should be sited in a section of duct at least 10 diameters from any bends or disturbances. It is very sensitive to its position in the cross-sectional area of the duct.

Computer

Generally an industrial unit should be used to generate graphics plus alphanumerics. A feature of this operating system is a disc which allows a programme to read or write data in the background while simultaneously allowing transfer of data to the computer memory. Process data is printed out as a hard copy.

The printer enables process data to be presented in such a way that the user can obtain a hard copy of alphanumeric and graphic symbols, tabulated and formatted to suit any experimental requirement. The paper can be positioned in the printer under command from the computer providing control of print width, decimal position, left and right margin control and many copies.

The computer and its accessories can be interfaced with the sensors using an analogue to digital converter. This interface is designed to accept data in one format and transmit data in another. The computer requires data to be presented in a correct and logical format.

Intratrace—a non-contact infrared digital thermometer

Any surface at a temperature above absolute zero emits heat in the form of radiated energy. At temperatures above 600°C some of this energy is visible but much of it is of longer wavelength than visible light (e.g. infrared) although it behaves in a similar way to visible light. The radiant flux from the surface is directly related to its temperature and it is this energy that the Infratrace measures. The value can be visually displayed in Centrigrade degrees or it can be relayed by a suitable interface to a computer and processed. It may also be used to measure and record temperatures through glass by using the correct emissivity setting.

Telemeter

A short range telemetry system can be used to measure strains and temperature. It consists of an oscillator and a discriminator. A possible requirement is the measurement of shaft torque on the coating pan. The oscillator and its battery are connected to a suitable strain gauge bridge fixed to the shaft. The earth side of the battery is connected to the shaft, and the output from the oscillator taken to a metal band fitted around the shaft, but insulated from it. The metal band acts as the plate of a capacitor, and a high-frequency electric field is generated between the band and the surrounding metal objects. By using a stationary high-impedance probe, it is possible to extract a signal from the field, coupled to the oscillator without actual contact with the shaft.

The signal obtained by the probe is fed to the discriminator to recover a voltage analogue of the shaft torque, which is shown on the meter. The amplitude of the signal from the probe varies as the shaft rotates, but as the system is frequency modulated, there is no error as long as the signal does not fall below a minimum value, usually referred to as the threshold level. The discriminator is operated from the mains.

The oscillator is a solid-state high-frequency modulated model specifically developed for the telemetering of millivolt signals from strain gauge bridges on rotating shafts without the use of slip rings. It can provide a full-scale deflection (7.5%) for an input of 5 mV. The unit is designed and the specification based on the use of a fully active bridge using 1000 Ω strain gauges with a gauge factor of 2. The unit provides a 5 v D.C. supply to energize the bridge.

The discriminator is a pulse-containing frequency modulation model operating at a centre frequency of 22 kHz. The demodulated signal is displayed on a meter. It can be used with a UV recorder from a 50 Hz mains supply.

6.3   COATING VARIABLES

The processing parameters for coating can be divided into two groups: independent and dependent.

6.3.1   Independent variables

Four independent variables can be considered to have a direct effect on the quality of the coated tablet. These are:

● spray rate
● inlet drying air volume
● inlet air temperature
● spray atomizing pressure.

The objective must be to obtain a satisfactorily coated tablet with the minimum coating time. This means optimizing the spray rate with the other three parameters. In a dynamic system such as this it is difficult to record all the operating parameters without the use of a computerized recording system. It is also difficult to reproduce exactly conditions for each experimental run due to variations in such in-house systems as steam supply and compressed air. An examination of a set of results generally shows variations in parameters such as atomizing presssure, temperature and air flow.

An example of these results is shown in Table 6.1.

6.3.2   Dependent variables

Data can also be obtained for those dependent variables which result from the value of the settings for the independent variables

● dew point of exhaust air
● outlet air temperature

Table 6.1 Summary of the independent operating parameters

Run no. s: sealed u: unsealed Coating pan	Independent variables			
	Spray rate (kg^{-4}/s)	Atomizing air pressure (kN/m^2)	Air flow $(10\ m^3/s)$	Inlet air temperature (°C)
01u	4.0			90
02u	3.2			87
03u	2.8		500–650	77
04u	5.0	428–524		59
05s	4.5			60
06s	6.8		788–902	75
07s	6.5			91
08s	16.7			76
09s	9.3		944–991	75
10s	10.5	414		78
11s	11.2			63
12s	8.0			80
13s	9.2		802–826	74
14s	6.8			89
15u	10.0			72
16u	11.2	434–490	916	71
17u	7.3			68
18s	7.0		127–151	68
19s	7.0			59
20s	6.3	345		68
21s	7.7	345		69
22s	7.7	345		68
23s	6.3			90
24s	6.5			59
25s	6.5			61
26s	8.0	448–483		61
27s	10.2		840–963	59
28s	9.2			59
29s	10.2			50
30s	10.0	579		50
31s	5.7	579		50

- tablet-bed temperature
- coat quality.

An example of these types of results is shown in Table 6.2.

6.4   ENERGY CONSIDERATIONS

This worked example is designed to show what energy is required during the coating process when two different types of equipment are used.

6.4.1   Energy balance

A comparison of the energy requirements for heating the drying air in a 1500 mm diameter pan and a 450 mm diameter fluidized bed film-coating column (see Table 6.3) suggests that the coating pan was excessively inefficient in its use of the hot air for drying purposes. The following analysis does tend to support this criticism superficially, but it does not take account of the improvement in product quality achieved by using the side-vented coating pan.

If the cost of coating 1 000 000 tablets (344 kg) of product in the 1500 mm model is considered and the following parameters apply where C_p is the specific heat of air at constant pressure (kJ/kg K), and T is its temperature (K), ΔT is the rise in

Table 6.2   Summary of the dependent operating parameters

Dependent Variables			Dependent Variables		
Dew point outlet air (°C)	Outlet air temp. (°C)	Tablet-bed temp. (°C)	Dew point outlet air (°C)	Outlet air temp. (°C)	Tablet-bed temp. (°C)
18.8	42	39	21.0	34	30
15.3	46	43	22.9	39	34
13.3	41	38	18.0	34	29
15.9	31	27	20.4	39	37
18.6	41	39	20.7	39	34
21.4	47	39	21.0	39	33
22.4	59	48	11.8	66	64
25.1	41	28	15.0	45	40
23.0	41	32	17.2	44	43
6.3	36	29	16.0	43	42
20.8	32	24	19.0	41	40
22.4	44	36	18.3	42	41
22.6	37	26	17.8	32	27
20.8	47	38	16.1	38	37
21.5	35	26	14.5	36	34
21.0	32	23			

Table 6.3 Energy balance: comparison of a 1500 mm diameter coating
pan and a 450 mm fluidized bed coating column

	1500 mm coating pan	450 mm column
Drying air volume (m³/h)	8500	2000
Drying air mass (kg/h)	9010	2120
Inlet air temperature (K)	333	344
Outlet air temperature (K)	313	326
Temperature drop (K)	20	18
Spray rate (kg/h)	23×10	3.2×10
Energy drop (kJ/h)	$9010 \times 0.25 \times 20 \times 4.2$ $= 189 \times 10^3$	$2120 \times 0.25 \times 18 \times 4.2$ $= 40.1 \times 10^3$
Batch load (kg/h)	140	50
Energy to evaporate water (kJ/h)	$23 \times 620 \times 4.2$ $= 59\,900$	$13.2 \times 620 \times 4.2$ $= 34\,372$
Energy loss (kJ/h)	$(189 - 59.9) \times 10^3$ $= 129.1 \times 10^3$	$(40.1 - 34.3) \times 10^3$ $= 5.8 \times 10^3$
Energy loss (kJ/kg) tablets	9.2×10^2	1.2×10^2

temperature (K), G is the flow of air (kg/h) and Q is the quantity of heat (kJ/h) the
tablet bed temperature is 40°C and the air temperature is assumed to be the same
on leaving the pan before it passes through the exhaust fan.

The exhaust fan has a power of 20 h.p. or equivalent to $12\,800 \times 4.2$ kJ = 53 760
kJ; 85% of this energy is transferred in the form of heat to the exhaust air, i.e.
$11\,000 \times 4.2 = 46\,200$ kJ.

To calculate the temperature rise (ΔT) of the exhaust air due to this energy:

$$Q = 46\,200 \text{ kJ} \qquad\qquad G = 9010 \text{ kg/h}$$
$$C_p = 1.05 \text{ kJ/kg K} \qquad\qquad \Delta T = ?$$

$$Q = G\,C_p.\Delta T \qquad\qquad \therefore \Delta T = \frac{Q}{GC_p} = \frac{46\,200}{9010 \times 1.05} = 4.8\text{K}$$

$$\therefore \Delta T = 4.8 \text{ K}$$

This value is required to determine the heat content of the air being exhausted to
the atmosphere.

If the temperature of the incoming air is 333 K and the ambient temperature is
293 K, then the temperature rise is 40 K.

Total energy required:

$$Q = GC_p.\Delta T = 9010 \times 0.25 \times 4.2 \times 40$$
$$Q = 38 \times 10^4 \text{ kJ/h}$$

To this is added the energy transferred from the exhaust fan.

Processing time = 2.5 hours
Total energy   = $95 \times 10^4 + 11.6 \times 10^4$ kJ
                = 106.6×10^4 kJ

If the cost of 1 kilowatt hour (kWh) of electricity is approximately £0.03 (1 kWh = 3.6×103 kJ), then:

$$\text{Total cost} = \frac{106.6 \times 10^{-4}}{3.6 \times 10^3} \times 0.03 = £8.88$$

The cost of coating one batch of tablets in the 1500 model is approximately £9, assuming 100% utilization of the heat content of the drying air. This is 0.9p per 1000 tablets.

The energy lost is the difference between the energy content of the air at exhaust temperature and the air at ambient temperature. The process time is 2.5 hours.

$$Q = \frac{G \times C_p \times (317.8 - 293) \times 2.5 \times 4.2}{3.6 \times 10^3}$$
$$= \frac{9010 \times 0.25 \times 4.2 \times 24.8 \times 2.5}{3.6 \times 10^3}$$
$$= 163 \text{ kWh}$$

Cost = 163×0.03, where 1 kWh costs £0.03.

Total cost of lost energy = £4.9

This is equivalent to a loss of 0.49p per 1000 tablets or 55% of the total energy coating cost.

From this it can be seen that there is a potential saving from recovering energy from the exhaust systems. However, the use of higher volumes of air results in a faster process and a more elegant product. Moreover, saving in process operator time is much more cost-effective than reducing the temperature and volume of the drying air. There are, however, additional reasons for ensuring that excessively high drying air temperatures are not used. These are:

● Spray drying of the film coat before it is deposited on the tablet.
● Excessive loss of coating materials due to spray drying.
● Contamination of the exhaust system with large quantities of film coating due to the spray drying effect, resulting in increased maintenance costs.
● Excess coating material deposited on the pan walls.

6.5   ENERGY RECOVERY

This is an example of how to analyse, calculate and design a system to reduce energy losses through air exhaust ducts. Energy conservation is a major concern of all companies and tablet-coating systems use a large volume of drying air which is usually exhausted to atmosphere at temperatures between 35 and 60°C. Depending on the location of the plant and the temperature of the environmental air outside the plant, this air needs to be heated on the inlet side of the coating pan to between 50 and 90°C. This can mean that air close to 0°C may need to be raised by 90°C. Some of this energy can be recovered from the exhaust air by using a heat exchanger. Recirculation of this air through the drying process is not possible for two reasons:

- possible contamination of the product;
- high solvent or moisture content of drying air.

In the general case, air exhausted to the outside from equipment and buildings is replaced by air from outside. The differences in energy levels (enthalpy) between exhaust air and outside air represents an energy loss.

Typical examples of equipment used where energy losses through an air exhaust system occur are: tray dryers, fluid bed dryers, coating pans, coating columns and building heating/cooling systems and dust control systems.

The most important factors for determining the energy losses are: air quantity, temperature and relative humidity. For a given process or room conditions these factors are usually fixed and cannot be changed without agreement with the research and process development departments. The only opportunity to conserve energy is, therefore, to look strictly at the exhaust system and evaluate a way to recover some of the energy content.

Two methods are available:

6.5.1 Recirculation of air

Generally for process equipment this is not possible because of cross-contamination as already mentioned and the change in relative humidity which will affect the process. For heating/cooling/dust control systems recirculation is possible. Evaluating changes in these systems requires an in-depth study.

6.5.2 Installing a heat exchanger between inlet and exhaust air.

This method is acceptable as it will not affect process and room conditions and is, therefore, usually justified when a 20% or more recovery in energy costs is realized.

The evaluation of a heat exchanger for a 1500 mm coating pan is given here as an example.

Calculation of energy loss

The following formula gives the yearly loss in kcal:

$$Q = 0.25 \times G \times (t_e - t_o) \times B_t \times B_n$$

G = exhaust air quantity (kg/h)
t_e = exhaust air temperature (°C)
t_o = average yearly outside air temperature (°C)
B_t = time that air is exhausted during one batch (hours)
B_n = number of batches per year.

(0.25 = C_p (specific heat of air at constant pressure))

The following conversion factors are frequently used:

1 ft^3/min = 1.7 m^3/h = 2.12 kg/h
1 kWh   = 860 kcal/h (1 Btu = 0.25 kcal)
1 h.p.   = 0.75 kW

Example
Energy loss for a 1500 mm coating pan:

Exhaust air = 5000 ft^3/min
Tablet bed temperature = 48°C
Time that system is running (heating up and spraying, 2^1/$_2$ h per batch).
Average yearly outside temperature = 14°C
Number of batches per year = 600.
Fan motor in exhaust duct = 20 h.p.

All parts of the installation: pan, fan, heater and ducting are insulated. This is required to reduce room air-conditioning loads and to prevent large fluctuations in building heating loads.

Exhaust air quantity:	$G = 5000 \times 2.12 = 10\ 600$ kg/h.
Exhaust air temperature:	Air is leaving pan with a temperature of 48°C. 85% of the fan energy is added to the exhaust air, increasing the temperature.
Fan energy:	20 h.p. = 15 kW = 15 × 860 kcal/h = 12 900 kcal/h. 85% = 0.85 × 12 900 = 10 965 kcal/h.
Temperature increase:	10 965 = 10 600 × 0.25 × ΔT. ΔT = 4.1°C. (0.25 is specific heat of air, kcal/°C/kg.)
Exhaust air temperature:	48 + 4.1 = 52.1°C.
Yearly energy loss:	$Q = 0.25 \times G \times (t_e - t_o) \times B_t \times B_n$ = 0.25 × 10 600 × (52.1 − 14) × 2.5 × 600 = 151 × 106 kcal/yr.
Energy costs:	£0.018/1000 kcal (estimated).
Yearly loss:	151 × 10^6 × 0.018 = £2718 per year

Heat exchanger
A well-designed heat exchanger will recover approximately two-thirds of the losses.

Energy recovery by heat exchanger:	2/3 × £2718 = £1812.
Pay out period:	6.2 years.

The heat exchanger can be justified when the capital costs are not more than 6.2 × 1812 = £11 234.

A scheme is shown in Fig. 6.6. The system is fitted with a heat exchanger and approximate temperatures are given.

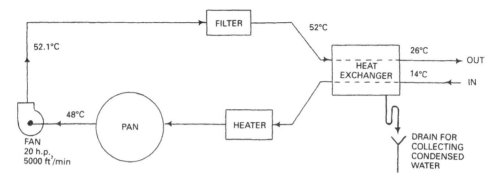

Fig. 6.6   Flow scheme for air supply system fitted with heat exchanger.

7

The coating process

Graham C. Cole

SUMMARY

In recent years tablet coating has undergone several fundamental changes. The original sugar-coating technique has been largely replaced by film-coating processes using organic solvents. The organic solvents are now being replaced by water because of the development of suitable polymers, improvements in the coating process, and legislation regulating the discharge of pollutants into the environment. This change has resulted in increased interest in equipment designed for film-coating based on cylindrical-shaped side-vented pans which allow the drying air to be drawn through the tablet bed. However, the process is complex and requires careful monitoring and control to ensure satisfactory results. The empirically derived conditions are not fundamentally understood and there are important differences in the operation of the commercially available equipment. This chapter discusses some of the theory behind the spraying process and describes the instrumentation and performance of these systems. It illustrates how considerable process improvements can be made by the application of heat and mass transfer theory and how changes in parts of the equipment can provide a reduction in the overall coating cycle.

7.1 PROCESS DEVELOPMENT OF AQUEOUS FILM COATING

Coating of tablets and pills is one of the oldest techniques available to the pharmacist and references can be traced as far back as 1838. The sugar-coating process was regarded as more of an art than a science and its application and technology remained secretive and in the hands of very few. Although a very elegant product was obtained its main disadvantage was the processing time which could last up to five days. Many modifications were advocated to improve the basic process such as air suspension techniques in a fluidized bed, the use of atomizing systems to spray on the sugar-coating, the use of aluminium lakes of dyes to improve the evenness of colour and more efficient drying systems. However, the process remained complicated. Generally, the sugar coating process resulted in the weight of the tablet being doubled, but the use of spaying systems enabled this increase to be dramatically reduced.

The first reference to tablet film coating appeared in 1930 but it was not until 1954 that Abbott Laboratories produced the first commercially available film-coated tablet. This was made possible by the development of a wide variety of materials, for example the cellulose derivatives. One of the most important of these is hydroxypropyl methylcellulose, which is prepared by the reaction of methyl chloride and propylene oxide with alkali cellulose. It is generally applied in solution in organic solvents at a concentration of between 2 and 4 %w/v: the molecular weight fraction chosen gives a solution viscosity of 5×10^{-2} Pa at these concentrations. Its properties have been discussed earlier by John Hogan.

Many advantages can be cited for film coating in place of the traditional sugar-coating process:

● Reduction in processing time, savings in material cost and labour.
● Only a small increase in the tablet weight.
● Standardization of materials and processing techniques.
● The use of non-aqueous coating solutions and suspensions.
● The tablets could be engraved with a code and house logo which remained legible after coating. Many sugar-coated tablets were printed with a house symbol, name of product, or code after coating. This was a difficult and costly process which added nothing to the value of the product.
● Film-coating processes are easier to automate.

During the period 1954–1975 the lower molecular weight polymers of hydroxypropyl methylcellulose with a solution viscosity of $3–15 \times 10^{-3}$ Pa did not receive much attention because of the cheapness of organic solvents and the ease with which the coating could be applied. There was also a belief that the lower viscosity grades produced weaker films which would not meet the formulation requirement for stablility and patient acceptability. However, there is now a trend towards aqueous film coating for the following reasons:

● The cost of organic solvents has escalated.
● A number of regulatory authorities have banned chlorinated hydrocarbons altogether because of environmental pollution.
● The development of improved coating pans and spraying systems has enabled these more difficult coating materials to be applied.
● Flameproof equipment is not required, which reduces capital outlay and a less hazardous working environment is provided for the operator.

Most of the early development work for aqueous film coating concentrated on the use of existing conventional coating pans and tapered cylindrical pans such as the Pellegrini. This pan is open at front and rear, and the spray-guns are mounted on an arm positioned through the front opening. The drying air and exhaust air are both fed in and extracted from the rear. The drying air is blown onto the surface of the tablets, but because of the power of the extraction fan most of the heat is lost with the exhaust air. Very poor thermal contact results and a poor coating finish is obtained. Modifications to introduce the drying air below the surface of the bed of tablets was only partially successful. The perforated rotary coating pan, which permits the drying air to be drawn co-current with the spray through the tablet bed and pan wall during film coating, offers better heat and mass transfer and results in a more efficient coating process and a more elegantly finished product.

There are several companies which offer equipment of this type; the Manesty Accelacota, the Glatt Coater, the Driam Driacoater and the Freund Hi-Coater are four of the best known. There are significant differences between them.

The early equipment such as the Accelacota suffered from the disadvantage that very few instruments were incorporated into the machine, or its ancillaries, for measuring the process parameters of film coating. For instance, the drying air flow measurement was taken from the exhaust fan rating. It was not possible to determine how much air was being introduced from the inlet side of the pan and how much was being drawn into the pan from the environment through leakage. The temperature of the exhaust air could be measured, but not its humidity. The spray rate was obtained by having the coating reservoir positioned on a balance, which gave only the average rate calculated over a period of several minutes. There was no measurement of tablet-bed temperature. Equipment currently available incorporates all of the fundamental instrumentation.

Fig. 7.1 is a flow diagram which illustrates the whole of the manufacturing process from mixing, granulating, compression, preparation of coating suspension, film coating of the tablets, packaging and storage of the product ready for sale. This book is concerned with the practical and theoretical aspects of coating. An example of the equipment used for this operation is outlined on Fig. 7.1 and a coating pan is shown diagrammatically in Fig. 7.2. Fig. 7.3 illustrates some types and shapes of tablets that can be coated.

7.2   THEORETICAL CONSIDERATIONS ON FILM COATING

Mike Aulton has discussed the basis of pharmaceutical technology relating to atomization and evaluation of films; in this chapter some chemical engineering fundamentals are considered.

7.3   THE MECHANISM OF THE TABLET COATING

Spray drying is widely used in the process industries to produce a range of heavy chemicals, food products, detergents, cosmetics and pharmaceuticals, particularly antibiotics. Some of the theoretical and practical concepts of spray drying can be applied to the aqueous film-coating process as applied to pharmaceutical tablets. One important difference between this process and conventional spray drying is that

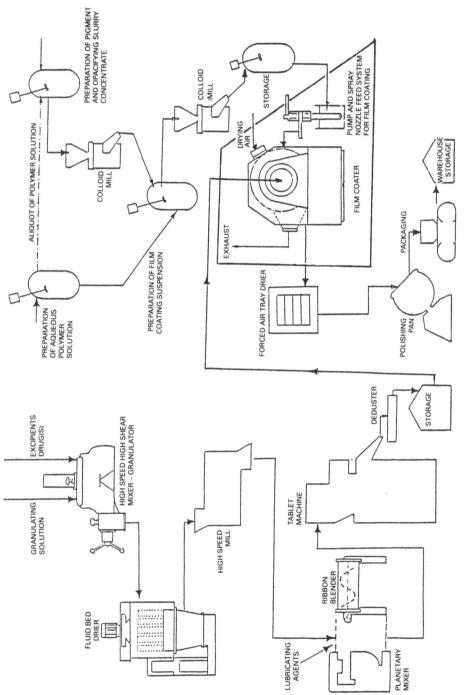

Fig. 7.1　Flow diagram for the film coating of pharmaceutical tablets.

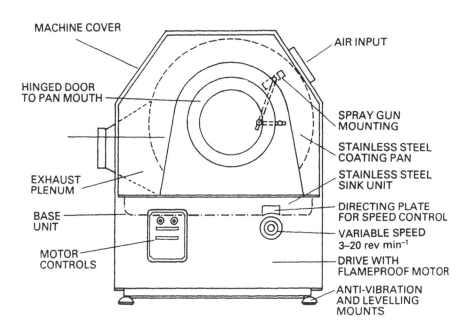

Fig. 7.2   Side-vented coating pan

the atomized coating suspension is not completely dried by the time it strikes the tablets. Final drying takes place extremely rapidly, however, when the partially dried droplets come into contact with the tablet surface.

The tablet coating process, as it occurs generally for film coating, can be broken down for convenience into stages. It is assumed here that the preparation of the coating suspension does not present any great difficulty. An examination of Fig. 7.1 shows a number of steps for its manufacture using colloid mills. The objective must be to produce a homogeneous mixture with all the solids—i.e. iron oxide, titanium dioxide, talc, etc.—as finely divided as possible. This produces an even colour dispersion and prevents blockages in the nozzle. The exact method of manufacture will depend on the ingredients in the formulation. The coating suspension must be atomized and the performance of the atomizing device is an important factor in the appearance of the final product. The size, trajectory and drying rate of the droplets as they move towards the tumbling bed of tablets also needs to be measured as a separate stage. The tablet bed itself is the location for the final drying; it is in some respects analogous to a packed bed humidifier, in that the air flows through the void space between the tablets in a mass transfer interaction with them, and it is important to know how closely the drying air will approach saturation in its passage through the bed.

These various stages are dealt with separately below.

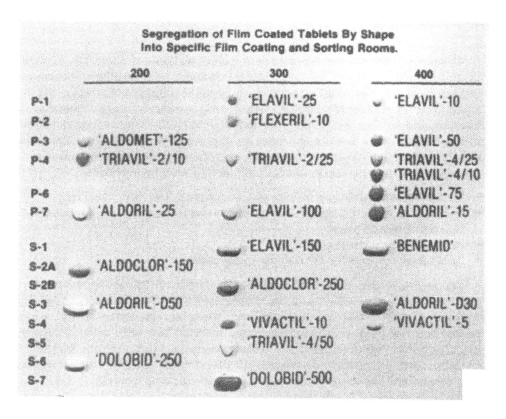

Fig. 7.3   Various types and shapes of film-coated tablets

7.4   ATOMIZATION

This is one of the independent variables of the process. The ideal spray is one of small individual droplets of equal size. Heat and mass transfers and drying times are the same for all droplets in the spray, ensuring uniform dispersion on the tablets.

When correct atomization is achieved, all droplets arrive on the tablet surface in the same state, and in one revolution of the drum will have dried to increment the film-coating thickness without overwetting.

The invention of the mechanism theory which is applicable to commercial atomization is credited to Lord Rayleigh who, in 1878, published a mathematical paper on the break-up of non-viscous liquid jets under laminar flow conditions. This was extended by Weber (1931) to include viscosity, surface tension and liquid density effects. Later Ohnesorge (1936, 1937) was credited with the following Reynolds number relationship: the tendency of the jet to disintegrate is expressed in terms of liquid viscosity (μ) , density (ρ), surface tension (γ), and the jet size (d_n). The liquid break-up is therefore expressed by the magnitude of a dimensionless number Z', which is the ratio of the Weber number, We, $[v_j\,(\rho d_n/\gamma)^{1/2}]$ to the Reynolds number:

$$Z' = \frac{\mu}{(\rho d_n \gamma)^{1/2}}$$

Although certain features are unique to particular types of atomizers, many of the detailed mechanisms of disintegration are common to most forms of atomizer. The most effective way of utilizing energy imparted to a liquid is to arrange that the liquid mass has as large a specific surface area as possible before it commences to break into drops. Thus the primary function of an atomizer is to produce thin liquid sheets. However, this is a simplification as all mechanisms tend to act simultaneously in commercial operations influencing the spray characteristics to some extent. It is postulated that the nozzle should fulfil the following requirements:

• be capable of producing a droplet size spectrum of low mean diameter;
• be able to handle a range of low-viscous suspensions with a solids content of between 8 and 20 %w/w;
• be of simple construction;
• have simple controls for altering the spray angle.

For the established types of film formers the quality of the coating is dependent upon the degree of atomization of the coating solution. If the droplets are all of a consistent size or have a very small size range, then the smoothness of the coating will be improved. This will enhance the appearance of the coated tablet. Consistent droplet size will result in a more even coating thickness, which, in turn, means that complete cover of the tablet is obtained with less coating material. Using less material reduces both the coating time and the quantity of heat required as there is less solvent to evaporate. The efficiency of the coating process is, therefore, very dependent upon the degree of atomization of the spray.

The high rate of evaporation possible with organic solvents enables high rates of application to be used. Under these conditions airless sprays give the best results and operate at liquid pressure of up to 1000 lb/in^2. To achieve high liquid pressures, air driven, double-acting piston pumps are normally used with ratios of 16:1–30:1, i.e. those where the maximum liquid pressure is in the range 16–30 times the air pressure applied to the air driven motor. The actual unit selected will depend upon the pressure of the compressed air supply available. Normally they contain two sets of seals manufactured from polytetrafluoroethylene (PTFE), one set on the piston and one at the throat. Their life can be short because of the abrasive nature of some of the materials in the coating solution, e.g. lake colours which contain aluminium hydroxide and pigments of iron oxide. An improved nylon seal with longer life can be used.

The rate of application of aqueous-based coating solutions must be much slower due to the latent heat of water being approximately three times that of the common organic solvents. When using these lower liquid flow rates airless sprays are not suitable. To lower the spray rate of an airless spray-gun either the pressure or the nozzle size must be reduced. If the liquid pressure is reduced the degree of atomization deteriorates, giving a poor quality of coating. If the nozzle size is reduced, problems can arise due to frequent nozzle blocking. There have been reported instances of the use of airless sprays for aqueous coating in large coating pans and a reduction in the number of spray-guns. However, this causes problems in obtaining an even thickness of film on the tablets. Air-atomized sprays are superior.

The coating solution is fed to the spray-gun at relatively low pressures, in the range 10–60 lb/in² depending upon the type of pump being used. Air driven, double-acting piston pumps, similar to those used with the airless sprays, but with pressure ratios of only 2:1 are quite suitable. As with the high-pressure pumps seal life can be a problem.

The action of the sugar syrup in forming the coating is quite different to that of the film coating. In the case of the common film formers, the droplet of coating usually reaches the tablets as a more concentrated solution than when it left the spray-gun, part of the evaporation of the solvent having taken place as it passes through the air. The small drop of solution dries very quickly, depositing a minute particle of film on the tablet surface. The solution does not go through a viscous flowable stage, or if it does the drying time is so short that the stage is passed through so quickly it has not time to spread. Consequently the thickness of this piece of coating is to a large extent dependent upon the size of the droplet and its concentration.

When sugar coating is applied the syrup reaches the tablet as a viscous solution which spreads over part of the tablet surface before drying. In addition, a certain amount of tablet to tablet transfer of the coating takes place. If the drying is allowed to take place too quickly the syrup will dry without spreading, giving a rough coating. It is, therefore, essential to obtain an even distribution of the coating before drying takes place.

Another reason for allowing the coating to spread is that it is difficult to deposit coating on the sharp edges of tablets.

The method of applying the coating must be aimed at obtaining an even distribution of coating over the surface of each and every tablet. In the manual method the operator uses his skill to distribute the coating as evenly as possible over the whole batch of tablets and then allows them to roll until he is satisfied the distribution is even before applying the drying air. Sprays obviously offer a means of covering the surface evenly and quickly, but a certain amount of rolling is still required before the distribution is even enough to dry to a smooth coat and to ensure a good rounding of the edges of the tablets.

For rapid coating concentrated solutions are used containing 66–80% solids. These solutions are usually too viscous for use with airless sprays (Fig. 7.4) and when air atomized sprays are used, the air impinging on the liquid results in a certain amount of crystallization taking place and nozzle blockages. The highly concentrated solutions are also likely to crystallize in the pipes, and these crystals can again cause nozzle blockages. The advantages of using sprays tend to be balanced out by the problems of operating them with highly concentrated solutions.

An alternative method is to use a distribution pipe designed with large nozzles of approximately 0.25 in. (5–7 mm) diameter which are not easily blocked by small crystals. The pipe is designed to give as even a distribution of the syrup over the tablet bed as possible. This method is slightly slower than using sprays but the loss

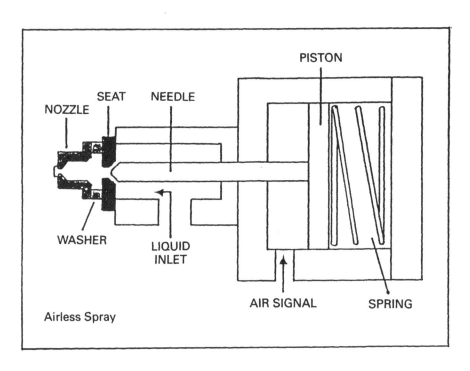

Fig. 7.4   Airless spray nozzle

of time in distribution of the syrup is compensated for by an elimination of the stoppages to clear blocked nozzles. It is also more suitable for automatic or semi-automatic operation.

Traditionally, for organic solvents both pneumatic and airless nozzles have been used for tablet film coating. However, for aqueous formulations there are serious difficulties with the airless system. In particular, the higher spray velocity and the denser spray cone causes overwetting, so that the tablets adhere to each other and to the walls of the coating pan. A more efficient system employs a two-fluid nozzle and air as the energy source to break up the liquid (Fig. 7.5). This method satisfactorily produces a spray of droplets having a high surface-to-mass ratio. A high relative velocity between liquid and air must be generated so that the liquid is subjected to the optimum frictional conditions. These conditions are generated by expanding the air to high velocity before it contacts the liquid or by directing the air onto thin unstable liquid sheets formed by rotating the liquid within the nozzle, thus providing a very efficient and rapid formation of droplets as small as 20 μm diameter. High- and low-viscosity liquids can be sprayed without difficulty. Because the flow rates and viscosity are low, rotation of the liquid within the nozzle is not essential for complete atomization.

Nukizama & Tanasawa (1950) have shown that the mean spray droplet diameter D produced by pneumatic atomization follows the relationship

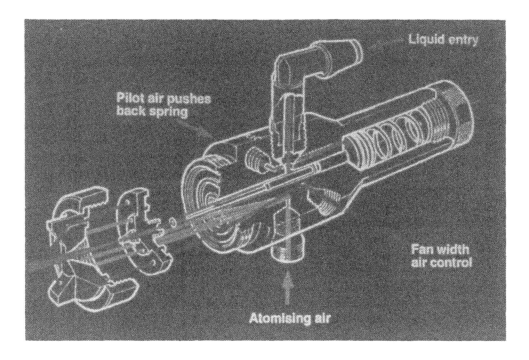

Fig. 7.5   Pneumatic nozzle for aqueous coating

$$D = \frac{A}{(\mu_{rel}^2 \rho)\alpha} + B\left[\frac{W_{air}}{W_{liq}}\right]^{-\beta}$$

where u_{rel} is the relative velocity of air and liquid at the nozzle head and W_{air}/W_{liq} is the mass ratio of air to liquid.

The exponents α and β are functions only of the nozzle design, while A and B are constants involving both nozzle design and liquid properties.

The mass ratio W_{air} to W_{liq} ranges from 0.1 to 10 and is one of the most important variables affecting droplet size. It has been reported that below 0.1 atomization deteriorates very rapidly and 10 is the limit for the effective ratio increase to create smaller sizes. Above 10 excess energy is expended without a marked decrease in the mean droplet size. It has also been reported that 5 μm droplets do not disintegrate into smaller sizes in the presence of high-velocity air, but experimental sampling has shown that particles as small as 1 μm can be present. From manufacturers' data for various nozzles, at a W_{air}/W_{liq} ratio of between 5 and 7.5 and an exit air velocity in excess of 300 ms^{-1} it is possible that droplets with a mean diameter of 20–30 μm would be obtained. The rationale for producing droplets of this size is to attempt to utilize the internal energy of the droplet as an aid to the evaporation of the droplet during its path from nozzle to tablet. Particles which are too small will be dried (spray drying) before striking the tablets, and therefore the coat will not adhere to the tablet surface. As the latent heat of vaporization of water is so large a combination of these energy sources can combine to dry the droplet completely immediately after striking the tablet.

Attempts to confirm these predictions can be made using two different approaches:

- photographic;
- impingement of particles onto microscope slides.

The photographic assessment of the droplet size and velocity distribution in an atomized spray presents no great problem when the size is 50 μm or greater but, below this, in-flight photography becomes more difficult and attempts to establish a dynamic method were inconclusive. Most previous workers, including Groenweg *et al.* (1967) and Roth & Porterfield (1965) found that 10–20 μm represented the lower limit of size that could be photographed. Ranz & Marshall (1951), however, using high-speed ciné, have produced shots of the thin sheets of liquid disintegrating into droplets.

Using the collection of droplets by impingement onto microscopic slides, Cole *et al.* (1980) clearly showed particles smaller than 5 μm. Similar results were obtained by a nozzle manufacturer (Schlick) using similar control parameters and measuring the particle size using a helium–neon laser and extracting the light energy from the droplet diffraction pattern. Some of these results are shown in Table 7.1.

7.5   THE DRYING OF DROPLETS TRAVELLING IN AIR

7.5.1   General theory

The evaporation of water from a spray of droplets containing dissolved and suspended solids involves simultaneous heat and mass transfer. With the contact between atomized droplets and drying air, heat is transferred by convection from the air to the droplets, and converted to latent heat during moisture evaporation. The vaporized moisture is transported into the air by convection through the boundary layer that surrounds each droplet. The velocity of droplets leaving the

Table 7.1 Droplet particle size spectrum

Particle size (μm)	Cumulative (%)	Histogram (%)
< 5.0	10.8	10.8
6.6	32.7	21.0
9.4	51.0	18.2
13.0	63.0	12.8
19.0	79.4	15.5
27.0	94.7	15.2
38.0	99.1	4.4
53.0	99.1	0

atomizer differs greatly from the velocity of the surrounding air and, simultaneously, with heat and mass transfer, there is an exchange of momentum between the droplets and surroundings. The rate of heat and mass transfer is a function of temperature, humidity and the transport properties of the air surrounding each droplet. It is also a function of the droplet diameter and the relative velocity between droplet and air.

The evaporation of spray droplets commences with moisture removal at a near-constant rate, with a constant droplet surface temperature and a constant partial pressure of vapour at the droplet surface (first period of drying) followed by a decline in removal rate until drying is complete (first and second falling rate drying periods). The rate declines rapidly once the droplet moisture content is reduced to a level known as the critical moisture content.

The majority of droplet moisture is removed during the first period of drying. Moisture migrates from the droplet interior at a rate great enough to maintain surface saturation, and the droplet attains the wet-bulb temperature of the air. The evaporation rate can be considered constant, although this is not strictly true. In a spray-drying operation droplet evaporation commences with the immediate spray-air contact, and the rapid transfer of moisture into the air is accompanied by reduction of the air temperature. Any decrease in air temperature reduces the driving force for heat transfer, and the evaporation rate can begin to fall off even though surface saturation is being maintained. The initial phase of droplet drying is the constant-rate drying period.

Moisture migration lowers the moisture level within the droplet, and a point is eventually reached when the rate of migration to the surface becomes the limiting factor in the drying rate. Surface wetness can no longer be maintained, and a falling-off in drying rate results. The rate of moisture migration is affected by the temperature of the surrounding air.

If the air temperature is so high that the temperature driving forces permit evaporation to commence at a rate at which migration of moisture cannot maintain surface wetness from the start, the droplet will experience little constant-rate drying. A dried layer will form instantaneously at the droplet surface. For tablet spraying this will reduce the adhesion properties of the suspension and produce an orange-peel effect on the surface of the tablet. It is important at this stage to ensure that any solids contained maintain an open structure to ensure that moisture can diffuse outwards from its centre at a constant rate. Any dried layer presents a barrier to moisture transfer and acts to retain moisture within the droplet.

In some spraying operations small craters or 'vacuoles' can form on the surface of coated tablets. Originally it was postulated that this was due to tablets sticking together because of overwetting from too high a spray rate or too low a temperature and volume of drying air. Increasing the temperature increases the occurrence but reducing the temperature can minimize this effect. It was considered that this was caused by moisture being trapped in the droplet due to the formation of an almost impervious outer layer, a 'case' hardening effect.

The actual evaporation time for droplets produced in air at constant temperature depends upon droplet size, chemical composition, physical structure, air flow and solids concentration. The actual time is the sum of the constant rate and the falling-rate periods until the desired moisture level is reached. The general drying characteristics are illustrated by a drying-rate curve, as shown in Fig. 7.6.

In phase AB, the drying rate increases as the droplet contacts the drying air. There follows a slight increase in droplet surface temperature, and the drying rate increases in the milliseconds required for heat transfer across the droplet–air interface to establish equilibrium.

In phase BC, there is dynamic equilibrium. Drying proceeds at a constant rate, which is in fact the highest rate achieved during the entire droplet evaporation. Saturation of the droplet surface is maintained by adequate migration of moisture from within the droplet to the surface.

At point C, the critical point is reached at which moisture transport within the droplet can no longer maintain surface saturation. Drying rate begins to fall, initiating the falling-rate drying period. This period is not well defined, as local areas of wetness may remain on the droplet surface. Phase CD continues until no areas of wetness remain.

In phase DE, resistance to mass transfer is wholly in the solid layer. Evaporation continues at a decreasing rate until the droplet acquires a moisture content in equilibrium with the surrounding air. Approach to the equilibrium moisture content E is slow. Droplet temperature rises throughout the two phases of the falling-rate period.

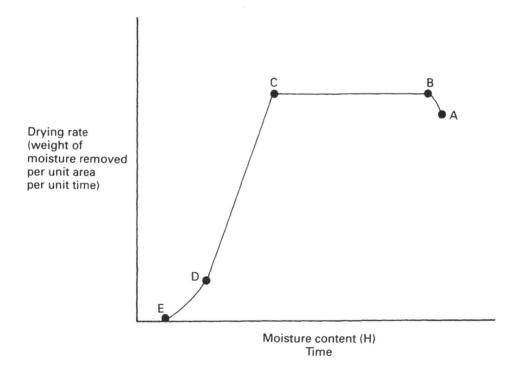

Fig. 7.6   Droplet drying-rate curve

Fig. 7.6 is diagrammatic and theoretical as drying curves in reality have no sharply defined points. Some of the drying zones may not even occur as shown.

Conclusions drawn from studies on the evaporation of pure liquid droplets form the basis for understanding the evaporation mechanisms of spray systems. The ideal case of evaporation of single pure liquid droplets can be modified to deal with the deviations in the basic theory necessary to include the presence of dissolved or insoluble solids.

The extent of moisture removal from a droplet depends upon the mechanism governing the rate of evaporation and the residence time during which evaporation takes place. The residence time depends upon the spray-air movement set up in the coating pan. For the greater part of droplet flow, the relative velocity between droplet and air is very low. The boundary layer theory states that the evaporation rate for a droplet moving with zero relative velocity is identical to that in still-air conditions. Thus the mechanism of evaporation for still air, based upon boundary layer theory, can be justifiably applied to many coating conditions.

7.5.2 Evaporation of single droplets

(a) Droplet evaporation under negligible relative velocity conditions
Experimental data in Coulson & Richardson (1980) have shown that heat transfer by conduction in still air surrounding a spherical droplet of radius r can be expressed as:

$$Q = 4\pi r k(T_1 - T_2)$$

where Q is the heat flow, $T_1 - T_2$ is the temperature difference between the particle and its surroundings and k is the thermal conductivity. This can be rearranged as:

$$\frac{Qr}{(4\pi r^2)(T_1 - T_2)k} = 1$$

If $Q/4\pi r^2 (T_1 - T_2) = h$, the heat transfer coefficient, then $hr/k = 1$ so hD/k, the Nusselt number (Nu), is given by

$$\frac{hD}{k} = \text{Nu} = 2 \tag{7.1}$$

Following the heat and mass transfer analogy in Coulson & Richardson (1980), a similar expression for mass transfer can be established using the Sherwood number (Sh). Mass transfer from spherical droplets to still air follows the law for molecular diffusion. By analogy with the heat transfer equation (7.1)

$$\text{Sh} = \frac{h_d D}{D_v} = 2 \tag{7.2}$$

where h_d is the mass transfer coefficient and D_v is the diffusivity.

The evaporation rate (dW/dt) in terms of mass transfer can be obtained from the equations for the rate of mass transfer from a saturated surface, if

$$h_d = \frac{2D_v}{D} \quad \text{and} \quad A = \pi D^2$$

and

$$\frac{dW}{dt} = hA(P_{WB} - P_W)$$

then, by substitution, this gives

$$\frac{dW}{dt} = 2\pi D_v D(P_{WB} - P_W) \tag{7.3}$$

The evaporation rate in terms of heat transfer can be expressed from the equations for the rate of heat transfer from a saturated surface:

$$\frac{dQ}{dt} = hA(T_a - T_s) \tag{7.4}$$

For dynamic equilibrium the rate of heat transfer is equal to the product of the rate of mass transfer (dW/dt) and the latent heat of vaporization (λ). By substituting $h = 2k/D$ and $dQ/dt = \lambda (dW/dt)$

$$\frac{dW}{dt} = \frac{2\pi D h_d}{\lambda}(T_a - T_s) \tag{7.5}$$

where T_a is the air temperature and T_s is the droplet surface temperature.

Conclusions can be drawn from equations (7.3) and (7.5) as to the characteristics of pure liquid droplet evaporation.

1. The evaporation rate is proportional to diameter not surface.
2. Absolute evaporation rates from large droplets are greater than from small droplets.
3. Initial evaporation is proportional to the square of the initial diameter.

The evaporation time can be deduced from a heat balance over a spray droplet and the following equation, derived from the heat and mass transfer analogy. By substitution of $h_d = h$ and $W = \pi D^3 \rho/6$ in equation (7.5),

$$dt = -\frac{\lambda\rho}{2h\,\Delta T}\,d(D) \tag{7.6}$$

ΔT is the mean temperature difference between the droplet surface and surrounding air. The term $-(\lambda\rho/2\Delta T)$ remains constant during the major part of the droplet's residence time in the coating pan, so that integration of equation (7.6) yields the evaporation time, t. (D_0 is the initial droplet diameter.)

$$t = \frac{\lambda\rho_1}{2\,\Delta T}\int_{D_1}^{D_0} \frac{d(D)}{h} \tag{7.7}$$

It is best to apply the logarithmic mean difference, but the arithmetic mean can be used with little error if $\Delta T_0/\Delta T_1$ is less than 2, where ΔT_0 and ΔT_1 are the temperature differences between droplet and air at the beginning and end of the evaporation period.

Equation (7.7) can be simplified further for negligible relative velocity conditions by putting $h = 2k/D$ so that finally

$$t = \frac{\lambda \rho (D_0^2 - D_1^2)}{8k \, \Delta T} \tag{7.8}$$

(b) Droplet evaporation under relative velocity conditions

Evaporation rates increase with increase in relative velocity between droplet and air due to the additional mass transfer allowed by the convection in the boundary layer around the droplet. The overall transfer coefficients for the transfer from a spherical droplet can be expressed in terms of empirical relations between the dimensionless groups where, for mass transfer,

$$\text{Sh} = 2 + K_1 \, \text{Re}^x \, \text{Sc}^y \tag{7.9}$$

and for heat transfer

$$\text{Nu} = 2 + K_2 \, \text{Re}^{x'} \, \text{Pr}^{y'} \tag{7.10}$$

Equations (7.9) and (7.10) reduce to equation (7.1) when the relative velocity is zero. There is much discussion over the power values of x, y, x', y', and the constants K_1 and K_2. Rowe *et al.* (1965) determined values of the above powers and constants for spherical droplets/particles, and, by comparison of data from other investigations, concluded

$$x = x' = 0.5 \tag{7.11}$$

$$y = y' = 0.33 \tag{7.12}$$

Equation (7.11) gives an average value and the value of x accepted generally for evaporation conditions in spray drying is 0.5. This is applicable to a Reynolds number range between 100 and 1000. Motion of small droplets in this range occurs only in the first fractions of a second of travel, and thus much of the evaporation occurs at a droplet Reynolds number far below 100. According to Rowe (1965), little importance should be attached to having an exact value for the power of Reynolds number. Various modifications of equations (7.9) and (7.10) have been made. The form most widely applied is the Ranz & Marshall (1951) equation.

$$\frac{h_d D}{D_v} = 2 + 0.6 \left[\frac{uD\rho}{\mu} \right]^{0.5} \left[\frac{\mu}{\rho D_v} \right]^{0.33} \tag{7.13}$$

$$\frac{hD}{k} = 2 + 0.6 \left[\frac{uD\rho}{\mu} \right]^{0.5} \left[\frac{C_\rho}{k} \right]^{0.33} \tag{7.14}$$

When applying the above equations, certain limitations must be taken into consideration:

1. Steady-state drag coefficients apply. It is convenient to apply the drag equations at steady state to the case of accelerating or decelerating droplets. In reality the drag coefficients (C_D) for accelerated motion can be 20–60% higher than for those at constant velocity.
2. Heat transfer to evaporated moisture is neglected. In this case drying conditions at high temperatures are not considered as the effect on the droplet is detrimental to the formation of a continuous and elegant film on the surface of the tablet. Reasons for this were discussed earlier.
3. The droplet internal structure is considered to be stable. Any internal circulation, oscillation or surface distortion of the droplet will increase heat and mass transfer rates due to variations in the thickness of the boundary layer.
4. The droplets are considered to be stable in the air flow and not subjected to any swirling action which would cause droplet rotation. Such rotation reduces the boundary layer and increases evaporation rates.

(c) Evaporation rate
Droplets released from an atomizer decelerate rapidly to become completely influenced by the surrounding air flow. During droplet deceleration considerable evaporation occurs. Equations by Frossling (1938) express evaporation during this period. The increase in evaporation rate due to droplet deceleration is represented in equations (7.15) and (7.16) by the second term on the right-hand side.
   Mass transfer

$$N = 2\pi DD_v \frac{\Delta P}{RT}(1 + 0.276\,\mathrm{Re}^{0.5}\,\mathrm{Sc}^{0.33}) \qquad (7.15)$$

Heat transfer

$$\frac{\mathrm{d}W}{\mathrm{d}t} = 2\pi DK\,\Delta T(1 + 0.276\,\mathrm{Re}^{0.5}\,\mathrm{Sc}^{0.33}) \qquad (7.16)$$

where N is the transfer rate and ΔP is the driving force in terms of partial pressures.
   Once droplet deceleration is completed and terminal velocity conditions prevail, the Frossling equation can be rearranged to obtain the weight of the droplet evaporated per unit length of travel ($\mathrm{d}W/\mathrm{d}l$):

$$\frac{\mathrm{d}W}{\mathrm{d}l} = 12D_v \frac{P\Delta P}{V_f D^2 \rho RT}(1 + 0.276\,\mathrm{Re}^{0.5}\,\mathrm{Sc}^{0.33}) \qquad (7.17)$$

where V_f is the terminal velocity. For aqueous droplet–air systems, equation (7.17) reduces to

$$\frac{\mathrm{d}W}{\mathrm{d}l} = 4.6 \times 10^{-7} \frac{\Delta H}{V_f D^2}(1 + 0.23\,\mathrm{Re}^{0.5}) \qquad (7.18)$$

where $\mathrm{d}W/\mathrm{d}l$ is the evaporation per metre length of fall, V_f is the terminal velocity, and ΔH is the difference between air input humidity and the saturated humidity at the same temperature.

A plot of equation (7.18) shows that dW/dl decreases rapidly with increasing droplet diameter. In a spray distribution, the smaller droplet sizes will dry more rapidly than the larger. This results in the possibility of overdried, small particles being present along with the larger particles of desired moisture content.

Certain significant conclusions can be drawn from these equations:

1. A slight reduction in droplet size causes a marked increase in the fractional evaporation.
2. If droplets are kept at a constant diameter by solids deposition, the resulting evaporation will act to reduce droplet density and hollow-dried particles will form. Hollow droplets fall at lower velocities. As the fractional evaporation is universally proportional to the droplet velocity and evaporation on a weight basis is equal, the fractional evaporation increases over that of a solid droplet at the same rate of fall by a factor equal to the ratio of the droplet volume to its hollow air space volume.
3. For small sized droplets, under 100 μm, evaporation during deceleration can be considered insignificant compared with the free-falling evaporation during the remaining residence time in the air.

(d) Evaporation time

By using this theoretical concept an example is given here of how process parameters may be evaluated in the early stages of a coating project.

The evaporation time, t, for a pure liquid droplet with a drop diameter of less than 100 μm under relative velocity conditions can be obtained from equation (7.8). The droplet is assumed to remain at its exit velocity temperature until it strikes the tablet surface despite the evaporating cooling effect and the heat transfer from the drying air. The effect of dissolved and suspended solids is not considered to have a significant effect on the evaporation time:

$$t = \frac{\rho\lambda(D_0^2 - D_1)}{8k\,\Delta T}$$

Take the following representative values for the process parameters:

Initial droplet diameter D_0	50 μm = 5×10^{-5}m
Outlet air temperature	313K
Inlet air temperature	343K
Density of aqueous suspension	1100 kg/m³
Latent heat of vaporization	2200 kJ/kg
Temperature of aqueous suspension	293K
Droplets evaporate completely to vapour	
Thermal conductivity of water k	0.0067 kW/m K
Mean temperature surrounding droplet	313K

then

$$t = \frac{1100 \times 2500 \times 10^{-12} \times 2200 \times 1000}{8 \times 0.0067 \times 30}$$

$$= 3.76 \text{ seconds.}$$

If the droplet had an initial diameter of 25 μm then the drying time would be 0.94 seconds.

This result is significant because it suggests that the droplet loses very little moisture in travelling from the spray nozzle, with an exit velocity of 300 m/s, to the surface of the tablet bed. If the distance in the test rig is 150 mm, the droplet's velocity is 1.23×10^{-2} m/s as measured by the flow of drying air through the coating pan. In the larger pans the distance is often empirically derived as 300–330 mm in order to achieve the best results. To some extent the results of the measurement of droplets impinged onto microscopic slides support these results and practical coating trials in pilot plants can start with this as a basis.

However, even allowing for the fact that it was not possible to determine the exact distance in which the particle reaches its terminal velocity, this equation shows that the drying time is proportional to the square of the droplet diameter. It had previously been shown by Prater (1982) that the dwell time for a single tablet in the spray zone varied between 0.091 s and 0.121 s and the time to reappear in this zone varied between 2 s and 243 s. It can be postulated, therefore, that atomization is more critical than was at first appreciated and that drying of the surface of the tablet is, in fact, occurring after the tablets move out of the spray zone. If the droplet diameter is too large then the excess moisture will not be removed by the time the tablet reappears in the spray zone, and the tablets will become too wet, resulting in an uneven surface and an inelegant product.

The velocity of the droplets and the drying distances can be verified using the photographic technique and the impingement of the droplet onto microscopic slides described earlier. A photograph is shown in Fig. 7.7 which illustrates the method, and from this it was possible to calculate the droplet velocity. The double-flash unit used, an argon jet with a minimum delay of 300 ns, enabled the velocity distribution and particle size to be clearly seen.

In this photograph the divisions at the bottom are 1 mm, the delay between the images is 50 μs, and the magnification is 32×. The smallest droplets are approximately 15 μm and the average size is 60 μm. The droplet velocity varies but is between 3 and 4 m/s.

The change in the form of the droplet as it moved further from the nozzle was also clearly shown on the microscopic slides. Close to the nozzle the drops were very aqueous in appearance, and although some spreading on impact occurs, many clearly defined droplets can be seen. As the distance from the nozzle increases, the droplets become more plastic in appearance and there is a critical zone in which they change their characteristics from aqueous to a semi-plastic form. This occurred between 28 and 32 cm from the nozzle.

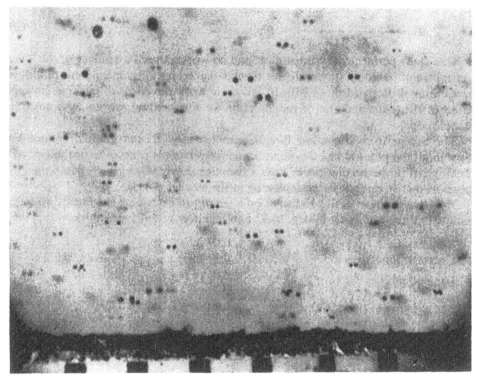

Size of droplet: 60 μm
Velocity: 3–4 m/s
Delay between images: 50μs
Division on scale: 1mm

Fig. 7.7   Photograph of spray

7.6   FLOW THROUGH A TABLET BED IN A SIDE-VENTED COATING PAN

There have been many attempts to obtain a general expression for the pressure drop and the mean velocity through packed beds in terms of the voidage and surface area as these terms can be easily evaluated. Alternatively, the surface area can be derived from the measurements of pressure drop, velocity and voidage. Correlations are then possible in terms of relating variations in the voidage to different shapes and sizes of tablets and the influence of voidage on the film-coating process.

If the voidage is considered to be a series of channels, then the Kozeny equation may be used

$$u = \frac{e^3}{K'' S_B^2 (1-e)^2} \cdot \frac{-\Delta P}{l} \cdot \frac{1}{\mu} \tag{7.19}$$

K'' is generally known as Kozeny's constant and a commonly accepted value for K'' is 5, although it does depend on porosity, particle shape and permeability.

The permeability coefficient B is given by

$$B = \frac{1}{K''} \cdot \frac{1}{S^2} \cdot \frac{e^3}{(1-e)^2} \qquad (7.20)$$

One study performed by the author and co-workers used a voidage of 40% as a general value based on the results for regular-shaped packings in columns published in Coulson & Richardson (1980). In this early work the effect of packing, and the effect of the shape and size of the tablet on the film-coating process, was not fully understood.

The change from streamline flow to turbulent flow is very gradual because the flow in all the pores is not the same. In the larger pores it becomes turbulent very rapidly but in the smaller pores stays streamline. Even at very high flow rates it is possible that streamline conditions exist in the smaller pores.

Experiments have been conducted on a test rig to determine the rate of evaporation within the bed using tablets 10.32 mm diameter and 4.5 mm thick.

Volume of air	0.09 m^3/s
Cross-sectional area	0.27 m^2
Velocity of air	$\dfrac{0.09 \text{ m}^3\text{/s}}{0.27 \text{ m}^2} = 0.3$ m/s
Surface area of one tablet	3.13 cm^2
Volume of one tablet	0.377 cm^3
Mass of one tablet	0.472 g
Density of tablet material	1.25 g/cm^3
Number of tablets per batch	17 000
Surface area of one batch	53 210 cm^2
Viscosity of air at 70°C	0.019 cP
Density at 70°C	$= \dfrac{29.0 \times 273}{22.4 \times 343}$
	$= 1.031$ g/dm^3
Thermal conductivity of air (k)	0.025 W/m K

Therefore, Reynolds flow number for one tablet

$$\begin{aligned} \text{Re} &= \frac{\rho l u}{\mu} \\ &= \frac{1.031 \text{ kg/m}^3 \times 0.01032 \text{ m} \times 0.3 \text{ m/s}}{0.019 \times 10^{-3} \text{ kg/ms}} \\ &= \frac{0.3 \times 10.32 \times 1.031}{0.019} = 168 \end{aligned}$$

Therefore the air flow is streamline.

The machine loading was 10 kg of tablets, the film-coating rate was 2.0 kg of suspension applied in 45 min at 7.5×10^{-4} kg/s containing 250g of polymer and solids therefore 1.75 kg of water was evaporated in 45 min equal to 6.5×10^{-4} kg/s. The mass of air passing through the side-vented pan was 0.09 kg/s. Therefore the increase in moisture content of drying air is $(6.5 \times 10^{-4})/0.09$ kg/kg, which is approximately equal to 7.2×10^{-3} kg/kg.

This is a very small increase and one result would be to permit the air to be recycled. The heat transfer coefficient is given by the equation:

$$h = \frac{Q}{4\pi r^2 (T_1 - T_2)}$$

where r is the radius of a sphere equivalent in volume and density to a tablet and Q is the heat flow. At a mass flow of 0.09 kg/s the heat flow is 4.7 kJ/s or 4.7 kW and a temperature difference of 30 K. Therefore

$$h = \frac{4.7}{4 \times 3.14 \, (5.16 \times 10^{-2})^2 \times 30}$$
$$= 4.99 \text{ kW/m}^2 \text{ K}$$

Now $hl/k = \text{Nu} = 2$, and by substituting appropriate values, we obtain

$$\frac{4.99 \times 10 \times 10^{-3}}{0.025}$$

which is approximately 2. Generally, the Nusselt group will deviate from 2 in forced convection systems. The value for thermal conductivity, k, here is for a temperature of 373 K which is not reached.

If we apply equation (7.14),

$$\frac{hl}{k} = 2 + 0.6 \left[\frac{ul\rho}{\mu} \right]^{0.5} \left[\frac{C_p\mu}{k} \right]^{0.33}$$

$$\frac{C_p\mu}{k} = \frac{4.2 \times 0.019}{0.025} = 3.19$$

$$\frac{hl}{k} = 2 + 0.6 \, (168)^{0.5} (3.19)^{0.33}$$

$$= 2 + 0.6 \times 12.6 \times 1.47$$

$$= 13.1$$

Therefore

$$h = \frac{13.1 \times 0.025}{10 \times 10^{-3}}$$
$$= 32.75 \text{ kW/m}^2 \text{ K}$$

and this shows considerable variation from the earlier result of 4.99 kW/m² K. If we consider the spray droplets in a steady state, for a 50 μ diameter droplet

$$\frac{hD}{k} = \text{Nu} = 2$$

$$h = \frac{2D}{k} \quad \text{where } k \text{ is the thermal conductivity of water vapour}$$

$$= \frac{2 \times 50 \times 10^{-6}}{0.0067} = 14.9 \text{ W/m}^2 \text{ K}$$

$$(k \text{ at } 303 \text{ K} = 0.0067)$$

If the droplet is 25 μ in size

$$h = \frac{2 \times 25 \times 10^3 \times 10^{-6}}{0.0067}$$

$$= 7.46 \text{ W/m}^2 \text{ K}$$

This suggests a linear relationship between the diameter of the spray droplet and the heat transfer coefficient.

The mass transfer coefficients are in the region of 1.5 kg/m^2 h for wet surfaces in the normal range of Reynolds numbers. The evaporation rate in the 600 mm side-vented pan was:

$$\frac{(1.5 \times 17\,000 \times 3.13)/10\,000}{60 \times 60} = \frac{1.5 \times 3.13 \times 1.7}{60 \times 60} \text{kg/s}$$

$$= 2.2 \times 10^{-3} \text{ kg/s}$$

This assumes that all the tablet surfaces are accessible and is a maximum value.

The following calculation is an attempt to explain the mass transfer of water vapour from the surface of the tablets in a 600mm pan in terms of the 'j-factor' for mass transfer (j_d), originally developed by Chilton & Coburn (1934), the mass transfer coefficient (h_d), and the treatment of the side-vented pan as a packed humidification column. Difficulties arise in the evaluation of mass transfer coefficients since this is a dynamic system and the composition of air flow will vary with distance from the wet surfaces and the physical properties are not constant and mean values must be used. An estimation of the number of theoretical transfer units (NTU) necessary to achieve satisfactory evaporation has also been calculated using additional data provided by Treybal (1955) for packed columns.

Flow of air through coating pan	0.09 kg/s
Area of tablet-bed surface	0.5 m^2
Mass air flow over tablet-bed surface	0.09/0.5 = 0.18 kg/m^2 s
Number of tablets used	17 000
Surface area of one tablet	3.13 × 10^{-4} m^2
Total surface of 17 000 tablets	5.32 m^2

The equivalent diameter (dp) of a sphere with this surface area using the Treybal (1955) formula:

$$\mathrm{d}p = \sqrt{\frac{3.13 \times 10^{-4}}{3.14}} = 1 \times 10^{-2} \text{ m}$$

Volume occupied by these tablets	0.01 m^3
Mass velocity of air through tablet bed	0.01 × 0.09 (m^3 × kg/s)
	= 9 × 10^{-4} kg/m^3 s
Viscosity of air (μ) at 333 K	0.019 cP
	= 1.9 × 10^{-5} N s/m^2 = 1.9 kg/m s^2
	(1 Newton = 1 kg/m s^2)
Diffusivity (D_v) of air at 333 K	3.05 × 10^{-5} m/s

The Reynolds number, Re, calculated previously is 168; 17 000 tablets occupy 0.01 m³, therefore,

$$\text{Total interface surface } (a) = \frac{17\,000}{0.01} \times 3.13 \times 10^4$$

$$= 532 \text{ m}^2/\text{m}^3$$

The molecular weight of air (L_m) is taken as 29. Therefore,

$$\text{Molar flow rate is} = \frac{9 \times 10^{-4} \times 1000}{29}$$

$$= 0.031 \text{ kmol/m}^2 \text{ s}$$

The Schmidt number is given by

$$\text{Sc} = \frac{1.9 \times 10^{-5}}{1.03 \times 3.05 \times 10^{-5}} \frac{\text{N s/m}^2}{\text{kg/m}^3 \text{ m}^2/\text{s}}$$

$$= 0.604$$

The j-factor, (j_d), from Treybal (1955) for a Reynolds number of 168 is 0.13. Therefore the mass transfer coefficient, h_d, is given by

$$h_d = \frac{L_m j_d}{(\text{Sc})^{0.67}} = \frac{0.13 \times 0.031}{(0.604)^{0.67}}$$

$$= 0.0056 \text{ kmol/m}^2 \text{ s}$$

$$= 5.6 \text{ mol/m}^2 \text{ s}$$

The water content of the drying air at 60°C and 60% relative humidity is 0.005 kg/kg and its maximum water content is 0.12 kg/kg (consult a psychrometric chart in *Perry's Chemical Engineers Handbook*, McGraw-Hill). It is necessary to convert this potential increase of 0.115 kg/kg into molar fraction

$$0.115 \text{ kg/kg} = \frac{0.115/18}{0.885/29 + 0.115/18}$$

$$= \frac{6.4 \times 10^{-3}}{3.05 \times 10^{-2} + 6.4 \times 10^{-3}}$$

$$= 0.173 \text{ mol/mol}$$

Therefore,

$$\text{Evaporation rate} = 0.173 \times 5.6$$

$$= 0.97 \text{ mol/s}$$

Molecular weight of water is 18. Therefore,

$$\text{Evaporation rate} = 0.97 \times 18 \times 10^{-3} \text{ kg/s}$$

$$= 63 \text{ kg/h}$$

This shows that the maximum amount of water vapour that can be absorbed by the drying air using a batch size of 17 000 tablets is 63 kg/h.

To determine the rate of drying of the free moisture within the tablet bed, the maximum rate (N_m) will occur if the air leaving the bed is saturated at the adiabatic-saturation temperature. If a is the interfacial area, Z_s is the average thickness of the tablet bed and N_{tg} is the number of gas transfer units in the tablet bed, then,

$$N_{tg} = \frac{j_d Z_s}{Sc^{0.67}}$$
$$N_{tg} = \frac{0.13 \times 532 \times 8 \times 10^{-2} \ m^2 \times m}{(0.604)^{0.67} \ m^3}$$
$$= 7.79$$

The number of theoretical gas units is 7.79. The maximum rate of drying (N_m) is given by

$$N_m = 0.13 \ (0.120 - 0.005) \ (N_m = j_d \ (H_2 - H_1))$$
$$= 0.13 \times 0.115 \ kg/m^2 \ s$$
$$= 0.01495 \ kg/m^2 \ s$$
$$= 53.82 \ kg/h$$
$$= 286 \ kg/m^2 \ h$$

If the temperature of the air leaving the tablet bed is expressed as T_s and its humidity is H_s, H_2 is the measured humidity of the air and H_1 is the humidity of the incoming air, then, to determine the actual drying rate (N) using Treybal (1955)

$$\frac{N}{N_m} = \frac{H_2 - H_1}{H_s - H_1} = 1 - \frac{H_s - H_2}{H_s - H_1}$$
$$= 1 - \exp(-N_{tg})$$
$$\frac{N}{0.015} = \frac{H_2 - 0.005}{0.120 - 0.005} = 1 - e^{-7.79}$$

$e^{-7.79} = 0.00055$, and $1 - e^{-7.79} = 1$, therefore, $N = N_{max}$. Therefore

$$\frac{N}{0.015} = \frac{H_2 - 0.005}{0.115} = 1$$
$$H_2 = 0.120$$
$$N = 0.120 \times 0.015$$
$$= 0.0018 \ kg/s$$
$$= 34.37 \ kg/m^2 \ h$$

These results suggest that the rates of evaporation could be increased 100-fold based on the available capacity of the drying air for absorbing water vapour. However, this does not take into account the elegance of the finish required on the tablet surface.

The number of gas transfer units available in a bed 160 mm thick is approximately 8. For satisfactory coating giving a pharmaceutically elegant tablet, 1.75 kg of water can be evaporated in 45 minutes experimentally and this indicates that as one unit is approximately 20 mm thick, all the evaporation of moisture takes place in this layer.

7.7 SOLVENT-BASED FILM COATING

Solvent-based film coating was the system of choice, but this has now given way to use of aqueous coating formulations. The most commonly used film former is hydroxypropyl methylcellulose (HPMC). The low viscosity grades (5–65 cP) are used together with a plasticizer and colour. Typically, these can be sprayed from a solvent system consisting of 60% methylene chloride and 40% ethanol. Typical operating conditions are:

Coating formulation:	
HPMC 15cP	300 g
Plasticizer (propylene glycol)	50 g
Colour (usually a 'lake')	qs
Methylene chloride	6.0 litre
Industrial methylated spirits (ethanol)	4.5 litre
Exhaust air flow rate	160–240 m^{-3}
Temperature	Approx. 20–25°C
Inlet air flow rate	130–150 m^{-3}
Temperature	50–65°C
Relative humidity	40–60%
Quantity	Approximately 0.4 litre of coating formulation per kg of tablets is required for minimum coverage
Batch size	150 kg
Pan speed	6–7 rev/min
Spray type	airless
Spray-guns	2
Nozzle size	0.4 mm orifice/60% spray angle, spray rate 1000 ml/min upwards (dependent upon tablets and evaporative capacity available)
Liquid pressure	50–80 kg/cm^2 (dependent upon solution viscosity)
Coating time	Between 40 min and 1 h.

Experience has shown that airless sprays give the best results. Adequate coverage of the tablet bed can be obtained by using 4 guns in a 300 kg capacity pan; 2 guns in a 150 kg capacity model, and 1 gun in a 75 kg and 15 kg capacity model. Normally the best pharmaceutically relevant coating is obtained by spraying continuously. However, in the model 15 the minimum spray rate from one standard spray gun would cause over-wetting unless a specially designed spray nozzle is used. To overcome this problem an intermittent spray cycle can be used.

Various types of nozzle have been used: 0.4–2.0 mm diameter orifice nozzles are fairly standard, and the usual reason for varying it is to prevent over-wetting or spray drying. Problems can arise when coating a small tablet which gives a very dense bed, with very small pore sizes and combined with fine intagliations on the tablets. The spray conditions quoted previously would have a tendency for infill of the lettering, ('intagliations'). Generally this is caused by the dense bed creating resistance to air flow and circulation and thereby reducing the evaporative capacity.

One method of preventing this is to reduce the droplet size. Increasing the liquid pressure may achieve the desired effect but may also increase the spray rate, leading to over-wetting. Alternatively the solution may be diluted, thus increasing the spray rate by reducing the surface tension. When the spray rate is reduced, the degree of atomization will also decrease, creating a percentage of large droplets which may cause the original problem to return. In addition, the increased coating time could result in the coating wearing off the tablets almost as quickly as it is applied. The best solution is to reduce the nozzle size and maintain the liquid pressure at its original setting.

Generally, where coating bridges the engraving on tablets, and where it is not due to special characteristics of the process or tablets, one of the following reasons may be the cause:

- the spray rate is too high;
- the droplet size is too large;
- the spray guns are positioned too near the tablet bed.

7.8 ALTERNATIVE FILM COATINGS

Apart from HPMC-based coatings, the side-vented pan has been used successfully for a wide range of solvent-based film coatings containing materials such as cellulose acetate phthalate (CAP), hydroxypropyl cellulose (Klucel), acrylic resins (Eudragit), and gum colophony.

CAP at a 1 %w/w concentration coats particularly well from a solvent system consisting of 73% methylene chloride, 23% acetone and 3% ethanol. Many variants are possible, and most companies using CAP coating have their own preferred solvent formulation. Experimental coating trials have shown that CAP coatings do not require hot air, and with certain solvent systems the use of hot air can prove to be a disadvantage.

7.8.1 Typical coating conditions for CAP

Coating formulation (150 kg batch of tablets)

CAP	5.4 kg
Diethyl phthalate	1.34 kg
Methylene chloride	54 litre
Acetone	19 litre
Industrial methylated spirits	2.7 litre
Pan speed	6–7 rev/min
Spray type	airless
Spray-guns	2

Nozzle size   0.4 mm orifice/60° angle
Spray rate   1250 ml/min
Liquid pressure   54–82 kg cm^{-2} (as required to obtain spray rate)
Exhaust air   140–160 m^{-3}
Inlet air   130–150 m^{-3}; 20°C (ambient); 40–60% relative
                            humidity
Coating time   1 h

7.8.2 Sugar coating

Previous attempts to sugar coat during the development of the side-vented pan were unsuccessful, largely because of the very rough coating produced by the high drying rates. Even when room temperature air was used for drying, the coating was still too uneven.

After a considerable amount of experimental work, a system of dosing, rolling and drying produced satisfactory results comparable to that achieved in the conventional coating pan process. The drying air was shut off immediately after the application of the sugar syrup was started, and kept shut off for a time after dosing was completed. During this period the sugar syrup was spread by tablet to tablet contact until the whole batch was evenly covered and the thin film of syrup just started to dry. At this point the drying air was switched on and the maximum drying rate used, leaving a smooth coat.

The air flow was stopped during the dosing and rolling period by closing a damper in both the inlet and exhaust ducts. Stopping the fan was found to be unsatisfactory for two reasons:

1. it took too long for the fan to slow down and stop;
2. even when the fan was stopped there was sufficient natural draught through the pan and ducting to cause some drying to occur, resulting in a slightly uneven coating.

Coating systems such as these are used with conventional pans. Here the drying time represents only about 30% of the total cycle time and, consequently, if the side-vented pan could reduce the drying time by as much as 50%, it represents only a 15% saving in the total cycle time. The advantages of the side-vented pan for sugar coating are given below:

- *Semi-automatic operation*: The side-vented pan can be adapted quite readily to semi-automatic operation. An excellent example of this is in the sugar-coating department of Ayerst Laboratories at Rouses Point, New York.
- *Dust-free operation*: Virtually eliminates tablets with 'pimples'.
- *Flexible operation*: The operating conditions are very flexible, and can apply to a wide range of different coating operations. In extreme cases it can be used for removing sugar coats with blemishes. The sink can be filled with water and the tablets gently tumbled through the water until sufficient coating has been removed. At this stage the sink is emptied and the tablets rapidly dried to prevent damage to the core.

- *Improved stability*: It has been reported that stability has been enhanced for some products coated in the side-vented pan compared with the same products coated in conventional pans. This may be due to a reduction in coating cycles and penetration of water into the core.
- *Low-temperature operation*: This is a distinct advantage where heat-sensitive tablets are to be coated, as ambient air can be used to dry the coating. This is also applicable to the confectionery industry in the coating of chocolate centres. It also saves energy.
- *Smooth coating*: An extremely smooth coating is achieved, even from the very early stages of coating. Excellent results have been obtained with a coating of only 50% of the core weight. Less could be used if it were really necessary. This is of little interest to companies wishing to copy existing products but can be attractive where new products are developed using sugar coating.
- *Evenness of coating*: At high speeds the sugar coating tends to follow the shape of the tablet. Normal or shallow concave tablets can retain their quite sharp corners after coating, even though the coating is smooth. If this is undesirable, a more rounded appearance can be obtained by extending the rolling time. At this stage the syrup is in a plastic state and will mould round the edges of the tablet.

7.9   AQUEOUS-BASED FILM COATING

The reasons for the introduction of aqueous-based film coating have been highlighted in the introduction, and will not be repeated here.

The big disadvantage of using water as a solvent for film coating is that it has a much higher latent heat of evaporation than most of the organic solvents (approximately three times that of ethanol: 539 kcal/kg cf. 204 kcal/kg).

The slower rate of evaporation gives rise to the possibility of water penetrating the surface of the tablet, which could result in either physical degradation of the tablet or deterioration of the active incredient. The side-vented pan, with its very high drying capacity, makes it an obvious choice for aqueous coating. During the last ten years techniques have been developed to such an extent that even extremely water-sensitive tablets have been coated without the penetration of water affecting the materials which comprise the core. Examples are aspirin, methyldopa, vitamin C.

In developing successful aqueous film coating there are a number of problems to be overcome. Most of the problems originate from the low evaporation rate of the water. This rate can be increased by increasing the air flow and/or its temperature. Increasing the air flow is not a simple solution. Time is required for the heat to be transferred to the aqueous phase and evaporation to take place, so that if the air flow is too high, heat is lost. In addition, increased air flow results in an increased pressure drop through the bed of tablets and the associated ducting, and thus requires more power. The costs of higher air flow, additional power required and the heat losses can increase without a significant reduction in the coating time. Consequently, there is an optimum air flow for each size of pan. Increasing the temperature of the air also helps, but this is possible only if the tablets are not heat sensitive. Results of many experiments have shown that the optimum inlet air temperature for most tablets lies in the range 50–80°C which maintains a bed temperature of approximately 40–45°C.

For an aqueous-based process the tablets must tumble in the pan for a longer period than would be necessary for a solvent-based process. The most critical part of the process is at the start when the tablets are without the protection of a coating. At this stage, tablets which are friable may suffer erosion of the surface and edges. It should be remembered that the pan is acting in a way very similar to a large ball mill. This is also a difficult time to apply the coating quickly as any excess liquid on the surface of the tablet will penetrate the tablet core, and overwetting can cause tablets to adhere to the pan walls and each other. The first stage of the coating process must, therefore, be a compromise between the need to apply the coating quickly and evenly to protect the tablet from abrasion, and slowly, to prevent water penetration and overwetting.

If the tablets are relatively hard, i.e. non-friable, or are not heat sensitive, then the coating process becomes relatively easy. Unfortunately, it is not always possible to produce tablets which will give the desired therapeutic effect and have the ideal physical properties. This was one of the major reasons for reducing the pan speed. While this helps to reduce abrasion it also reduces the frequency with which the tablets pass through the spray zone and increases the time they remain in that area. This, in turn, increases the possibility of overwetting the tablets, resulting in uneven coating and an inelegant tablet.

The use of the baffles certainly reduces this problem, but it is essential that the action is gentle and that it provides homogeneous mixing even at low pan speeds. The object is to keep the tablets rotating as they pass through the spray zone, thus preventing overwetting. Baffles also prevent the formation of a very slow-moving core of tablets in the centre of the bed, which have a tendency to receive less coating than the tablets travelling through the rest of the batch. It was found that the use of the baffles greatly assists in the coating of tablets which have a higher than normal friability. To minimize abrasion it is necessary for the baffle to be fully covered by the tablets. It is equally important to ensure that the pan is not over-loaded as this tends to reduce the efficiency of the baffles.

7.9.1 Development of a spraying system

The high degree of atomization which can be achieved from airless spray-guns makes them the ideal choice for applying film coatings containing organic solvents. The very small droplet size gives a large surface area per unit volume, allowing a high rate of evaporation, and produces a very even coating. It was, therefore, considered that they might also be suitable for aqueous coating. However, for aqueous coating the spray rate is much lower, and to reduce the spray rate by using an airless spray-gun requires either a lower liquid pressure or a smaller nozzle diameter. Reducing the liquid pressure leads to poor atomization and an uneven droplet size, and while reducing the nozzle size to a 0.07 mm diameter orifice obtained the required spray rate for aqueous coating, blocking of a nozzle became a serious problem. This nozzle size is suitable provided that soluble dyes are being used, but these are the exceptions rather than the rule as superior results for coloured films can be obtained by using insoluble aluminium lake pigments. With a nozzle size of 0.07 mm and incorporating these lake pigments into the coating formulations, repeated nozzle blocking occurs.

In the larger pans it was possible to reduce the number of spray-guns, but increasing the liquid flow per gun and covering a larger portion of the tablet bed, results in uneven tablet to tablet coating. This has meant that airless sprays are not generally used for aqueous coating.

Conventional air-atomizing sprays can give excellent atomization of a liquid provided that the atomizing air volume is kept high and the liquid flow rate is low. The liquid feed to this type of spray-gun is normally from a pressurized vessel (particularly for solvent solution), but this feed system did not provide the constant flow required for aqueous coating. The variations in flow rate results in variations in droplet size, and this manifests itself as an uneven coat or overwetting. Many methods for obtaining a consistent liquid flow can be used for atomizing sprays in aqueous coating, and the Manesty Co-Tab and Spray Tab Units are examples. The Spray-Tab unit is designed specifically for aqueous coating processes. These units achieve a consistent flow of coating solution suspension using a recirculating system. This system has given excellent results with a wide range of aqueous coating materials including methylcellulose, hydroxypropyl cellulose, hydroxypropyl methylcellulose, and the acrylic resin suspension, Eudragit L30D.

7.9.2 Method of operation
The operating conditions for the spray are critical. Some drying of the droplets takes place as they pass from the spray-gun to the tablets, resulting in a coating that has partly dried when it strikes the tablet. The liquid is more concentrated when it is deposited on the tablet surface, and this together with the rapid evaporation of the remaining liquid prevents absorption on the tablet surface. The position of the spray-guns in the pan is not extremely critical, but some care must be taken to ensure their correct operation according to the conditions being used.

The angle of the spray and its direction must be considered. Generally it is advisable to spray as far up the bed as possible to retain the tablets on the surface of the bed for the maximum time where a high evaporation rate exists. Tablets sampled from immediately below the spray zone will feel slightly tacky, but samples taken from the bottom of the bed, just before the tablets contact the pan and mix with the remainder of the batch, should have lost this tackiness. However, they will not be completely dry at this stage. If the tablets are still tacky at the bottom of the bed several options are possible:

- reduce the spray rate;
- increase the temperature and/or volume of drying air;
- check the angle of the spray produced and the air pressure used for atomization.

Tablets in this condition when mixed together will result in coating from one tablet sticking to another, and on separation a small portion of the coating is pulled off one of the tablets (commonly known as 'picking'). If 'picking' is allowed to take place a very inferior quality of coating is obtained. Final drying of the tablets takes place as they mix with the rest of the tablets in the bed. To complete the drying process before they pass again through the spray zone it is advisable not to have the spray directed at the very top of the bed as this portion of the bed is the least dense and the fastest evaporation takes place in this area.

Excellent coating results have been found by setting the direction of the spray approximately one-third of the way down the bed. The distance of the spray nozzle from the bed will vary slightly with the materials being used and the operating conditions, but is usually between 250 and 350 mm from the surface.

If the guns are too near the tablet bed overwetting may occur, and if they are too far away or if the temperature of the drying air is too high, spray drying occurs. This results in a loss of coating material through the exhaust system, blocked filters, and a build-up of material in the pan, plenum and ductwork. When the correct conditions are used the recovery in terms of weight of coating deposited on the tablets to weight of coating material used, can be very high. Eli Lilly have claimed recovery as high as 99%, and while this figure has undoubtedly been obtained, more usual results are in the region of 95%. Spray drying of the solution can occur if the correct conditions are not used, and this emphasizes the need for spray-guns to produce a very even droplet size. When a wide range of droplet sizes exist it will be difficult to establish optimum operating conditions.

Most of the process parameters are interrelated, and changes to improve one will affect at least one other. Fluctuating conditions will inevitably result in a poorer quality of coating. It is, therefore, essential to use equipment which will not only provide flexible operating conditions but must be capable of maintaining constant conditions once they have been optimized.

7.9.3   Operating conditions for aqueous-based coating
A typical set of operating conditions are given below:

Coating formulation	% by weight
Hydroxypropyl methylcellulose (15cP)	5.0
Polyethylene glycol (6000)	1.0
Colour (as solid matter)	1.25
Water	92.75
Atomizing air pressure	6.0 kg/cm^{-2}
Exhaust air flow rate*	140–160 m^{-3}
Temperature	38–42°C
Inlet air flow rate*	130–150 m^{-3}
Temperature	65–70°C
Relative humidity	40–60% at 15°C
Quantity	28 litres of suspension
Batch size	150 kg
Pan speed	3–6 rev/min
Spray type	air atomizing
Spray-guns	3

Spray rate	100 ml/min/gun (dependent on tablet shape and size)
Nozzle pressure	2.7 kg/cm^{-2}
Coating time	90 min

* Volume of air flow will depend on size of pan and batch size.

7.10 FUTURE DEVELOPMENT

7.10.1 Thermal efficiency

One area which is being investigated is the efficiency of the coating system as a whole. It is common practice in the USA for units to be purchased without ancillary equipment. The user normally designs and installs his own exhaust and inlet air systems. In Europe and most other areas there is a demand for a complete package. Ideally, this should be a custom-built system, each installation having its own design criteria. However, users in general have not attempted to optimize conditions, and once empirical operating conditions have been set they are then maintained without further investigation. Unfortunately, this has resulted in details of operating conditions, which are far from optimum, being circulated in the industry. The Accelacota in particular has been criticized on the grounds of poor thermal efficiency on the basis of this information. An examination of the results from several units from different manufacturers show that coating cycles are very similar; some use longer coating periods but with lower air volumes, while others increase the air volume to reduce the cycle. The cost of operating the process utilities is very similar.

REFERENCES

Rayleigh, Lord (1878) *Proc. London Math. Soc.* **10**.

Weber, C. (1931) *Angew, Z. Math. Mech.* **11**, 136.

Ohnesorge, G. (1936) *Z. Angew. Math. U. Math.* **16**, 355.

Ohnesorge, G. (1937) *Z. Vereins Deutscher Ingenieure* **81**(16).

Nukizama, S. & Tanasawa, Y. (1950) Defence Research Board, Dept. of National Defence, Canada. 10.M9.47 (393) HQ 2-0-264-01 March (trans. E. Hooch).

Groenweg, J. *et al.* (1967) *Brit. J. Appl. Phys.* **18**, 1317.

Roth, L.O. & Porterfield, J.G. (1965) *Trans. Am. Soc. Agric. Engrs* **8**, 493.

Ranz, W.E. & Marshall, W.R. (1952) *Chemical Engineering Progress* **48**, 3 (March).

Cole, G.C., Neale, P.J., Wilde, J.S. & Ridgway, M. (1980) *J. Pharm. Pharmac.* **32** (Suppl.), 92.

Coulson, J.M. & Richardson, J.F. (1980) *Chemical Engineering,* Vol. 1, Chap. 7 (rev. edn), Pergamon.

Coulson, J.M. & Richardson, J.F. (1980) *Chemical Engineering*, Vol. 1, Chap. 8 (rev. edn), Pergamon.

Rowe, P.N., Claxton, K.T. & Lewis, J.B. (1965) *Trans. Inst. Chem. Eng.* **43**, T14.

Frossling, N. (1938) *Beitr. Geophysics* **52**, 170.

Prater, D.A. (1982) Ph.D. Thesis, Bath University, pp. 110–117.

Coulson, J.M. & Richardson, J.F. (1980) *Chemical Engineering*, Vol. 2, Chap. 4 (rev. edn).
Chilton, T.H. & Coburn, A.P. (1934) *Ind. Chem.* **26**.
Treybal, R.E. (1955) *Mass Transfer Operations*, Chaps 3 and 12, McGraw-Hill.

LIST OF SYMBOLS

Parameter	Symbol	Units of measurement
Coefficient of discharge for droplet in atomisation	C_D	–
Constant	A	Relationship between nozzle design and liquid to be sprayed
Constant	B	Relationship between nozzle design and liquid to be sprayed
Constant	K_1	Derived constant for mass transfer equation
Diameter of tablet	l	m
Density	ρ	kg/m^3
Drying rate	N or N_{max}	$kg/m^3 \, s$
Diffusion coefficient	D_v	$m^2 \, s$
Dispersion factor	α	Function of nozzle design
Droplet diameter	D	m
Droplet size group	β	Function of nozzle design
Heat transfer coefficient	h	$W/m^2 \, K$
Humidity of drying air	H_1	kg/kg
Humidity of exhaust air	H_2	kg/kg
Humidity of air at maximum saturation	$H_s \, (H_{max})$	kg/kg
Interfacial surface % volume	a	m^2/m^3
Kozeny constant	K''	Generally given the value of 5
Latent heat of vaporization	λ	kJ/kg
Liquid jet velocity	V_j	m/s
Nozzle orifice diameter	d_n	m
Number of gas transfer units	N_{tg}	–
Mass	W	kg
Mass transfer coefficient	h_d	m/s
Nuzzelt number (Nu)	hD/k	–
Partial pressure of water vapour in surrounding air	P_W	N/m^2
Permeability coefficient in the Kozeny equation	B	m^2
Prandtl number (Pr)	C_p/uk	–
Ratio of the Weber number (We) to the Reynolds number (Z')	$\mu/(\rho d_n r)^{\frac{1}{2}}$	–

Reynolds number (Re) (droplets)	$uD\rho/\mu$	–
Reynolds number (Re) (tablets)	$ul\rho/\mu$	–
Saturated vapour pressure of water vapour at droplet wet surface	P_{WB}	N/m^2
Schmidt number (Sc)	$\mu/\rho D_v$	–
Sherwood number (Sh)	$h_d d/D_v$	–
Specific heat at constant pressure	C_p	J/kg K
Surface area per unit volume of bed	S_B	m^2/m^3
Surface area per unit volume of particle or packing	S	m^2/m^3
Surface tension	γ	J/m^2
Tablet bed thickness	Z_s	m
Tablet diameter	1	m
Temperature	T_a, T_s, T_1, T_2	K (°C)
Temperature difference	ΔT	K (°C)
Terminal velocity	u_t	m/s
Thermal conductivity	k	W/m K
Total heat transferred	Q	kJ/kg
Vapour pressure of water at temperature of the saturated droplet surface	P_{WB}	N s/m^2
Velocity	u	m/s
Viscosity	μ	N s/m^2
Voidage	e	–
Weber number (We)	$V_j\,[(\rho d_n/\gamma)^{\frac{1}{2}}]$	–

8

Coating pans and coating columns

Graham C. Cole

SUMMARY

This chapter provides some examples of the type of equipment that is currently available. It is not exhaustive, but will highlight the main features that should be considered when evaluating and selecting appropriate units together with ancillary equipment for spraying and control of the coating process.

8.1 CONVENTIONAL COATING PANS

It is not proposed to discuss in detail the use of conventional coating pans as these are being phased out with the preference for more sophisticated pans and systems.

Various methods have been used to improve the coating characteristics in this type of pan which was originally designed for sugar coating. Some examples are shown in Figs. 8.1–8.3.

The modifications made to sugar-coating pans were an attempt to utilize existing equipment and while successful for solvent-based film-coating systems, they do not have the advantages of side-vented pans when aqueous film coats are applied.

8.2 MANESTY ACCELACOTA

The Accelacota is used as a model against which all other manufacturers' units are compared. That is not intended to imply any preference, but as a means of providing a road map through the maze of information available.

The data quoted is intended as a guideline to indicate the range and size of the Accelacotas and the most suitable ancillary equipment available. Margins of safety

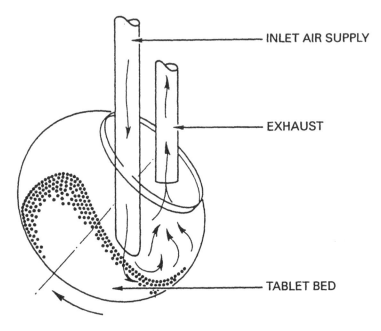

Fig. 8.1   Standard coating pan.

have been included to allow for a range of operating conditions. They should not be considered as specific nor should they be compared with other manufacturers' quoted data. Where comparisons are to be made, these should be related to the particular coating conditions. Like must be compared with like.

Four sizes of Accelacota are available:

- Model 10, operates with a batch size of 8–18 kg.
- Model 75, operates with a batch size of 40–90 kg.
- Model 150, operates with a batch size of 80–180 kg.
- Model 350, operates with a batch size of 250–450 kg.

The essential features are illustrated in Figure 8.4.

The Accelacota has a horizontal rotating cylindrical drum, the curved surface of which is uniformly perforated. The ends of the cylinder are conically dished, so that tablets in the drum are inverted and also mixed laterally during the coating operation. There are baffles to assist the mixing process. Drying air enters the drum through the perforations on the side remote from the tablet bed, and is drawn through the bed by the exhaust fan located in the exhaust duct connected to the plenum positioned under the tablet bed. This plenum has a mouth that fits closely to the outside of the perforated curved surface of the drum.

The angles of the front and rear sides of the pan are 56° and 61° respectively, which was originally intended to ensure complete mixing of the tablets from the top of the bed to the bottom and from front to rear. However, it was found that this was insufficient to ensure homogeneous mixing and baffles were fitted. Generally,

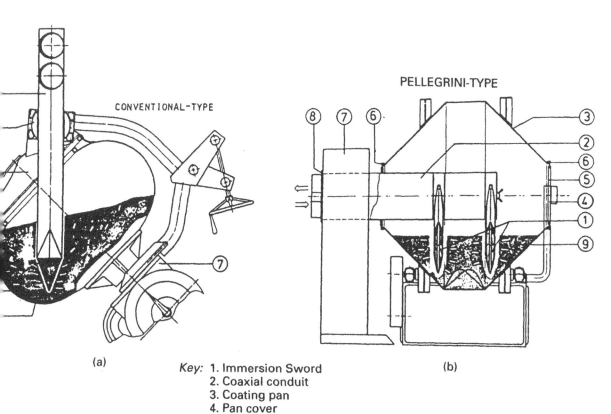

CONVENTIONAL-TYPE

PELLEGRINI-TYPE

(a)

(b)

Key: 1. Immersion Sword
2. Coaxial conduit
3. Coating pan
4. Pan cover
5. Clear control cover
6. Silicone seal
7. Stand
8. Coaxial conduit adjustment
9. Coating bed
10. Base unit fitted with Rollers

Fig. 8.2 Standard coating pan and a Pelligrini pan using the Glatt immersion–Sword system.

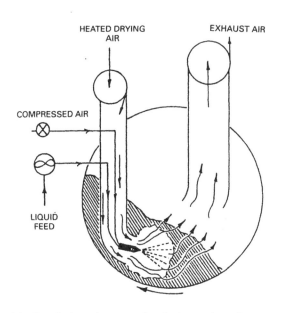

Fig. 8.3 Standard coating pan using the immersion tube system.

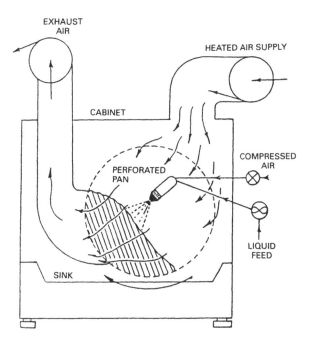

Fig. 8.4 Manesty Accelacota.

the baffles are of the same shape but of different size for each model and can be easily removed or replaced with those of a different design depending on the physical characteristics of the tablet to be coated, e.g. friability.

The batch size for each particular model will depend upon the bulk density of the tablets. Maximum loading will be achieved with tablets made from a high-density material or from small tablets which will have a high packing density. Exceeding these maximum loadings can cause damage to the drive mechanism.

Minimum loadings are found by experience and depend on size and shape of the tablets. If the units are used with batch sizes below these levels, then it is likely that problems will be encountered due to a large portion of the baffles being exposed above the tablet bed. In addition, the exhaust plenum will not be completely covered and this can result in the drying air bypassing the tablets before entering the exhaust duct.

Shape can affect the coating process in a number of ways. Tablets shaped as squares can cause sticking problems and the formation of 'twins'. Logos across the centre of bi-convex tablets result in damage to the intagliations. It is, therefore, an aspect of tablet design which should be appreciated by both marketing and formulation departments. Small tablets produce a very dense bed in the coating pan which tends to reduce the batch size and increase the coating time.

For sugar coating it should be remembered that the maximum loads refer to the weight of the coated tablets and not to the weight of the cores. Therefore, when pan loadings are optimized both the weight of the core and coated tablet need to be taken into consideration.

Having decided upon a batch size, coating times can be estimated from the following:

1. *Sugar coating.* Approximately 6–7 h are required to double the core weight. Thicker or thinner coatings will take proportionally longer or shorter. Coating time is directly proportional to the weight of coating applied. This time is typical but very much shorter times can be obtained with certain coating formulations and favourable tablet shapes. Care must be exercised when comparing these times with those quoted by different equipment manufacturers as they may be quoting times for favourable rather than average conditions. Considerably longer may be needed to finish the coating to produce an elegant product with a high gloss.

2. *Solvent-based film coating.* From 30 to 90 min: 30 min is usual where a very thin transparent coating is applied (this type of coating would be used to prevent dusting rather than as a protective coat) but normal thicknesses require 45–60 mins. When coating a batch of small tablets (less than 10 mm diameter) which has a high-density bed, the time could increase to about 75 min. The longest coating time would occur when thick coatings are being applied to small tablets.

3. *Aqueous-based film coating.* Coating times range from 45 min to 3 h with a typical time being about 90 min. The lowest and highest times apply for a variety of reasons similar to those given for a solvent-based coating.

These times have been generalized and apply to all models. In practice, however, if a particular coating formulation is used under similar conditions in a range of different sizes, the times tend to increase slightly for the larger pans.

When evaluating the suitability of a particular model for a coating process, allowances must be made for loading, unloading, cleaning and maintenance. For the Accelacota the following loading and unloading options are available

- manual;
- Accelascoop;
- pneumatic transfer;
- automatic unload.

The time required for each operation will depend upon the method used. The manual process can be considered the worst case. The following times are typical:

	Loading	*Unloading*
Model 10	2–3 min	5 min
Model 75	4–5 min	8 min
Model 150	5–6 min	10 min
Model 350	10–20 min	30–40 min

The Accelascoop is available for the 75, 150 and 350 models and this attachment significantly reduces the unloading time. Further improvements in productivity can be achieved by using a conveyor rather than a container. Containers should be designed to hold multiples of the capacity of the Accelascoop.

Mechanical or pneumatic loading and unloading systems can be designed to meet specific requirements.

The Accelacota models 150 and 350 are available with automatic unload. This material handling option allows for the automatic discharge of tablets, through an inward-opening flap in the pan, into a product container or onto a conveyor.

Automatic unload may be operated manually or linked to a control panel as part of a fully automatic coating system. This concept is illustrated in Fig. 8.5.

8.2.1 Cleaning

Two options are available, the manual method and an automatic washing system called the Auto Wash (Fig. 8.6).

All Accelacotas are fitted with a sink below the coating drum which is used either as a unit to hold the various cleansing agents or to collect washings from a clean-in-place system. This is partially filled with water, solvent or cleansing agent and the drum rotated through this solution. Where manual systems are used, water (or solvent) can be sprayed onto the internal surface and collected in the sink and discharged into an effluent system.

The clean in place (CIP) system (Auto Wash) can be fitted to both the 250 and 350 models. Designed to operate inside the pan only, or in the pan interior, cabinet, and inlet and outlet ducts, strategically positioned nozzles ensure thorough cleansing of the coating area and surrounding zone. Washing can be linked to either a manual or a fully automatic control panel to form part of the complete coating

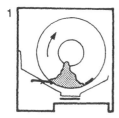
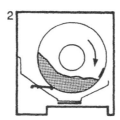
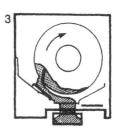

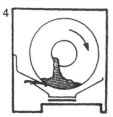

1. Tablets are loaded through the pan mouth, either manually or mechanically, prior to the coating cycle commencing.
2. Coating cycle commences and the tablets are coated.
3. After the coating cycle the coated tablets are discharged, through an inward opening flap in the drum, into a product container or onto a conveyor. The automatic wash cycle commences upon completion of tablet discharge from the drum.
4. The drum is reloaded for next coating cycle. The Accelacota unload feature may be operated manually or linked to a control panel as part of a fully automatic coating cycle.

Fig. 8.5   Automatic loading and unloading system.

system. It should be remembered that the wash cycles need to be carefully formulated and validated. The absence of active ingredients or excipients from the rinse water is not accepted by the FDA as evidence that the equipment is clean. Swab tests will need to be taken from strategic points in the system and analysed.

Coatings that are water soluble can be hosed off the inside of the pan and drained through the sink. Alternatively, the sink can be filled and the pan rotated through it to dissolve material that has adhered to the pan walls.

Cleaning after a sugar-coating process can be achieved in approximately 30 min in the best case, but coatings that contain materials which cause strong adhesion to the pan will take longer. Allowing one hour for cleaning would be quite generous, but it must be remembered that cleaning is an essential part of cGMP (current Good Manufacturing Practice) and cannot be short-circuited.

8.2.2   The air flow system
A typical schematic layout is shown for free standing models in Fig. 8.7, which illustrates the coating pan, hot air unit, fan unit (exhaust), damper controls and interconnecting duct work.

(a)   Exhaust air
It is essential to have some means of drawing the air through the bed of tablets. In its simplest form this consists of an exhaust fan and ducting to carry the air from the plenum to the fan and from the fan to the atmosphere. The optimum quantity of air will vary with the evaporation rate required; the total pressure drop will depend upon the resistance to air flow of the tablet bed, the resistance of the exhaust ducting, and any additional equipment such as filters and solvent recovery system that may be fitted. It should be remembered that the exhaust air will contain a

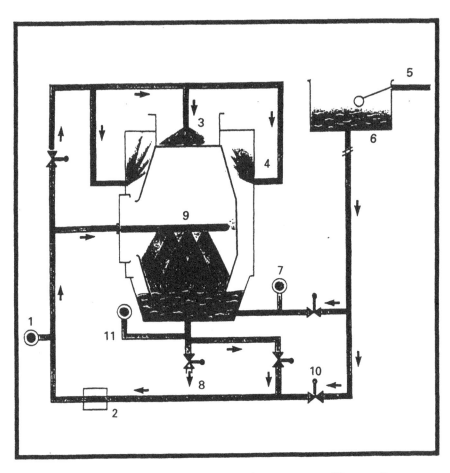

1 Provision for injection   4 Cabinet spray nozzles   8 Water waste
  of releasing agents (optional)   5 Mains supply   9 Drum spray nozzles
2 Pump   6 Header tank (customer supply)   10 Valve
3 Duct spray nozzles   7 Level pressure switch   11 Sink empty pressure switch

Fig. 8.6   The Manesty Auto Wash system.

percentage of particulates ranging in size from submicron to 200–300 μm and levels
of solvent. Additionally conditions will not always be constant. The type of coating
may change, the batch size may vary and the inlet air conditions may also vary. An
oversize fan is therefore used and a damper is incorporated into the exhaust ducting
to adjust the air flow for particular conditions. It is essential to have a control and
instrumentation system that will modify the condition of the air as it enters the
coating pan, depending on the local climatic conditions.

Sugar coating
For this process it is necessary to stop the air flow at various stages during coating.

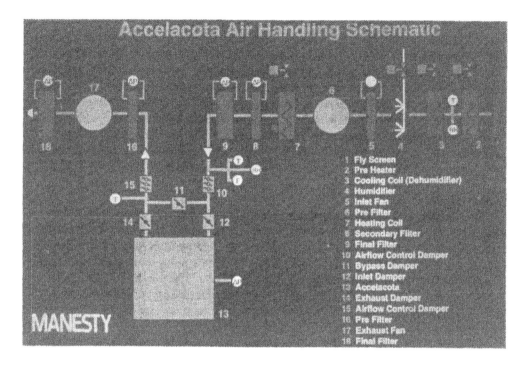

Fig. 8.7   Schematic of complete air flow system.

This can be achieved by closing the damper completely. Stopping the fan has been found to be an unsatisfactory means of shutting off the air flow because natural convection takes place through the ducting and this will affect the quality of the coating.

The Model 10 contains an exhaust fan and damper unit built into the cabinet which requires connecting to an external exhaust duct and filter system. Models 75 and 150 incorporate a free-standing exhaust unit which contains the fan, motor, starter and the damper valve. The damper valve can be manually preset to a partially or fully open position to regulate the air flow and can be moved from the preset position to the fully closed position by a pneumatic signal. The equipment is housed in a cabinet with a sound-absorbing lining to reduce the noise of the fan. These units are suitable for standing alongside the appropriate model or mounting remotely and using interconnecting ductwork. An overrated fan is used which allows for longer lengths of ducting to be used when necessary. The required volume of air can be regulated by means of a damper valve.

The Model 350 requires a much larger air volume and flow. The size of the fan and the unit housing the fan and starter would be too large and expensive to be conveniently sited alongside the Accelacota. It is essential to design a properly balanced system. The use of qualified heating, ventilating and air-conditioning engineers to achieve this is the best option. The fan and starter and a section of ductwork containing the damper valve and assistance with the ducting layout can be obtained from Manesty for integration into the facility.

To prevent atmospheric pollution a filter must be fitted in the exhaust ducting, and it may be necessary to use a more powerful fan to overcome the resistance of the filter as its efficiency is reduced during the coating process. This will affect the coating, resulting in a reduction of the rate of evaporation, a reduction in the spray rate and longer coating times. It is, therefore, advisable to fit some form of pressure drop indicator to the filter. A simple manometer with alarm can be sufficient to warn the operator that conditions are changing and that the filter requires cleaning. Alternatively, a more elaborate filter system with automatic cleaning could be employed. Alternatives to filters are discussed in Chapter 9.

(b)   Inlet air
In the simplest case, and for the smallest pans, the drying air can be drawn into the pan from the coating room. However, the suitability of the air will depend upon the type of coating process being carried out and the temperature and relative humidity of the air. It is unlikely to be suitable unless the coating is an organic solvent-based film and the air is conditioned to about 30% to 35% r.h. at 20–22°C. Even if these conditions are met the additional load which the coating process will place on the air-conditioning system for the building should be evaluated before deciding to use localized environmental air.

Generally, an inlet air system is required. This normally consists of a filter to remove coarse particles from the air which may be drawn from outside the building: a fan; a heat exchanger; a fine filter to prevent product contamination and a damper to regulate the air flow. In theory the exhaust fan should draw all its air from the inlet system. This would necessitate the coating pan being sealed, but if the door is opened to examine the tablets the inlet system would be by-passed. It is, therefore, preferable to install a fan with just sufficient power to overcome the resistance of the filters, heat exchanger and ducting.

A hot air unit incorporating a fan, heat exchanger and filter, together with fan starter and the damper valve for the 10, 75 and 150 models are suitable for standing alongside the appropriate model and can be connected by a short length of ducting. Alternatively, they can be remotely sited. In the case of the larger 350 model a separate fan, heat exchanger and filter are incorporated into the inlet air-ducting system.

8.3   GLATT PERFORATED COATING PANS

Glatt manufacture a wider range of coating pans than Manesty. These start with the laboratory coater with a capacity of 2.5 litres (1–2 kg) up to the GC 2000 with a capacity of 1250 litres (620–1000 kg). In general terms the concepts are similar but Glatt have developed the interchangeable pan option much further and they also provide more sophisticated automated washing systems.

The laboratory coater GC 300 provides an easy to clean option and a built-in data-processing system. The pan can be easily removed for washing purposes. Fig. 8.8 illustrates this operation.

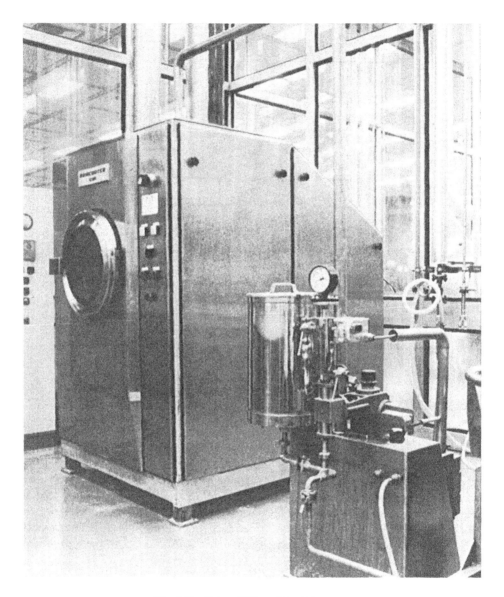

Fig. 8.17   Driam 1200 model coating pan.

Fig. 8.8   Glatt Coater GC300.

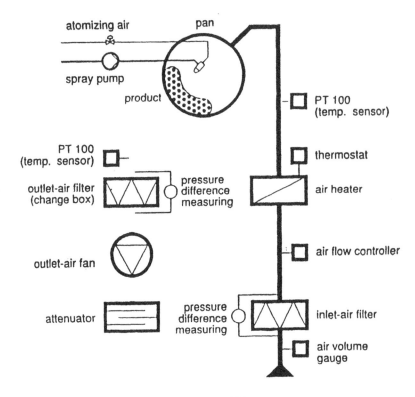

Fig. 8.9   Data acquisition system.

The process parameters monitored by its data acquisition system are illustrated in Fig. 8.9. This concept has been further extended to some of the larger laboratory models shown in Fig. 8.10. The advantage of this type of system is that options for coating pellets and various sizes of tablets can be incorporated onto one machine by having pans with different size perforations. The downside is the need to have a clean storage area available and a means of changing the pan from one size to another. However, advantages in cost, floor space, cGMP and the different process development options clearly outweigh any disadvantages.

8.3.1   Loading and unloading

These operations are illustrated in Fig. 8.11. Manual loading, semi-automatic or automatic options are available and are controlled as shown in Fig. 8.12.

Several items of equipment are required. In the semi-automatic operation it is necessary to have a lifting device to raise the product container to a height where it can be inverted into a funnel or similar transfer chute to convey the tablets into the coating pan. In automatic systems the tablets are usually transferred from an intermediate bulk container (IBC) which may be moved by an automated guided vehicle (or fork lift truck) or conveyed pneumatically from a silo to the coating pan. The illustrations in Fig. 8.11 shows a silo feeding tablets into the coating pan.

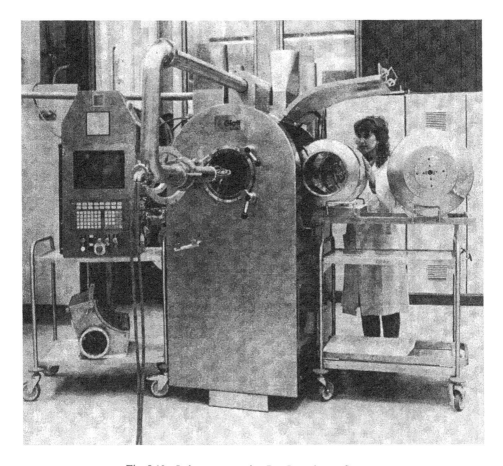

Fig. 8.10   Laboratory coating Pan Interchange System.

Discharge

There are many variations of ways of unloading coating pans. Glatt uses a variation of the Accelascoop device as one method. This requires fitting a specially designed scoop and reversing the coating pan motor to discharge the tablets into a container. Alternatively a flap can be incorporated into the pan and the tablets discharged into a mobile trolley or large funnel before being conveyed pneumatically to an IBC or silo.

Cleaning

A schematic is shown in Fig. 8.13. The cleaning system consists of a spray nozzle integrated into the coating spray arm for spraying the entire drum interior and a set of separate nozzles used to clean the pan exterior. The cleaning liquid is collected in a tray below the coating pan. This permits the coating pan and baffles to be immersed and rotated through the cleansing agent. After completion of the cleaning process the solution is drained and the drum is rinsed. The cleaning of the spray

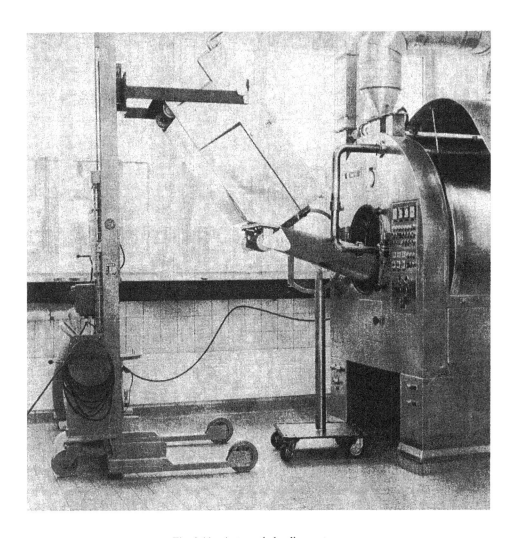

Fig. 8.11   Automatic loading system.

nozzles and supply tubing is included in the cleaning process. Usually water pressure is sufficient for cleaning; however, where high-pressure water is needed, a pump can be fitted.

Spray system

All spray systems need to be designed around the requirements of the coating solution to be sprayed and the tablet substrate. A schematic of the Glatt system is shown in Fig. 8.14 and the actual arrangement in Fig. 8.15.

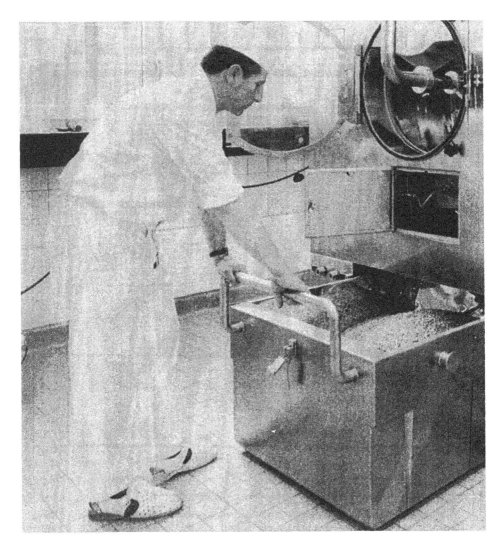

Fig. 8.12 Automatic Control System for loading.

8.4 DRIAM

Driam claim that their unique system of controlling the drying air and reversing the flow at critical stages of the coating process provide advantages particularly when coating friable tablets. The interchangeable perforation sections enable a wide range of tablets, pellets and granules to be coated. Driam claim that:

1. Products are handled more sympathetically as drying air is introduced from below into the pan, giving rise to a fluid bed action. This separates the tablets and provides an envelope of air around the product separating it both from other products and the pan walls.

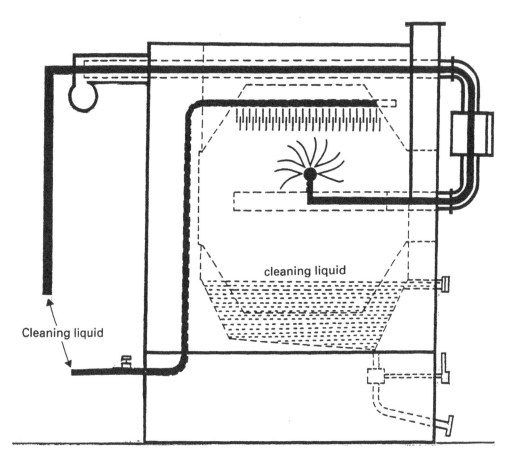

Fig. 8.13   Glatt cleaning system.

2. The direction of the way the air is introduced can be reversed, the previous air inlet becoming the air exhaust and vice versa. For example, when polishing is required after coating, the polishing agent is introduced into the pan and the direction of the air is reversed. To achieve a good polish it is necessary that the tablets rub against each other and the pan walls, and this process is improved by low air pressure.

3. This method results in good mixing of the tablets which, combined with the close control of spraying, gives a homogeneous coating.

4. The air requirements are substantially lower when compared with other manufacturers' units. In conventional pans the air often strikes the product and is exhausted without any drying effect. This cannot happen in the Driacoater, and consequently, with lower air requirements, there is a saving in energy costs.

Driam manufacture a range of nonagonally shaped coating pans with capacities of between 5 kg and 600 kg. The laboratory model, DRC 500/600 Vario, is equipped with an interchangeable pan which provides the flexibility of different operations:

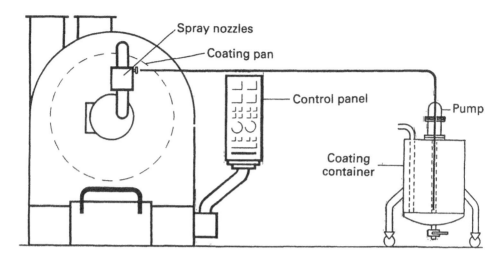

Fig. 8.14   Schematic of Glatt spray system.

- a range of capacities of 5 to 30 kg;
- a range of perforation inserts from 0.2 to 3.0 mm.

In the Varico combination unit it is claimed that the load can be reduced to 2.0 kg for coating in a similar way to the Driacoater 500 which was designed as a single unit for small batches of tablets of between 2 and 6 kg.

The Driam differs from the Accelacota and Glatt coaters in the shape of the coating pan and the way the air is utilized in the drying process. This is shown in Fig. 8.16. On the outside of the drum covering the perforated areas, there are the air flow channels with removable covers. At the rear of the pan the air channels are connected to the air distributor. This distributor guides the drying air through the air channels and the perforations into the product. The direction of air flow is reversible.

- *Direct Air Flow*: Air is supplied through the perforated areas at the top of the pan and through the product bed, and the air exhausted through the perforated areas under the product.
- *Reverse Air Flow*: Air is supplied through the perforated areas at the bottom of the pan and through the product bed. It is exhausted through the perforated areas at the top of the pan or through the hollow shaft at the rear.

In contrast to the production machines, the laboratory unit is a complete and self-contained piece of equipment with built-in air supply and exhaust, steam heating, spray system, a completely contained cleaning system with pump, and all control and monitoring instruments. The unit is mobile, requiring little space, and is operational after connections have been made to electric power, steam and compressed air supply. The air volume and the differential pressure in the drum are adjusted by the air control dampers in the air supply and exhaust system. A built-in temperature control stabilizes the pre-set air supply temperature. The casing, the drum and all parts in contact with the product are of 304 stainless steel. A special stand is

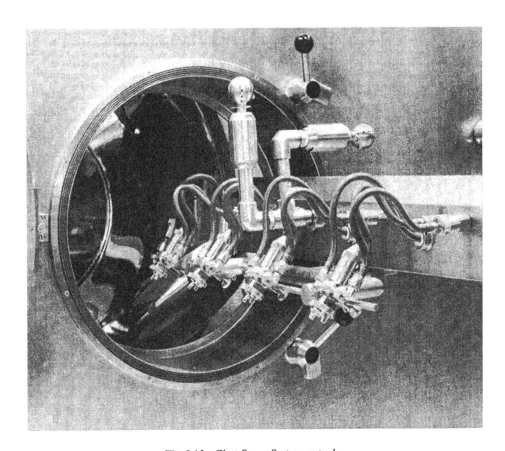

Fig. 8.15   Glatt Spray System, actual.

available to change the coating pans in the 500/600 Vario model. The control cabinet is fitted with gauges to monitor:

- temperature of the air supply;
- temperature of the exhaust air;
- the differential pressure in the coating pan;
- the air volume in cubic metres per minute (m^3/min).

Controls and switches are available for:

- drive;
- spraying;
- air supply;
- air exhaust;
- heater;
- cleaning pump;

- atomizing air;
- temperature control;
- emergency stop;
- compressed air;
- time control (generally an option for sugar coating only).

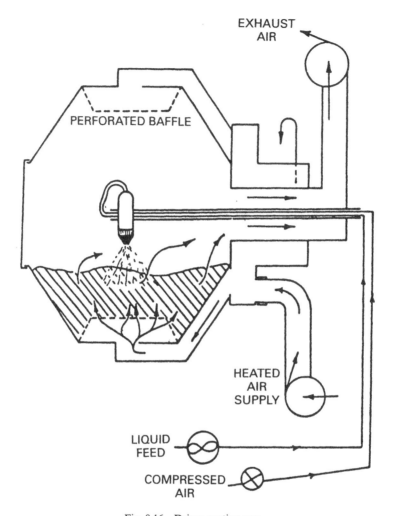

Fig. 8.16   Driam coating pan.

The Driacoater 500/600 Vario comes with various options.

Type	Batch Capacity
500/016	5 kg
600/016	10 kg
500/031	10 kg
600/031	20 kg
600/046	30 kg
Drum diameter	500–600 mm
Speed range	5–27 rev/min
Perforated inserts	0.2–3.0 mm

The following production models are available:

Model No.	900	1200 1600/600/1 1600/1.25
Drum diameter (mm)	900	1200 1600/600 1600
Batch sizes	60	120 300 500 600

The suffix 1 and 1.25 relates to the depth of the drum in metres.

A model 1200 with associated control cabinet and coating reservoir is shown in Fig. 8.17.

8.4.1 Cleaning

As with all coating pans, attention to cGMP requirements is an essential part of an evaluation programme to assess the suitability of the equipment for pharmaceutical production. The cleaning of these pans is shown schematically in Fig. 8.18. The process operates in four phases:

1. cleansing of the inside of the pan;
2. cleansing of the outside perimeter;
3. cleansing of the air channels;
4. cleansing of the sink.

As in all cGMP operations, a check by Quality Assurance is an essential requirement. For inspection the side panels can be opened to offer access to all parts of the equipment. The air channels can be removed manually for swab and visual inspection.

8.4.2 Loading and unloading

On early Driacoater production models, loading of tablets was manually through the front of the unit. To unload, a chute was fitted to the front of the pan, the rotation of the pan reversed and the tablets discharged into an appropriate container. Options are available for rear loading, depending on the particular requirements.

8.5 SIMILAR COATING PANS

Other side-vented coating pans, which are very similar to the Glatt Coater and the Accelacota, are manufactured by Dumoulin in France and by Freund in Japan who manufacture the Hi-Coater. The Hi-Coater was originally designed to overcome the patents on the Accelacota held by Eli Lilly, the inventors. It has four perforated panels linked to air ducts that are in constant contact with the exhaust ducts. It is illustrated in Fig. 8.19.

Capacities range from 500 g load up to the HCF 200, claimed to hold 700 kg. Loading and unloading can be achieved through the front of the unit and by a flap in the pan which discharges into a mobile container under the machine or onto a conveyor.

8.6 PELLEGRINI COATING PANS

These pans are marketed by GS Technology of Bologna, Italy, who supply the

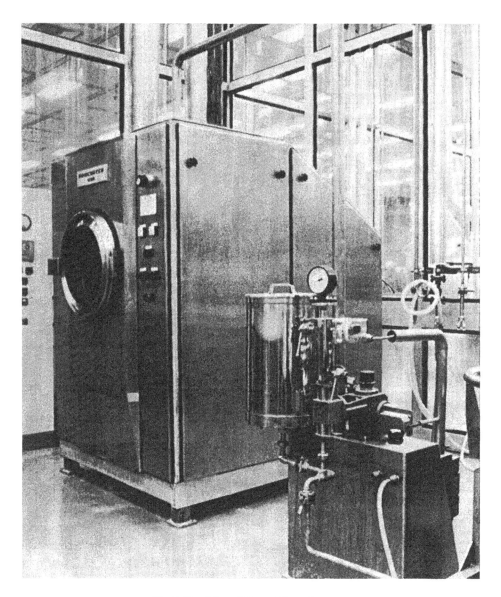

Fig. 8.17   Driam 1200 model coating pan.

expertise in air handling spray systems, controls and coating technology. Pelligrini are the fabricators of the pan.

These are non-perforated pans with capacities from 10 to 1000 litres. Originally developed for sugar coating, they use baffles which give a very even distribution of the drying air through the tablet bed or pellets. An advantage of this type of pan is that it can be used for coating a large range of particulate sizes from less than a

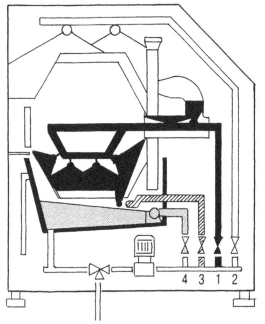

High capacity cleaning system
with built-in cleaning pump

Cleaning phases:
1 Drum inside by cleaning spray arm
2 Drum outside with air distributor
3 Air channels inside
4 Rinsing of cleaning container

Fig. 8.18   Driam auto cleaning system.

millimetre to tablets of all shapes and sizes. It is claimed to be the best statistical mixer for coating available.

The GS control and coating systems can be fitted to any coating pan, be it Accelacota, Glatt, Driam, Hi-Coater, etc. This control, it is claimed, results in dramatic decreases in coating times, particularly for sugar.

For film coating, GS have a special reciprocating piston pump, the speed of which is automatically controlled from the bed temperature. For sugar coating, a modified GRACO pump is used.

The type of spray-gun, nozzle configuration and position above the bed is critical in all coating processes. These are all either fully interchangeable or adjustable in the GS system.

Drying is effected through perforated baffles immersed in the bed of cores, similar to the immersion–Sword technique, giving a very even distribution of drying of air and allowing a very low differential pressure to be employed which reduces attrition considerably.

Two computerized systems are available which can be fitted to existing equipment: COMREC monitors and records all process parameters; COMAUT monitors, records and controls the entire process. A full printout, graphical representation and statistical analysis is obtained either through COMREC or COMAUT.

A typical system is shown schematically in Fig. 8.20.

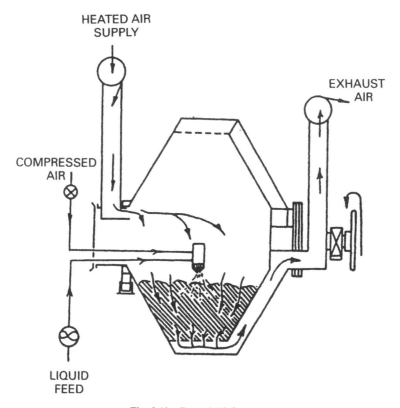

Fig. 8.19 Freund Hi-Coater.

8.7 THE BUTTERFLY COATING PAN

These pans have capacities ranging from 15 litres up to 1200 litres and are manufactured in Germany by Huttlin. Originally developed for sugar coating, they are claimed to be suitable for all current types of film coatings, and in particular for larger tablets.

The Butterfly pan (Fig. 8.21) has a special pan cross-section with inward-sloping sides. The cross-section of the pan containing the product area is shaped like a trapezium. In contrast to all other sugar-coating pans this pan has its largest breadth at the biggest cross-section and its smallest breadth at the smallest cross-section. Therefore, even with maximum load the height through which the product falls is relatively small.

Intensive product movement is achieved which provides optimal mixing. In the interior of the pan there are no blades or other baffles to mechanically stress the product.

Spray coating is effected at the point where the product is moving at constant speed in the narrow section of the pan.

The loading and evacuation of the tablets (or pellets) is performed tangentially from the sides of the pan through segments in the wall. This is a unique system which provides a very efficient handling process.

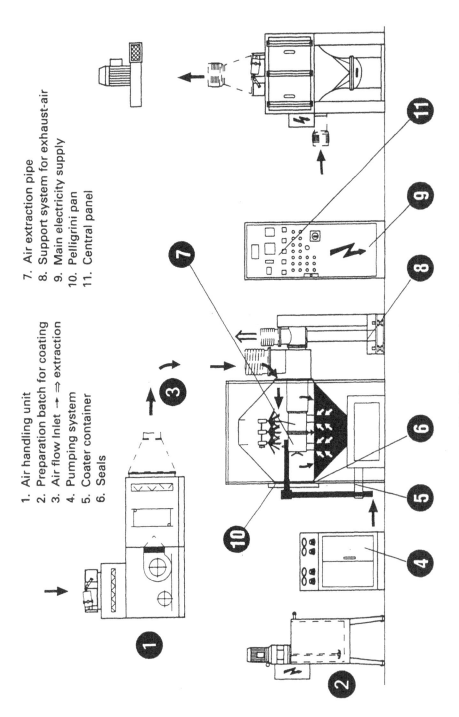

1. Air handling unit
2. Preparation batch for coating
3. Air flow Inlet → ⇒ extraction
4. Pumping system
5. Coater container
6. Seals
7. Air extraction pipe
8. Support system for exhaust-air
9. Main electricity supply
10. Pelligrini pan
11. Central panel

Fig. 8.20   GS control system.

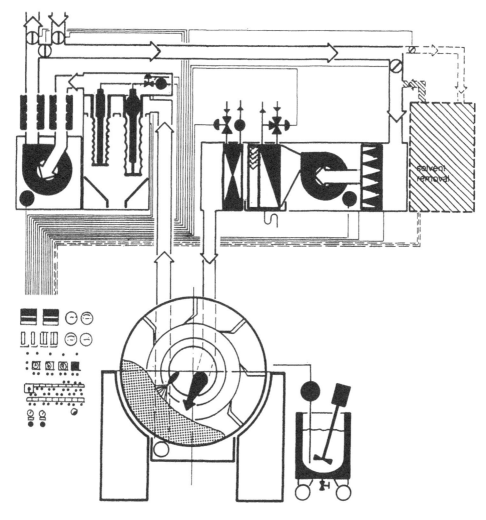

Fig. 8.21   The Butterfly Coater.

The side walls of the pan (which can be removed for cleaning) are attached by means of a simple fastener enabling the pan walls to be dismantled and the coating pan thoroughly cleaned. As with the other types of coating pans, automatic control systems are available to monitor and optimize the process parameters.

8.8   COLUMNS: FLUIDIZED BED

As was mentioned in Chapter 1, fluidized bed coating columns were used in the early days by Abbott Laboratories based on the Wurster process and latterly by Merck to coat tablets using air sprays and solvent-based formulations. The Merck formulation was converted to an aqueous system with some difficulty and current processes now use side-vented pans.

The laboratory column shown in Fig. 8.22 is ideal for coating 15–20 tablets or 10–50 g of pellets.

One of the problems that exists in the earlier stages of formulation is the very small amounts of drug available. This column can be used to coat varying loads depending on the diameter of the column. It can be built with interchangeable columns. The important criteria are:

- a pump capable of delivering 0.1 ml of coating consistently and accurately;
- a controllable source of drying air;
- a nozzle of 0.25 mm diameter.

This model can be built from parts of a spray drier and a portable air handling unit.

Commercial models are available from companies such as Glatt and Niro Atomisers. They are more sophisticated and provide options for fluid bed drying of materials, spray granulation and other options. Their control systems are able to monitor and record all the relevant process parameters.

The type of column used by Merck in the manufacture of ALDOMET is shown schematically in Figure 8.23.

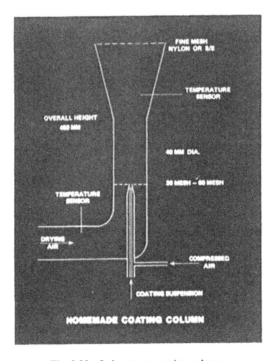

Fig. 8.22   Laboratory coating column.

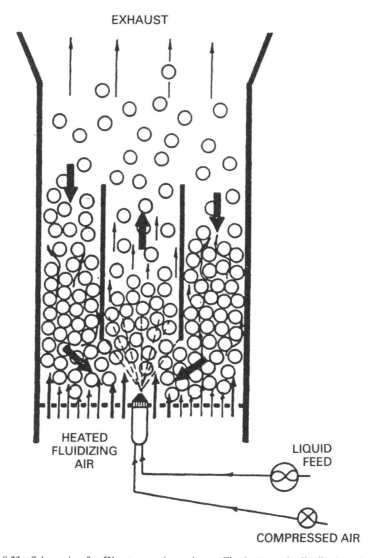

EXHAUST

HEATED
FLUIDIZING
AIR

LIQUID
FEED

COMPRESSED AIR

Fig. 8.23 Schematic of a Wurster coating column. The bottom air distribution plate is
designed to assist the flow of particles during coating.

This is the most efficient way of utilizing the drying capacity of the air.
Unfortunately the tablets must be robust as they are subjected to considerable physical stress and this has largely led to the switch to side-vented pans.

The earliest fluid-bed coating equipment was based on the Wurster design.

A moving bed of tablets continuously passes up the central column and, as a
result of the effect of the expansion chamber at the top which reduces air velocity,
the tablets drop back to the bottom between the walls of the inner and outer
chamber. The concept of the equipment is based on a single spray gun situated in

the centre of an air-distribution plate. The geometric proportions of the inner and outer columns are such that a continuously moving column of tablets passes through the spray path with every tablet capturing some of the coating and at the same time, ensuring that little or no solution reaches the wall of the inner column.

The Vector Corporation offer a range of fluid bed coating equipment together with a range of control options from manual through to a fully automatic operation. A coating pan option would use CompuTab and the fluid bed option CompuFlo control system respectively. Fig. 8.25 illustrates their laboratory multifunctional system based on the Wurster Column principle.

The configuration of the bottom plate with the larger perforations on the perimeter encourages the flow of tablets, as shown in Fig. 8.24. A modification of this system has been marketed under the name of the Combi Cota by Niro Atomiser who manufacture three models with capacities 2 to 62 litres. The difference here is that the spray is downward onto the centre of the bed and the perforated plate is dished, as shown in Fig. 8.25. This, it is claimed, does not subject the tablets to the same physical stress as a conventional Wurster type column.

8.9   TABLET-COATING EQUIPMENT EVALUATION

The manufacturers of tablet and particulate coating equipment offer an impressive

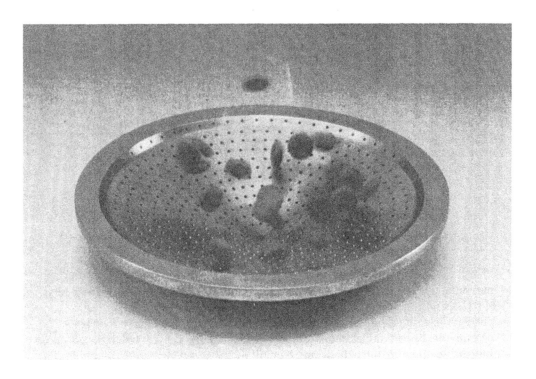

Fig. 8.24   Combi Coater disked perforated air distribution plate.

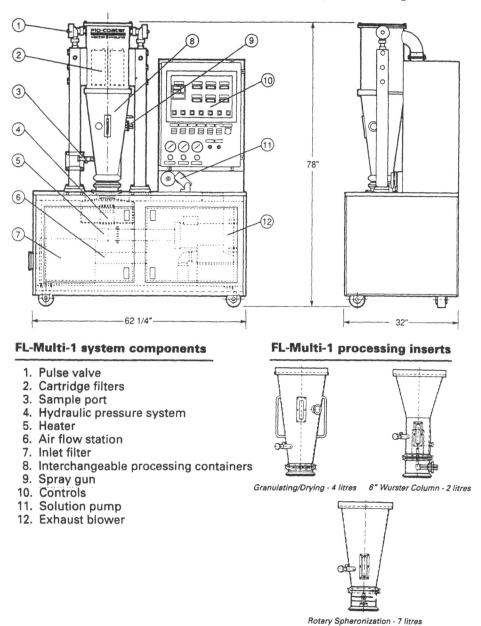

FL-Multi-1 system components

1. Pulse valve
2. Cartridge filters
3. Sample port
4. Hydraulic pressure system
5. Heater
6. Air flow station
7. Inlet filter
8. Interchangeable processing containers
9. Spray gun
10. Controls
11. Solution pump
12. Exhaust blower

FL-Multi-1 processing inserts

Granulating/Drying - 4 litres   6" Wurster Column - 2 litres

Rotary Spheronization - 7 litres

Fig. 8.25   FL-Multi-1 Multi-functional Fluid Bed System. Vector Corporation.

range of machines with varying degrees of sophistication and automation. Even the standard coating pan, which relied on the skill of the operator for sugar coating, has been improved to comply with the requirements of GMP and the equipment needs to be evaluated with this as one of the fundamental requirements. It is probably true to say that all the major manufacturers recognize this as of major importance.

However, many still lack the ability to supply the necessary documentation without considerable prompting from the customer.

It may also be true that these major companies all provide equipment that will coat your particular product (tablet, pellets, granules) but differ in the way this is achieved. It then needs to be established what the differences are in terms of performance, cost, GMP, documentation, delivery and maintenance.

To evaluate this equipment, a test programme should be developed that will highlight the critical requirements of the dosage forms to be coated. For example, for an enteric-coated tablet it is essential that all the tablets have almost identical coats applied to them otherwise the tablets will fail the pharmacopeia test (or in-house test) and the lot or batch will be rejected.

In the industry today, greater emphasis is placed on material-handling systems and automation. The tests devised should consider these aspects together with the fundamental question, do we require a fluidized-bed coating column or a coating pan?

Essentially the programme should be divided into two parts: pharmaceutical appraisal and mechanical appraisal. The programme will identify the objectives and answer such questions as:

- What capacity (output) is required?
- Is the equipment required for laboratory, process development or production purposes?
- Is it proposed to establish a standard range of units from laboratory through process development to production? (If this approach is adopted, then alternative equipment should be evaluated to ensure a back-up position when or if problems develop with the preferred supplier.)
- Does the equipment comply with current Good Manufacturing Practice (cGMP)?
- What validation problems exist?
- What is the effect of coating different types and shapes of tablets?
- What are the safety aspects?

The initial tests should be conducted to derive basic pharmaceutical and mechanical data such as optimum shapes of tablets, coating times and drying air-handling requirements.

If tablet-coating equipment is considered, it can be divided into four parts:

1. the coating pan;
2. the system that applied the coating;
3. the air-handling system;
4. the monitoring and control systems.

Many parameters need to be recorded and some form of automatic sensor reading and recording system is very useful to provide a printout of the results of the trial.

Once it is decided to perform a full-scale trial, then these trials should be divided into a number of phases which subject the machine to both ideal and non-ideal operating conditions. A log should be maintained to record faults that develop, and from this time/event log a general indication of the machine's performance can be derived.

To carry out the test, load up the machine with each shape of tablet or particulates and in turn coat under ideal conditions, applying the following criteria for the appraisal of the equipment:

1. Uniformity of weight between individual tablets after coating for a definite time interval.
2. Uniformity of weight between groups of tablets (same time intervals as in 1).
3. General appearance of coated tablets.
4. Need for polishing.
5. Proportion of rejects.
6. Time spent clearing operating faults (blocked nozzles).
7. In-process control of coated weights (if fitted).
8. Maintain a time event log.

The machine should then be run under non-ideal conditions.

1. Pan: Reduce load to a low level in the pan, and check the weight variation of the coat.
2. Examine the effects of changing the drying air temperature and, if possible, the humidity.
3. Vary the speed of the machine over as wide a range as is possible.
4. Estimate the amount of dust produced, the smooth running or vibration of the machine, and examine for overheating of motor.
5. List any modifications that are required.
6. Consider the noise level near the machine, the extent to which moving parts are protected and how easy it is to load and unload the machine.

If the equipment is fitted with an automatic weight control system, then Phase 1 should be repeated to check the performance of this system. Only checks on the weight of the coated tablets are required, but a time/event log should be kept.

The most fundamental of all these tests is checking the weight of the coated tablet. For manually operated tested systems, this is relatively simple and checks can be in line with an appropriate monograph in the USP, BP or EC pharmacopeias (or other pharmacopeias depending on the country of origin) or the company's own corporate specifications. Determination of elementary statistics such as mean weight, standard deviation and coefficient of variation can be used to evaluate the samples. Where the equipment under evaluation has a high output then the experimental plan is more complex and there are other variables which will apply.

8.9.1 Pharmaceutical evaluation

Having decided on the system to be tested (pan or column), experimental materials will be required. Further questions need to be answered.

1. What coating formulations will the equipment use? For example:
    (a) sugar;
    (b) film (aqueous or organic).

2.   Will the coating provide standard, enteric or sustained release characteristics?
3.   What shape are the tablets?

Many of these variables can be studied using a placebo or blank tablets (active ingredients are very costly and, depending on the location of the tests, GMP considerations may prevent sale of the product.) However, no simulated system can exactly reproduce the active formulation and the final trial will require at least one batch of actives to be coated in the equipment of choice before a final decision is made.

The following experimental plan is designed to evaluate a tablet coater:

1.   Define location and environmental controls available.
2.   What system will be used to record process parameters? For example:
     (a)   manual;
     (b)   computer.
3.   What parameters are being recorded? For example:
     (a)   temperature;
     (b)   humidity;
     (c)   pan speed;
     (d)   spray rate, etc..
4.   Is the location a validated GMP facility?
5.   What tablet parameters are being measured or tested? For example:
     (a)   friability;
     (b)   coating uptake;
     (c)   moisture content;
     (d)   dissolution.
6.   What sampling plan is being used?
7.   What is the most critical aspect of the test programme? For example:
     (a)   appearance;
     (b)   quality of coat applied per tablet.

8.9.2   Mechanical evaluation

Simple machines are generally the best to operate and maintain. All equipment manufactured by the leading companies can achieve a pharmaceutically elegant product; however, certain products perform better on some types of machines than on others. It is not always possible to define the scientific basis for this and it is better to test the product on a number of different types to determine the best performance.

One of the main areas of mechanical concern for a tablet-coating operation is how quickly and easily a change may be completed and the machine cleaned ready for the manufacture of a different product. In addition, the main emphasis during evaluation must be on the following areas:

●   lubrication systems;
●   access for maintenance;
●   noise level;

- mechanical and electrical documentation;
- materials of construction finishes and standards, particularly product contact surfaces;
- maintenance required;
- instrumentation systems;
- equipment specifications;
- ease of cleaning;
- safety (how well is the operator protected from moving parts and what inter-locks are provided?);
- services required;
- cost of basic unit, spares and change parts;
- dimensions (footprint and height clearance required) and weight;
- type of air-handling system available and its control;
- type of exhaust air system;
- loading and unloading systems;
- after-sales service provided by manufacturer or agent

All of these items need to be evaluated in the overall appraisal.

8.9.3   cGMP and validation

No equipment evaluation is complete without an assessment of cGMP and valida-tion requirements. Validation is expensive and the documentation supplied for the equipment should be examined for details on:

- specifications
- materials of construction used for product contact
- maintenance schedules and manual
- operating manual
- diagnostic fault analysis
- calibration of instruments
- documentation of control system.

316L (low carbon content) stainless steel is the most commonly used material where products are in contact and is readily accepted by regulatory agencies as the material of choice. Painted surfaces are now being replaced universally by stainless steel cladding and this improves both the appearance and the cleaning operation.

Some loading and unloading of equipment requires the use of a vacuum and the effectiveness of this sytem should be tested to ensure consistent performance. Separate dust extraction may be required and an assessment of the way in which the filters are installed, how easily they can be changed, and their cost, should be deter-mined as part of the engineering/GMP evaluation.

Companies that supply excellent equipment are not always so efficient in provid-ing simple but detailed operating instructions for the machine. It must be borne in mind that a standard operating procedure (SOP) will be required, and assimilating badly written or poorly translated documentation can be lengthy, and expensive.

Calibration of instruments must be addressed to ensure that they are easily maintained in their operating range and it is important to differentiate between critical and convenience instruments. Critical instruments must be calibrated in their operating range against known traceable standards for validation. Examples would be the temperature sensor for measuring the bed temperature required to ensure that the tablets do not reach a temperature which may affect the stability of the active ingredient or its dissolution. Critical instruments are defined as those likely to affect the quality of the finished product. Convenience instruments are those required to provide data for production operations and management purposes, e.g. a timer which records the time taken to coat a batch of tablets.

8.10   EXPERIMENTAL PLAN

In tablet-coating equipment evaluation one of the most important aspects is to define the experimental plan. It may be that some preliminary test work is required to determine what are the most critical operations on a particular machine. This can be achieved using a placebo material before proceeding to the plan proper. It should be remembered that faults do not always show up on large capacity equipment until it has been operating for several hours and reaches a steady state operating temperature.

Placebo formulations do not necessarily behave as products containing active formulations and a final trial will be required using the product. The size of this trial will depend on cost and whether the material used can be sold. These trials are best conducted in registered premises to ensure all cGMP requirements are met.

It is also worth discussing with other users (companies that use the equipment under consideration) their particular preferences and experiences. (Many pharmaceutical manufacturing companies will discuss their use and assessment of the performance of various types of equipment.)

The following check list may be useful in developing an experimental plan:

1. Define objectives:
   (a)   comparison of new equipment against existing (same supplier);
   (b)   higher capacity required;
   (c)   new product requires tablet coating.
2. Define formulations to be used:
   (a)   placebo: the physical characteristics required;
   (b)   product containing actives;
   (c)   coating.
3. Define tests:
   (a)   on tablet core;
   (b)   on coated tablet.
4. Define location:
   (a)   in-house;
   (b)   at equipment suppliers;
   (c)   other.

5. Define personnel expertise requirements for tests:
   (a) formulation pharmacist;
   (b) quality control/quality assurance;
   (c) engineering support;
   (d) others.
6. Validation/cGMP input requirements
7. Cost:
   (a) manhours;
   (b) materials:
       (i)   placebo;
       (ii) product;
       (iii) coating types.
   (c) other:
       (i) transport;
       (ii) total cost of test programme.

9

Environmental considerations: treatment of exhaust gases from film-coating processes

Graham C. Cole

SUMMARY

Solvents such as acetone, methylene chloride, chloroform, ethanol and methanol must be prevented from entering the environment. Two options are available: convert all the processes to aqueous-based formulations or recover all the solvent by the use of an appropriate system. Recovery is expensive and is generally the reason for pharmaceutical companies to convert coating formulations to aqueous systems or formulate aqueous coating for all new products.

Where this is not possible, a solvent recovery system must be used. Some options are discussed in this chapter together with systems for removing particulates from the exhaust gases.

9.1 INTRODUCTION

No coating process is 100% efficient in terms of the amount of solids incorporated into the coating and the amount actually deposited on the tablets. Some losses will always occur. The efficiency of the process is very difficult to measure as the tablets themselves may lose weight by abrasion and by loss of moisture from the core during the coating process. Weighing the tablets before and after coating will not, therefore, give an absolute measure of the weight of coating deposited. Various workers have devised methods of measuring the amount of coating applied and have claimed efficiencies of 85–95% and even higher. Some of the coating material will be deposited on the pan and some will escape with the drying air in the exhaust system.

Material can be lost from the tablets in several ways. If the tablets are not dedusted before they are loaded into the pan, the dust on them will be removed by the tumbling action, intertablet friction and the exhaust air. If tablets are left rolling in the pan for any length of time without application of sufficient coating, then the frictional effects of the tablets being in contact with each other and the pan will result in some weight loss. This material will be removed with the exhaust air.

In addition to the particulate solids in the exhaust air, the solvent (organic or aqueous) used to apply the coating will be present. For sugar coating or aqueous-based film coating it is not necessary to remove the water from the exhaust gases, but where organic solvents are used they must be removed to prevent environmental pollution. If they can be recovered in a usable form, not necessarily for coating, cost savings can be achieved which will offset the cost of plant used for their recovery.

The total quantity of heat used in the coating process is relatively small and its value will depend upon the cost of the fuel used and the efficiency of the heating system. However, if some of this heat can be recovered in combination with solvent recovery it can further improve the economics of the total coating process.

9.2 CYCLONES

The simplest and cheapest method to remove solid particles present in the exhaust gases is the cyclone. Air enters this equipment tangentially at the top and is forced to spiral downwards into the bottom section. As the dust particles in the air have a much greater mass than the gas molecules, the centrifugal force exerted on them is much larger and they are thrown against the wall of the cyclone. The particles pass down the wall of the cyclone with the air and are collected at the bottom. The gas then flows up the centre of the cyclone in a much smaller spiral and escapes at the top. The solid particles which collect at the bottom of the cyclone are continuously removed by means of a rotary valve or via an air lock with automatically operated flap valves. Typical examples of centrifugal separations are shown in *The Chemical Engineers Handbook* (Perry & Chilton).

This equipment has the advantage that it is cheap to build and install, it has no moving parts and therefore it requires little maintenance. However, it is not totally efficient. Cyclones are usually only suitable for removing particles larger than 50 μm and many particles smaller than this are present in coating exhaust gases.

For the particle to be removed from the air stream its centrifugal force must be greater than the drag of the air which tends to carry it away. To increase the centrifugal force, the diameter of the cyclone must be reduced and this will in turn increase the pressure drop across it and hence the power required to drive the air through.

Some manufacturers now produce high-efficiency cyclones and these are usually operated as a series of small units to obtain the required capacity without introducing an excessive pressure drop. These can be suitable for removing in excess of 95% of all particles larger than 5 μm.

It is difficult with this type of equipment to specify exactly what its performance will be unless trials are conducted using specific operating conditions. Sometimes it is possible to obtain much higher efficiencies than those predicted by theoretical calculations. Particles can agglomerate in the cyclone, resulting in the removal of a much larger percentage of the small particles.

Efficiency can also be affected by changes in the air volume; one common cause of a reduction in efficiency is leakage of air into the cyclone at the discharge point.

9.3 FABRIC FILTERS

These are probably the most commonly used method of removing dust particles from airstreams. The design of the units varies considerably from one manufacturer to another. The filter elements are either in the form of bags or candles. The main object of the design being to make the maximum surface area of cloth available for filtration in the minimum space but in such a way that the whole of the surface area of the cloth is exposed to the contaminated air.

A wide variety of fabric types is available which enables the most appropriate type of filtration to be selected. This type of filter is capable of 99% efficiency and can remove particles down to submicron size. The performance of the filter varies very little with air flow rate; but the surface of the fabric will gradually become coated with the particles being removed from the air, resulting in a pressure drop across the filter. Magnahelic gauges or monometers are generally used to monitor filter performance. Any resistance to air flow in the exhaust will reduce the air flow through the coating pan, and in turn affect the coating process. It is, therefore, necessary to monitor the air flow and control it to ensure consistent coating conditions.

Most filters of this type are fitted with a means of automatically cleaning the filter surface. This can either be by mechanical shaking or by reverse air flow through the fabric to remove the particles adhering to the surface. Obviously filtration cannot take place while the cleaning is proceeding. As it would be detrimental to the coating process to stop the air flow each time the filter is cleaned, a method of maintaining the air flow must be devised. One solution is to arrange the filter in, for example, three subsections. In this case, two sections would filter the air while the third was being cleaned, with each section in turn being automatically shut down and the exhaust air from the coating process directed to the other two. Ultrasonic frequencies can also be used to separate dust particles from the fabric. Fig. 9.1(5) illustrates the use of ultrasonics and the cleaning of filters by mechanical shaking Fig. 9.1 (1–4).

One recent development which has improved the cleaning of filters is the introduction of a fabric which is coated on one side with a 'plastic' membrane. The surface coated with plastic has a very small pore structure compared with that of conventional material. This prevents the particles penetrating the surface of the material and the particles much less tendency to adhere to the surface of the filter. It is consequently easier to clean. It also allows the filter to operate for long periods with a lower pressure drop (i.e. near to new fabric conditions) than is possible with traditional filter cloths.

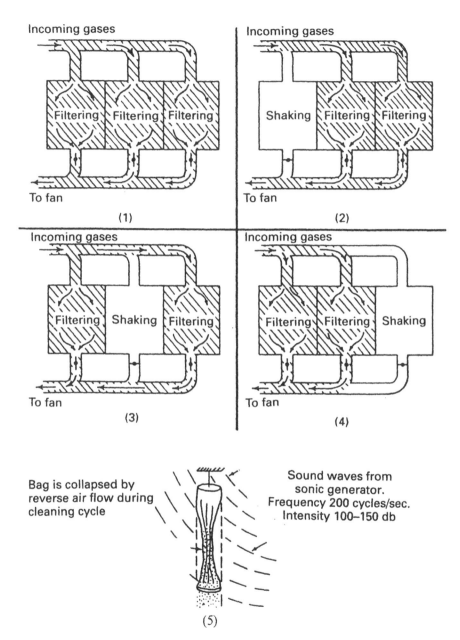

Fig. 9.1 Fabric bag cleaning with reverse air flow and ultrasonic vibration.

Fabrics have the advantage that they can be chosen to form the filter so that the required degree of filtration is obtained. They are also resistant to attack by organic solvents should they be present in the exhaust gases. Their main disadvantage is their physical size.

9.4   WET SCRUBBERS

A simpler and cheaper piece of equipment than the cloth filter is the wet scrubber. This type of equipment takes many forms but it essentially consists of a two-stage process taking place in one piece of equipment. At first the exhaust air is mixed with water from a spray, to ensure that the solid particles are wetted or captured by the drops of liquid. The air is then turned 180° and passed into a much larger diameter chamber to reduce its velocity. In this stage the larger drops fall back and the smaller ones are removed by the mist eliminator.

The design of the first part is critical and differs considerably from one manufacturer to another. The objective here is to ensure maximum particle/water contact and the highest level of solids removal. If good contact is achieved, a moderate proportion of submicron particles and over 90% of particles as small as 5 μm can be eliminated.

The design of the second stage is equally important and again designs vary widely. The danger in this part of the equipment is that any small droplets of water which do pass through the mist eliminator will carry some solid particles, thus reducing the efficiency of the unit.

The main advantages are:

● Its small size – considerably less that that required for the equivalent fabric filter.
● Low maintenance costs.
● Low power consumption.

Its main disadvantage, if in fact it is a disadvantage, is the method of disposing of the solution/slurry which collects in the base of the unit. It is usual to operate the unit on a closed system, i.e. the water is not continuously run to waste. If the water was continuously run to waste the cost of the water used could be quite considerable. After several batches of tablets have been coated, it is necessary to dispose of the solution/slurry—which may contain a certain amount of active material—using a specifically designed treatment system or a specialist waste disposal company. If scrubbers are used in conjunction with a sugar-coating process, the dilute sugar solution which collects in the scrubber is an ideal medium for bacterial growth. It is, therefore, essential that it is cleaned regularly. In fact scrubbers have been referred to as units which turn an air pollution problem into a water pollution problem.

An added advantage compared to cyclones and fabric filters, the wet scrubber can also remove organic solvents from the exhaust gases. This applies particularly to water-soluble solvents such as alcohol.

9.5   CYCLONE SCRUBBERS

One of the ways of improving the efficiency of a water-washing system for solids removal is to combine the advantages of the cyclone with that of the simple scrubber. The design of this equipment also varies widely. Water can be introduced at the top, bottom or even on the central axis. The wet cyclone offers some advantages for certain types of gas cleaning, but it is doubtful if this type of equipment could offer any substantial advantages over a simple scrubber for the cleaning of exhaust gases from a tablet-coating plant.

9.6 ELECTROSTATIC PRECIPITATORS

Another type of gas cleaning used is electrostatic precipitation. It is very good for removing small particles from gas streams. Electrostatic precipitators are capable of efficiencies as high as 97–98% for particles down to 0.05 μm and are suitable for very large gas volumes. However, their installation and running costs are much higher than for any of the other equipment described and there could be dangers when inflammable solvents are used.

9.7 REMOVAL OF ORGANIC SOLVENTS

Some organic solvents can be removed by washing the exhaust air. However, the type of wet scrubber already described is not designed to obtain the best results for the maximum removal of solvents. Other problems occur if solvents such as methylene chloride are being used. Methylene chloride will, to some extent, decompose to produce a dilute solution of hydrochloric acid, which is corrosive. To overcome this problem one European pharmaceutical company has made the decision that all their organic solvent-based coating will be carried out without the use of methylene chloride which has been replaced by ethanol. This enables the exhaust gases from the coating plant to be removed by washing with water.

9.8 GAS ABSORPTION TOWERS

For the highest efficiency of solvent removal the equipment must ensure maximum exposure of gas and liquid surfaces to each other. This can be done in three ways.

1. The liquid can be broken up into a number of slow-moving films which are dispersed through the gas.
2. The liquid can be broken up into as small a droplet size as possible and dispersed into the gas steam.
3. The gas can be broken up into small bubbles that are passed through the liquid.

As with all types of gas cleaning equipment the design varies widely from one manufacturer to another. Often more than one of these concepts are combined in different parts of the equipment.

One system which could be suitable for use with exhaust gases from a coating plant consists of two towers, a short fairly large diameter tower and a much taller tower with a smaller diameter. In the first tower water is sprayed as very fine droplets to remove some of the solvent. In the second tower the gases flow upwards through a series of trays against a downward flow of water.

So much has been published on the design of these absorption towers and there are so many possible designs for the internal structure that it is not possible to deal with all the variations. If this is considered an option then a specialist company should be consulted.

The main advantage of this type of cleaning process is that it is probably the cheapest means of efficiently removing solvents such as alcohol. Its main disadvantage is that the solvent is lost as the solution is normally too dilute for economic recovery.

9.9   CARBON ABSORPTION SYSTEMS

A carbon absorption plant consists of two or more towers each containing a bed of active carbon. Any solid particles are first removed from the exhaust gases as these tend to block the carbon bed. The gases are passed through the first tower or the first set of towers depending upon the total quantity of gases to be treated. The solvent molecules are absorbed onto the carbon. This continues until a significant amount of solvent can be detected in the gases leaving the tower, i.e. the carbon bed has become saturated with solvent; here the gases are diverted to the second tower where absorption of the solvent continues. The first tower is then stripped of solvent by passing steam through the carbon bed. The steam/solvent vapours are condensed and the solvent/water mixture collected. The carbon bed is dried and cooled ready for a second pass of the exhaust gases. The size of the plant is to some extent governed by the time of the stripping, drying and cooling stages, in other words by the number of towers or the size of tower that is required to absorb the solvent vapour until the first unit can be brought back into use.

For tablet coating, which is frequently a batch process with a period between batches, it might be possible to use just one tower. If the time between batches is sufficient for stripping, drying and cooling to take place, or if the tower has a capacity to absorb the solvent from several batches before stripping, then a one-tower system would be suitable which would reduce the capital cost of the plant.

The major disadvantage of this system is that the collector contains a mixture of solvents or solvents and water. It is usually necessary to distil this mixture before the solvent can be reused and this requires additional plant and higher capital investment. If a solvent mixture has been used which cannot be completely separated by distillation, for example, an azeotropic mixture, then the problem is more complex.

Various reports on the economics of operating this type of plant in connection with film coating give different results. Early reports said that the value of the solvent recovered offset the operating costs of the plant but the capital cost had to be considered as the cost of complying with antipollution legislation. More recent reports indicate that it is possible to obtain a return on the capital invested but this depends on the quality of the solvent recovered.

9.10   CONDENSATION SYSTEMS

The alternative method of recovering the solvents is by condensation. A very interesting paper was published recently in *Die Pharmaceutical Industrie* by Koblitz,

Bergbauer-Ehrhardt of Sandoz, Nürnberg, concerning this particular method. The experimental system they are using has many advantages over carbon absorbers. The exhaust gases leaving the coating pan are first filtered and then passed through an air to air heat exchanger, where they are cooled from about 45–50°C to about 7–8°C. The gases then pass into a condenser and cool in two or three stages to –30°C. It can be shown from vapour pressure calculations that at this temperature 98% of the solvent vapour will be condensed. The liquid is collected and here it is in a form that can be reused without further treatment.The cold gases are then passed through the other side of the first exchanger, where they cool the air leaving the coating plant before it enters the condenser and, in turn, are warmed by that air. The exhaust gases then pass to a reheater. The reheater and condenser are linked by a heat pump so that at least some of the heat removed is replaced. The gases are then returned to the coating pan via a final heat exchanger which is used to raise their temperature to the required level.

This type of plant is expensive to install, but apart from preventing any pollution of the atmosphere, it recovers the solvent in a usable form and reduces the heat input resulting in savings in operating costs.

One difficulty which can occur with this system is the control of any water which enters the system. If ethyl alcohol in the form of Industrial Methylated Spirit is used it will contain water. This water, as well as any entering the system from any other source, is likely to form ice on the heat exchanger surface of the condenser, thus reducing the effectiveness of the condenser.

For companies that require a fully engineered recovery system, Glatt offer two systems—based on closed loop and fluid bed vacuum—for solvents such as acetone, methylene chloride, ethyl alcohol (ethanol), methyl alcohol (methanol) and isopropyl alcohol.

An example of a closed loop system for solvent recovery is shown in Fig. 9.2, and an example of a Glatt vacuum fluid bed dryer coater is shown in Fig. 9.3.

There are various ways in which water can be removed, and these systems probably offer the most cost effective ways of operating an organic solvent-based film-coating process.

Ten years ago it looked possible that aqueous-based film coating could take over completely and that organic solvent-based coating could gradually die out, and this is generally true. However, quite a number of companies have at least one product which must be coated from an organic solvent-based coating and it will be necessary to ensure that all of the particulates and solvents from this product are prevented from entering the environment. Once the equipment is installed for solvent recovery, and if it is as economic to operate as condensation appears to be, then there is no reason why other products should not be coated from organic solvent-based solutions.

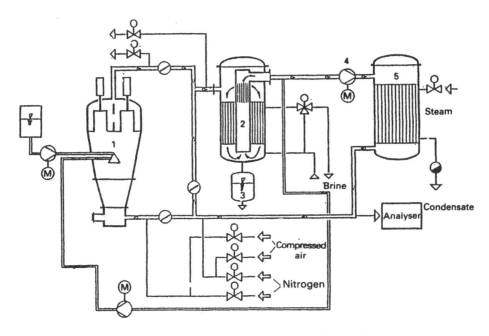

Fig. 9.2 Closed loop solvent recovery system (Glatt). 1. Fluid bed coating column,
2. Condenser, 3. Solvent container, 4. Blower, 5. Gas heater.

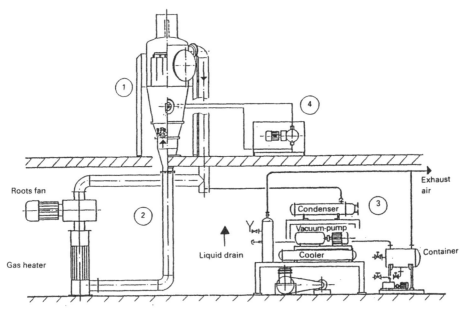

Fig. 9.3 Fluid bed coating column with condensate solvent recovery. (Glatt)
1. Coating column, 2. Fan and heater for fluid bed air, 3. Vacuum pump and condenser,
4. Pump.

10

Automation of coating processes

Graham C. Cole

SUMMARY

Current Good Manufacturing Practice (cGMP) and the demands of the regulatory authorities world-wide requires greater care in the design of manufacturing facilities, the selection of materials used in their construction, their layout, the equipment used in the preparation of tablets to be coated and the coating operation. It is claimed that robotic systems will eventually take over all processing tasks! (Kanig & Rudic,1986). This chapter will discuss automation concepts and suggestions based on cGMP (DHSS, 1983) in two areas:

- the design and layout of the building
- the control and transfer of materials between the various unit operations.

An examination of Fig. 7.1 (Chapter 7) shows the general requirement, and this chapter will describe how automation of this process can be achieved.

10.1 INTRODUCTION

Since 1970 the explosion in the development of the microprocessor, the programmable controller and personal computers has provided tools to make substantial productivity improvements in manufacturing systems. Many of the major pharmaceutical products in the oral solid dosage field are now produced using automated plants. Merck's ALDOMET manufacturing facility is well known and a well-documented example (Lumsden, 1982; Fig 10.1). This process uses fluidized bed coating columns. Figs 10.2 and 10.3 show schemes that uses both side-vented and conventional pans.

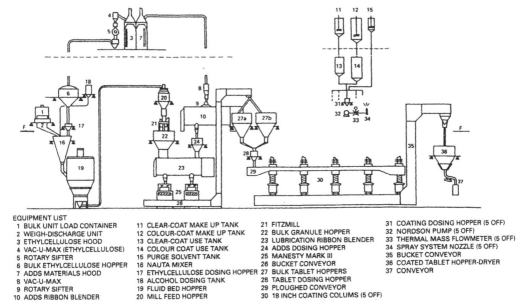

EQUIPMENT LIST

1 BULK UNIT LOAD CONTAINER	11 CLEAR-COAT MAKE UP TANK	21 FITZMILL	31 COATING DOSING HOPPER (5 OFF)
2 WEIGH-DISCHARGE UNIT	12 COLOUR-COAT MAKE UP TANK	22 BULK GRANULE HOPPER	32 NORDSON PUMP (5 OFF)
3 ETHYLCELLULOSE HOOD	13 CLEAR-COAT USE TANK	23 LUBRICATION RIBBON BLENDER	33 THERMAL MASS FLOWMETER (5 OFF)
4 VAC-U-MAX (ETHYLCELLULOSE)	14 COLOUR COAT USE TANK	24 ADDS DOSING HOPPER	34 SPRAY SYSTEM NOZZLE (5 OFF)
5 ROTARY SIFTER	15 PURGE SOLVENT TANK	25 MANESTY MARK III	35 BUCKET CONVEYOR
6 BULK ETHYLCELLULOSE HOPPER	16 NAUTA MIXER	26 BUCKET CONVEYOR	36 COATED TABLET HOPPER-DRYER
7 ADDS MATERIALS HOOD	17 ETHYLCELLULOSE DOSING HOPPER	27 BULK TABLET HOPPERS	37 CONVEYOR
8 VAC-U-MAX	18 ALCOHOL DOSING TANK	28 TABLET DOSING HOPPER	
9 ROTARY SIFTER	19 FLUID BED HOPPER	29 PLOUGHED CONVEYOR	
10 ADDS RIBBON BLENDER	20 MILL FEED HOPPER	30 18 INCH COATING COLUMS (5 OFF)	

Fig. 10.1   ALDOMET manufacturing and coating process (MSD).

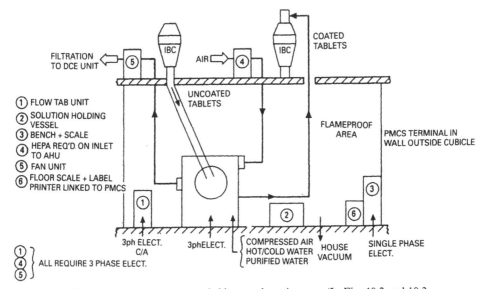

Fig. 10.2   Feed system to automated side-vented coating pan. (In Figs 10.2 and 10.3 —
IBC: Intermediate Bulk Container; AHU: Air Handling Unit; PMCS: Process
Monitoring Control System; ELECT: Electricity; ph: Phase; C/A: Compressed Air; DCE:
Dust Control Equipment).

The purpose here is to consider some of the ideas for automated coating systems
that are incorporated into these plants, and to look at what has been achieved with
products that are not produced in large volumes and, therefore, require a more

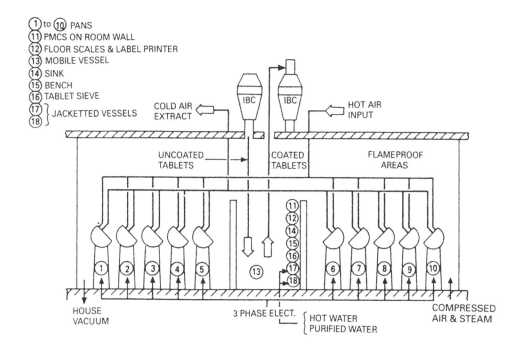

①to⑩ PANS
⑪ PMCS ON ROOM WALL
⑫ FLOOR SCALES & LABEL PRINTER
⑬ MOBILE VESSEL
⑭ SINK
⑮ BENCH
⑯ TABLET SIEVE
⑰} JACKETTED VESSELS
⑱}

Fig. 10.3   Automated feed system to standard coating pan.

flexible approach. The key driving forces towards providing better utilization of assets are:

- the rising cost of labour relative to productivity increases
- the high cost of energy and raw materials
- poor material-handling facilities
- the high cost of quality control
- inefficient use of manufacturing equipment
- short runs and a variable product mix.

It has been suggested that, in any productivity increase over the next decade, almost 60% will be provided by new and existing technology, 25% will be provided by capital and 13% by labour management (Morley, 1984).

All of these pressures are dependent on control. It is the control of the process, inventory, information flow, materials handling and the utilization of plant which is the essential part of automation.

Generally, to do this efficiently requires the use of a microprocessor or computer. Depending on the complexity of the operation, the number of parameters to be recorded and the degree of control required, there are a number of systems that can be used.

10.2   SYSTEMS

For the application of computer control to the coating process, some of the possible alternatives available are highlighted here. There are three main possibilities:

1. A data acquisition system;
2. A distributed control system;
3. A centralized computer system.

Each system is briefly described with points to consider when evaluating each of them and finally suggestions and conclusions on the final choice. It is not an exhaustive list but more a discussion to assist in making the basic decisions.

10.2.1 Data acquisition system

Fig. 10.4 shows the layout of a data acquisition system. These are normally small devices for low levels of inputs only, but some have limited computing power. They can also be used to provide printouts of the information gathered, similar to that described in Chapter 6. They do not provide any plant control and have only limited processing of information capacity. Some can be linked to high-powered computers which would store data or manipulate it, depending on the degree of automation required.

The field inputs have to be cabled back to a control location such as a control room and the system interface requires safety protection.

Advantages:
● Small and cheap.

Disadvantages:
● No control provided.
● Limited data processing.

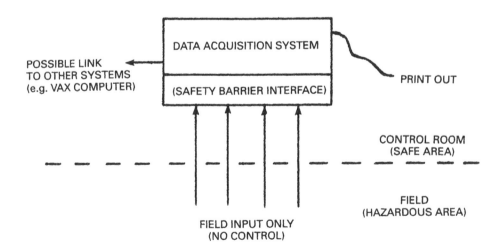

Fig. 10.4   Data acquisition system.

- Limited number of inputs.
- No data storage.
- Long lengths of field cabling required.
- No local operator interface.

10.1.2 Distributed control system

Fig. 10.5 illustrates the layout of a distributed control system. In a distributed system not only are the hardware items geographically distributed, but the functions of processing, power and software are also distributed.

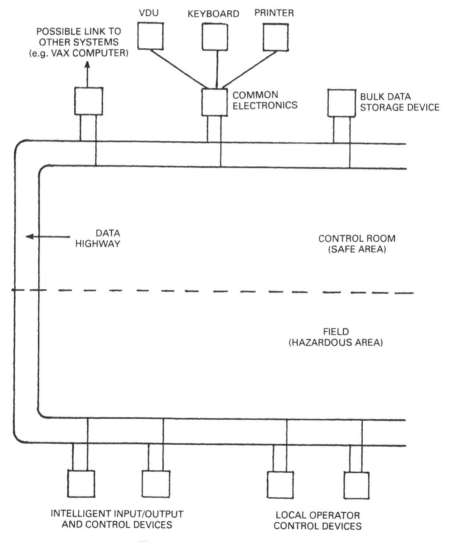

Fig. 10.5   Distributed control system.

Each hardware item performs a specific task and information is passed between the various hardware items using a dual data highway. This dual highway provides good security for communications.

The field devices, such as the input, output and control devices, must be protected by suitable housing and safety equipment for use in a hazardous area, particularly if flammable solvents are used in the coating process.

Computer type functions are distributed throughout the process area using smaller microprocessor devices. It can support local operator control devices located in the plant area providing these are adequately protected.

This system can provide process control for continuous variables such as atomizing air pressure and tablet-bed temperature and batch or sequence control. It can be linked to other devices such as an existing in-house computer.

Advantages:
- Batch, sequence operations and continuous control is available.
- Data logging and data storage are available.
- Calculations on the stored data can be performed.
- Logs and reports can be generated.
- Local operator interfaces can be provided.
- Batch and sequence control can store and use many different recipes and values, and the system can be used to optimize process control.
- System is easily expandable and very flexible.
- Short field cable lengths.
- High security of control as all functions are distributed.

Disadvantages:
- System more suitable for plants with greater than 500 loops.
- High cost due to its large capacity.
- Local plant equipment must be protected in safe enclosures.

10.2.3   Centralized control system
Fig. 10.6 shows the layout of a centralized computer control system. This is very similar to the distributed control system. It can perform all the same functions, but they are centralized within a computer system. The computer would normally be the process control manufacturer's standard.

Advantages:
- Same as distributed system.
- System size tends to be intermediate between the systems illustrated in Figs 10.4 and 10.5.

Disadvantages:
- Long lengths of field cabling required.
- System operation dependent on one device (the computer) thus a redundancy of a back-up computer may be required to increase reliability.

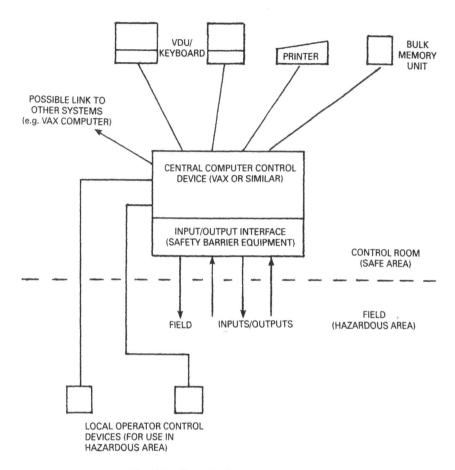

Fig. 10.6   Centralized computer system.

Ideally the type of system required for a coating plant should have the following capability:

- Data logging and process control of various parameters, temperature; spray rates.
- Batch control is required with various recipes and sequences.
- Optimization of batch control parameters.
- Flexibility to change the process, size of batches, product, etc.
- Local operator interface in hazardous area.
- Interface to field devices suitably protected against hazardous area (intrinsically safe circuits, etc.)
- Operator control/display within the control room via VDU/keyboard/printer devices.
- Calculations and optimization of sampled and/or measured variables for analysis.

- Printouts and logs required.
- System size relatively small (150 loops approximately).

Either the centralized or the distributed control system would be suitable for a film-coating facility, depending on the number of coating pans which, in turn, is related to the number of variables to be measured or recorded.

A number of additional options are also possible:

- A dual processor computer to provide back-up security for control and data storage.
- Links to an in-house computer can be accommodated if a separate system is used. This data can be passed to the in-house system for processing or display if required.
- Inventory control could be added.
- In a potentially hazardous plant, it may be worth considering a separate emergency shutdown system for increased safety.

In general, however, the centralized system is preferable to the distributed system for the following reasons:

- It is smaller and cheaper.
- System input/output interface is simpler while the distributed system requires special housings.
- It allows the possibility to use an existing computer.

A typical centralized control room is shown in Fig. 10.7.

Most process control and data logging manufacturers use their own computers and their software structure may not be comparable with the in-house computer software. However, the necessary interface can be provided, but this is always difficult and should be avoided if possible.

10.3   INSTRUMENTATION

Examples of the instruments necessary for automation were examined in Chapter 6. Here the instrumentation will not only control the process but will assist in moving materials from one unit operation to the next. A further example is shown in Fig. 10.8.

10.4   FACILITY DESIGN AND EQUIPMENT REQUIREMENTS

There are many different types of tablets that can be coated, ranging from a cosmetically coated tablet to those that use the osmotic pump principle to release the drug. Examples were illustrated in Fig. 7.3 (Chapter 7).

In the development and implementation of any automated tablet-coating process there are a number of objectives that must be addressed:

1. What types of product are to be handled?
    (a) Are they highly potent?

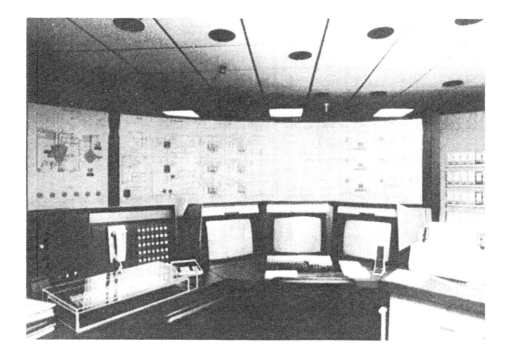

Fig. 10.7   Centralized control room.

(b)   Can they cause allergic reactions in the operators?
(c)   Are they mutagenic?

Current Good Manufacturing Practice suggests there are two overriding considerations that take precedence. These are:

(i)   total containment of the product within a closed system;
(ii)   providing a barrier between the product and the operator, i.e. total protection.

2.   Are these products beta-lactams, e.g. penicillin? If this is the case, then a separate manufacturing facility must be designed.
3.   What quantities and mix of products are required? There may be relatively small quantities of a number of products required rather than large quantities of individual products. In one case, flexibility of the operation is the main objective requiring a multiplexity of services, whereas a single dedicated production line can save on materials handling, personnel, and special conditions (protection from light and oxygen).

A five-year forecast of requirements will be needed as there may be new coated-tablet products coming through from Research and Development and some older products may be declining in volume. These factors should be assessed in the design

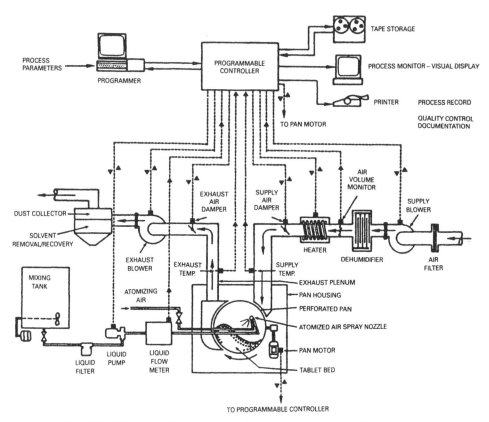

Fig. 10.8   Schematic of an instrumented and computer-controlled coating pan.

of a facility, the refurbishment of an existing operation or in selection of new equipment for development and production purposes.

10.5   PROCESS CONCEPT

To design the facility requires an understanding of the overall tablet-coating process. The building and building services provide the envelope around the process and the process operation must be performed in areas designed to conform to cGMP. It will also need a validation programme.

For any tablet-coating operation there are four essential requirements:

1.   a supply of tablet cores;
2.   a supply of coating materials;
3.   the process equipment;
4.   a building to house the equipment, raw materials and finished product.

A flow diagram should be developed, as shown in Fig. 11.2. (Chapter 11). All or some of these operations take place whether in a laboratory or on a production scale. For efficient and accurate operations the following stages must be assessed:

1. storage of raw materials—warehousing
2. raw material dispensing
3. process operations
4. packaging.

10.5.1 Warehousing

In all companies, the size of the inventory is critical to the efficient operation of any plant. More and more companies are employing Just-in-Time (JIT) concepts to minimize stock levels and ensure that First In First Out (FIFO) principles apply. A typical flow diagram is shown in Fig. 10.9. In addition, storage space must be available for raw materials and finished stock. The simplest way of handling all these requirements is by installing a computer-controlled materials management system. This records incoming goods, allocates location, and notifies internal departments of the arrival of these goods. The status of the material can be controlled using the computer and with limited personnel access the Quality Control Department can provide means of quarantining the materials until they are passed for production use or sale.

10.5.2 Dispensary

A schematic example is shown in Fig. 10.10. The size and equipment required will depend on the scale of the operation and the nature of the materials being dispensed.

All balances will be selected on the basis of their sensitivity and range of weights required. For example:

Balance 1   0.010 kg (sensitivity 0.01 mg)
Balance 2   10.0 kg (sensitivity 500 mg)
Balance 3   50.0 kg (sensitivity 1.0 g)

In some cases a floor balance may be installed for larger quantities up to 200 kg. It should be remembered that the cost of balances increases with their sensitivity. These balances will need to be located in cubicles in the dispensary, so that there is no danger of cross-contamination and different products can be weighed out simultaneously. An area should be provided for the short-term storage requirements of materials used in large quantities and an adjacent area should be provided for materials used in small quantities, i.e. colours and surfactants.

Each cubicle should be equipped with laminar air flow to ensure maximum protection for the operator, minimize dust contamination of the surrounding area and cross-contamination.

Each dispensary should be equipped with suitable dust masks, air supplied suits, safety showers and eye wash stations, to ensure the maximum safe handling of the materials. Carefully designed HVAC (heating, ventilating and air conditioning) and dust extraction systems are major requirements.

10.5.3 Process

The next stage in the material-handling procedure is to transfer the batch of raw

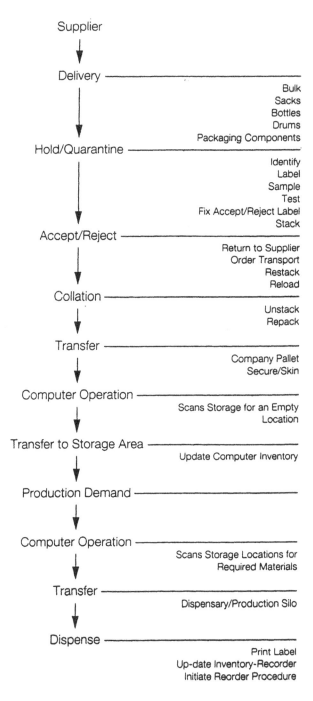

Fig. 10.9   Flow diagram for storage of materials.

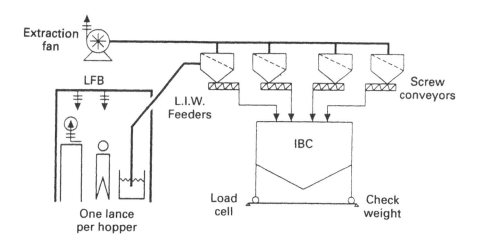

L.I.W.   Loss in weight feeders
L.F.B.   Laminar flow booth
I.B.C.   Intermediate bulk container

+||► Air flow

Fig. 10.10 Schematic diagram for an automated pharmaceutical dispensary.

materials to the production area for preparation of the powder mix ready for tablet core manufacture and raw materials for the preparation of the coating.

The layout of the process area will depend on the material-handling concept. If pneumatic transfer is used for an automatic transfer operation, then the IBC can be linked to the blender/granulator/dryer/mill and the blender to the tablet machine or an intermediate bulk container (IBC; see Fig. 10.11).

Figs 10.2 and 10.3 show an automated feed and receiving system for tablet-coating equipment. Units are linked to a process monitoring and control system (PMCS). For an automated system, coated tablets can be stored in an IBC until released to packaging; the IBC can be positioned above the packaging unit and the coated tablets are then gravity fed into the blister packer or securitainer filling unit.

The objective in all these operations should be to minimize manual transfer and reduce exposure and contact of the product to the operator and the environment.

10.5.4 Layout and design of facility

A typical layout is shown in Fig. 10.12. Process areas require high-quality finishes to maintain cGMP standards. Traditionally pharmaceutical secondary manufacturing facilities have been designed on the basis of single rooms or cubicles for each stage of the manufacturing process. Transfer of materials has been accomplished using a large drum or mobile trolley. Today the industry is investing in more automatic transfer systems for material handling in an attempt to reduce costs and improve yields. This results in a more integrated manufacturing unit. Computer integrated manufacturing (CIM) is becoming more widely used in the pharmaceuti-

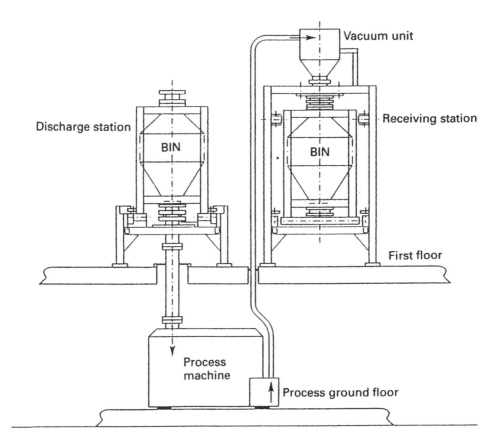

Fig. 10.11   Automated materials handling.

cal industry to reduce labour costs, improve efficiency and increase yields. It also reduces the size of the building and the high cost areas within that building for each manufacturing operation. The objective is to remove the service functions outside the process area into a lower grade technical area. This means that process utilities can be serviced without interfering with manufacturing operations as illustrated in Fig. 10.13. A comparison with Fig. 10.14 shows how the expensive process space has been reduced.

All these drawings have been numbered to indicate the grading of each area, e.g. 1, 2 or 3. These gradings refer to the quality of the air required in each area and the quality of the finishes required. Areas marked 3 will require minimum standards and areas marked 1 the maximum. Figs 10.15, 10.16 and 10.17 illustrate the concept required for an automated facility. The traffic floor (Fig. 10.17) is designed with a pathway for the movement of IBCs for feeding and receiving the product from the process equipment on the floor below (Fig. 10.16). An alternative process based on fluid bed granulation is shown in Fig. 10.18. This was built by SmithKline French (now part of SmithKline Beecham).

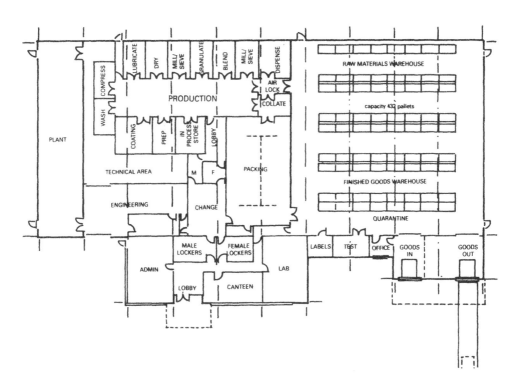

Fig. 10.12   Typical layout for a tablet-coating process.

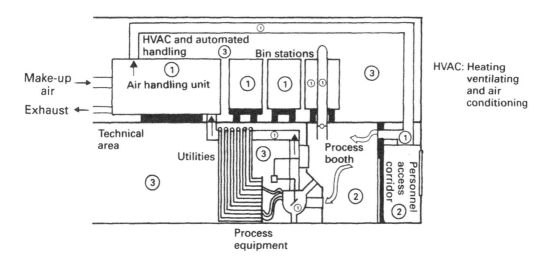

Fig. 10.13   Detailed section through an automated manufacturing facility.

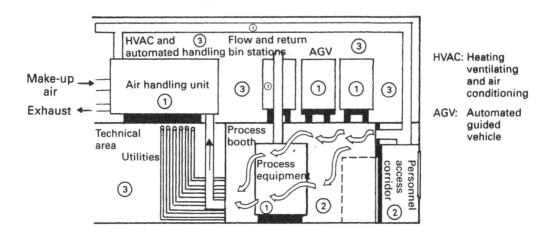

Fig. 10.14   Detailed section (contained equipment) through an automated manufacturing facility.

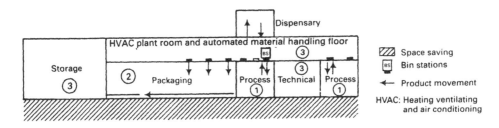

Fig. 10.15   Section through automated and non-automated facility showing flow of material.

The most difficult problem is how to transfer tablets (core and coated) between each unit of equipment. To a certain degree the system chosen will depend on the extent of damage that occurs and this relates to the robustness of each part of the tablet. It will also depend on how much deterioration the Quality Assurance Department can accept and write into the specifications. Older products can withstand little mechanical shock, whereas modern formulations have been developed using current materials which provide a greater degree of robust handling.

To transport tablets various systems have been tried, all with limited success. These are:

● bucket conveyors;
● fluidized bed transfer system;

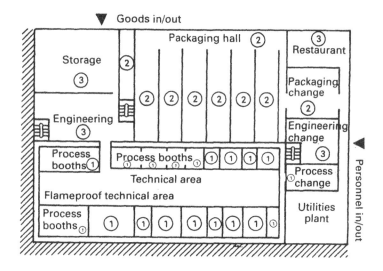

Fig. 10.16   Ground-floor layout for an automated facility.

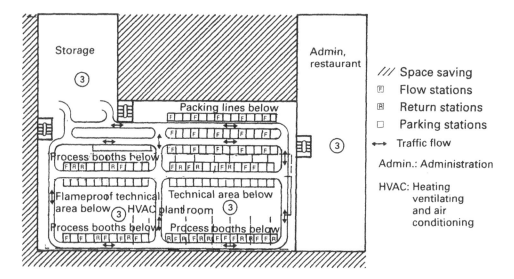

Fig. 10.17   First-floor layout for an automated facility.

- a mixture of perforated plates with a layer of fluidizing air;
- pulse air systems;
- vacuum systems;
- spiral vibrating chutes.

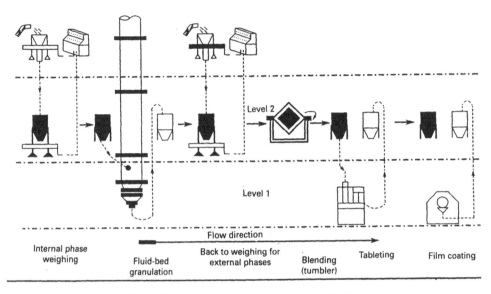

Fig. 10.18   Flow diagram for an automated facility.

REFERENCES

DHSS (1983) *Guide to Good Manufacturing Practice* 1983 (The Orange Guide), Department of Health and Social Security.

Kanig, J.L. & Rudic, E.M. (1986) The basics of robotic systems, *Pharm. Tech.* June

Lumsden, B. (1982) *Industrial Powder Technology Conf., London*, 24–25 November.

Morley, R.E. (1984) The rate of control in automation trends and perspectives *Pharmaceutical Engineering*, Jan–Feb.

11

Validation of tablet coating processes

Graham C. Cole

SUMMARY

Validation is a concept that means different things to different people. This chapter will highlight all the activities that are necessary to ensure that all aspects of the coating process are fully documented from design through to operation, to provide compliance with regulatory requirements.

'If it hasn't been documented, it hasn't been done.'

FDA

11.1 INTRODUCTION

The FDA defines validation as: 'Establishing documented evidence which provides a high degree of assurance that a specific process will consistently produce a product meeting its predetermined specifications and quality attributes.' Validation has also been defined as the activity performed to demonstrate that a given utility, system, process or piece of equipment does what it purports to do. The primary means of accomplishing this end is the scientific study designed to specifically permit the determination as to whether the entity under scrutiny in fact:

- meets or exceeds the specifications of its design;
- is properly built, shipped, received, stored, installed, operated and maintained;
- is suitable for its intended application;
- is in accordance with principles established and generally accepted by the scientific community;
- conforms to basic cGMP design criteria;

- will satisfy the concerns of regulatory bodies;
- is capable of consistently producing a product that is fit for use;
- will meet objectives established for productivity, safety and quality.

The EC has adopted very similar cGMP criteria.

This scientific study is generally detailed in a validation protocol. A well-designed validation programme properly supported by senior management will accrue considerable benefit to its sponsor. Not only will regulatory obligations be fulfilled, but also processes will be optimized, productivity improved and downtime reduced. In short, a validation programme with a sound scientific base and proper experimental design is simply good business if taken seriously and executed conscientiously.

Among the most relevant of the regulatory issues from the Code of Federal Regulations, Volume 21, that should be considered in the assembly of any validation programme are the following:

Part 58   Good Laboratory Practice For Non-clinical Laboratory Studies.
Part 210   Current Good Manufacturing Practice in Manufacturing, Processing, Packing, or Holding of Drugs; General.
Part 211   Current Good Manufacturing Practice for Finished Pharmaceuticals.

It is also necessary to take into consideration the various guidelines and manuals published by the EC, FDA, NIH and OSHA, e.g.

The Rules Governing Medicinal Products in the European Community. Vol. 4: *Guide to Good Manufacturing Practice for Medicinal Products*, 1989.

GMP regulations state what must be done, but do not attempt to explain how to do it; Guides and Guidelines do that. Since GMPs represent substantive law, they can be established only by due process. FDA Guides and Guidelines, on the other hand, can be written and made effective at any time, with or without public notice or hearings; but, they are not legally binding on the industry. In the USA, a person, a pharmaceutical firm, or the whole industry, can write its own guidelines if it so elects.

Obviously a compliance guideline is not very valuable unless all parties involved are in general agreement. Consequently, with regard to validation in the US, the last 13 years have seen a remarkably cooperative and widespread effort by members of the regulatory sector, the industrial sector, academia and, most recently, even the vendor sector, to establish meaningful guidelines.

11.2 SCOPE

The validation requirements are identified in the Documentation Master Plan for a facility. This Plan is considered necessary to explain all the constituent parts that are listed in the introduction and provide all the validation team members with a 'bible' so that they all 'sing from the same hymn book'. The Master Plan explains the GMP type documentation required and has the effect of producing similarity/ uniformity of documentation.

11.3 MASTER PLAN

The Master Plan serves a dual purpose:

1. It is a document which may be presented to regulatory bodies to convey the level or understanding of the company responsibilities concerning the validation programme along with plans to discharge that responsibility.
2. It is a guide to those administering and performing validation activities. The Master Plan will address and include, but need not necessarily be limited to, the following topics:

- Approvals.
- Introduction.
- Scope.
- Glossary of terms.
- Preliminary drawings/facility design.
- Process descriptions.
- Rooms and room classifications.
- Description of utilities.
- Description of process equipment.
- Automated systems.
- Equipment history files.
- Construction documentation.
- Description of required protocols.
- Lists of standard operating procedures (SOPs).
- Required document matrices.
- Validation schedules/construction schedule/integrated schedule.
- Protocol outlines/summaries.
- Environmental monitoring.
- Analytical testing procedures.
- Calibration programme.
- Training programme.
- Preventive maintenance programme.
- Change control programme.
- Document control programme.
- Manpower requirements.
- Key personnel.
- Protocol examples.
- SOP examples.

As part of the 'Validation Schedules' portion of the Master Plan, the typical schedule outline in Fig. 11.1 should be developed to show a completion date depending on the company's specific requirements. It is a living schedule and will evolve with time.

At this stage it is necessary to highlight some of the areas that should be addressed in the validation programme, even though the process under consideration is tablet coating. All validation programmes have common features and these are addressed under the following headings in the Master Plan.

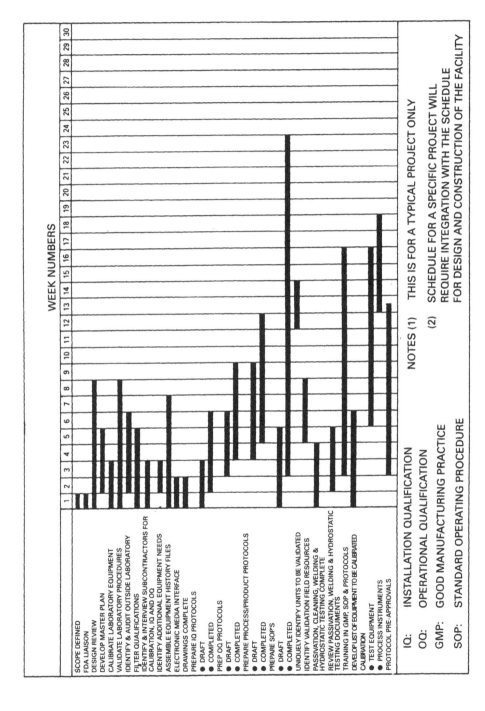

Fig. 11.1 Schedule for validation of coating processes from Cole, G.C. (1990) *Pharmaceutical Production Facilities: design and applications*, Ellis Horwood.

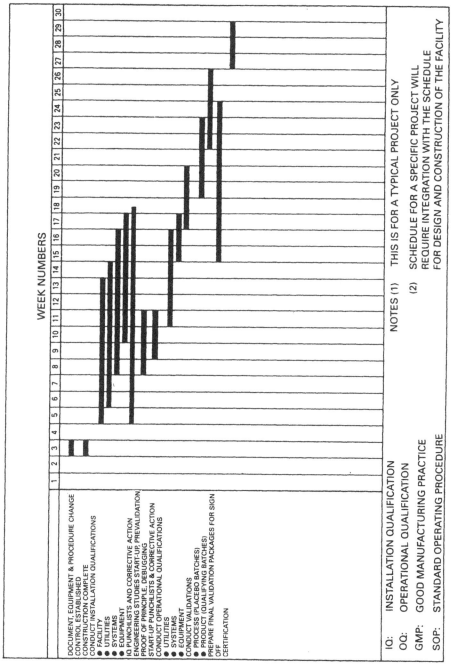

Fig. 11.1 (continued)   Schedule for validation of coating processes from Cole, G.C. (1990) *Pharmaceutical Production Facilities: design and applications*, Ellis Horwood.

Approvals

The approval of this Validation Master Plan will be the joint responsibility of a number of functional areas in the company's facility. Examples:

- Manufacturing.
- Engineering.
- Quality Assurance.
- R&D.
- Safety.
- Site Manager.
- Regulatory Affairs.
- Validation Manager.

The completion of this stage indicates review of the contents by the relevant disciplines and approval by responsible individuals.

Glossary of terms

This is not an exhaustive list but highlights some of the terms relevant to coating processes that must must be defined.

Acceptance criteria: The product specifications and acceptance/rejection criteria, such as acceptable quality level and unacceptable quality level, with an associated sampling plan, that are necessary for making a decision to accept or reject a lot or batch (or any other convenient subgroups of manufactured lots).

Action levels: Levels or ranges which, when deviated from, signal a potential drift from normal operating conditions; these ranges are not perceived as being detrimental to end-product quality.

Audit: An audit is a formal review of a product, manufacturing process, equipment, facilities or systems for conformance with regulations and quality standards.

Calibration: Comparison of a measurement standard or instrument of known accuracy with another standard or instrument to detect, correlate, report, or eliminate by adjustment any variation in the accuracy of the item being compared.

Certification: Documented statement by qualified authorities that a validation event has been done appropriately and that the results are acceptable. Certification is also used to denote the acceptance of the entire coating operation and the manufacturing facility where it takes place, as validated.

Change control: A formal monitoring system by which qualified representatives of appropriate disciplines review proposed or actual changes that might affect validated status and take preventive or corrective action to ensure that the system retains its validated state of control.

Computer validation: This is particularly relevant to automated coating systems. The validation of computers has been given a particular focus by the FDA.

Three documents have been published for agency and industry guidance. In February 1983 the agency published the *Guide to Inspection of Computerized Systems in Drug Processing*; in April 1987, the *Technical Reference in Software Development Activities* was published; on 16 April 1987 the agency published

Compliance Policy Guide 7132 in Computerized Drug Processing: Source Codes for Process Control Application Programmes.

In the inspection guide, attention is called both to hardware and software; some key points being the quality of the location of the hardware unit as to extremes of environment, distances between CPU and peripheral devices, and proximity of input devices to the process being controlled; quality of signal conversion, e.g. a signal converter may be sending inappropriate signals to a CPU; the need systematically to calibrate and check for accuracy of I/O devices; the appropriateness and compatibility within the distributed system of command overrides (e.g. can an override in one computer controlled process inadvertently alter the cycle of another process within the distributed system?). Maintenance procedures form another matter which interests the agency during an inspection. Other matters of concern are methods by which unauthorized programme changes are prevented, as inadvertent erasures, as well as methods of physical security.

Hardware validation should include verification that the programme matches the assigned operational function. For example, the recording of multiple lot numbers of each component may not be within the programme, thus second or third lot numbers of one component may not be recorded. The hardware validation should also include worse case conditions, e.g. the maximum number of alphanumeric code spaces should be long enough to accommodate the longest lot numbering system to be encountered. *Software validation* must be thoroughly documented—they should include the testing protocol, results, and persons resonsible for reviewing and approving the validation. The FDA regards source code—i.e. the human readable form of the programme written in its original programming language, and its supporting documentation for application programmes used in any drug process control—to be part of the master production and control records within the meaning of 21CFR, Parts 210, 211 (Current Good Manufacturing Practice Regulations). As part of all validation efforts, conditions for revalidations are a requirement.

Concurrent validation: Establishing documented evidence that the process, which is being implemented, can consistently produce a product meeting its predetermined specifications and quality attributes. This phase of validation activities typically involves careful monitoring/recording of the process parameters and extensive sampling/testing of the in-process and finished product during the initial implementation of the process.

Critical process variables: Those process variables that are deemed important to the quality of the product being produced.

Drug product: A finished dosage form—for example, coated tablet, capsule, solution, etc.,—that contains an active drug ingredient generally, but not necessarily, in association with inactive ingredients. The term also includes a finished dosage form that does not contain an active ingredient but is intended to be used as a placebo.

Dynamic attributes: These are classified into *functional*, *operational* and *quality* attributes (see below).

EC: European Community.

Edge of failure: A control or operating parameter value that, if exceeded, may have adverse effects on the state of control of the process and/or on the quality of the product.

Facilities: Facilities are areas, rooms, spaces, such as receiving/shipping, quarantine, rejected materials, approved materials warehouse, staging areas, process areas such as coating make-up and finishing rooms, etc.

FDA: Food and Drug Administration of the USA.

Functional attributes: Functional attributes are such criteria as controls, instruments, interlocks, indicators, monitors, etc., that are operating properly, pointing in the correct direction, valves which permit flow in correct sequence, etc.

Good Manufacturing Practices (GMPs): The minimum requirements by law for the manufacture, processing, packaging, holding or distribution of a material as established in Title 21 of the *Code of Federal Regulations*, Part 211 for finished pharamceuticals.

Installation qualification protocol: An installation qualification protocol (IQ) contains the documented plans and details of procedures which are intended to verify specific static attributes of a facility, utility/system, or process equipment. Installation qualification (IQ), when executed, is also a documented verification that all key aspects of the installation adhere to the approved design intentions and that the manufacturer's recommendations are suitably considered.

Operational attributes: Operational attributes are such criteria as a utility/system's capability to operate at rated ranges, capacities, intensities, such as revolutions per minute, spray rate per minute, kilos per square centimetre, pounds per square inch, temperature range, etc.

Operation qualification protocol: A operation qualification protocol (OQ) contains the plan and details of procedures to verify specific dynamic attributes of a utility system (air supply to coating pan) or process equipment (coating pan) throughout its operating range, including worse case conditions. Operation qualification (OQ), when executed, is documented verification that the system or subsystem performs as intended throughout all anticipated operating ranges.

Processes: Processes are those activities which are repeated frequently such as: spray coating; preparation of coating solutions (suspensions); pH adjustment, including the preparation of solutions which are used for adjusting the pH; cleaning in place (CIP), and the preparation of CIP solutions; the various piping adjustments required to direct the coating solutions, sanitizing/sterilizing in place (SIP) and supportive activities; any sterilization of product, component, garment, equipment, etc.; and any electromechanical or computer-assisted processes associated with them.

Process equipment: Process equipment are such items as scales, load cells, flow meters, coating pans, mixers, reaction/process/storage vessels, centrifuges, filters, driers, packaging equipment including electromechanical or computer-assisted instruments, controls, monitors, recorders, alarms, displays, interlocks, etc., which are used in the manufacture of pharmaceutical products.

Process parameters: Process parameters are the properties or features that can be assigned values that are used as control levels or operating limits. Process parameters ensure the product meets the desired specifications and quality. Examples might be: Pressure at 5.2 lb $in^2(g)$, temperature at $37 \pm 0.5°C$, flow rate at 10 ± 1.0 GPM, pH at 7.0 ± 0.2.

Process variables: Process variables are the properties or features of a process which are not controlled or which change in time or by demand; process variables do not change product specifications or quality.

Process validation: Establishing documented evidence which provides a high degree of assurance that a specific coating process will consistently produce a product meeting its predetermined specifications and quality attributes.

Process validation protocol: Process validation protocol (PV) is a documented plan and details of procedures to verify specific capabilities of process equipment system through the use of simulation materials, such as the use of placebo tablets in a coating process, a nutrient broth in the validation of an aseptic filling process, or the use of a placebo formulation in a tablet coating process. Here the term process validation (PV) will be used to include the use of the product as the material to validate the process.

Product validation: A product is considered validated after completion of three successive, successful, full-lot size attempts. These validation lots are saleable.

Prospective validation: Validation conducted prior to the distribution of either a new product, or product made under a revised manufacturing process, where the revisions may have affected the product's characteristics, to ensure that the finished product meets all release requirements for functionality and safety.

Protocol: A protocol is defined as a written plan stating how validation will be conducted.

Quality assurance: The activity of providing evidence that all the information necessary to determine that the product is fit for the intended use is gathered, evaluated and approved. The Quality Assurance Department executes this function.

Quality attributes: Quality attributes refer to those properties of the product of a utility/system, such as: resistivity of a water solvent, particulate matter, microbial and endotoxin limits of water for injection.

Quality control: The activity of measuring process and product parameters for comparison with specified standards to ensure that they are within predetermined limits and therefore, the product is acceptable for use. The Quality Assurance Department executes this function.

Retrospective validation: Validation of a process for a product already in distribution based upon establishing documented evidence, through review/analysis of historical manufacturing and product testing data, to verify that a specific process can be consistently produced meeting its predetermined specifications and quality attributes. In some cases a product may have been on the market without sufficient premarket process validation. Retrospective validation can also be useful to augment initial premarket prospective validation for new products or changed processes.

Revalidation: Repetition of the validation process or a specific portion of it.

Specifications: Document which defines what something is by quantitatively measured values. Specifications are used to define raw materials, in-process materials, products, equipment and systems.

Standard operating procedure (SOP): Written procedures followed by trained operators to perform a step, operation, process, compounding or other discrete function in the manufacture or production of a bulk pharmaceutical chemical, biological, or drug product.

Utilities/systems: Utilities/systems are buildings, mechanical equipment and include such things as heating, ventilation and air conditioning (HVAC) systems, process water, product water (purified water, USP), water for injection (WFI), clean steam, process air, vacuum, gases, etc. They include electromechanical or computer-assisted instruments, controls, monitors, recorders, alarms, displays, interlocks, etc., which are associated with them.

Validation: Establishing documented evidence which provides a high degree of assurance that a specific process will consistently produce a product meeting its predetermined specifications and quality.

Validation programme: The collective activities that are related to validation.

Validation protocols: Validation protocols are written plans stating how validation will be conducted, including test parameters, product characteristics, production equipment, and decision points on what constitutes acceptable test results. This definition is provided by the FDA of the USA. A maximum of four protocols are possible. They are protocols for installation qualification, operation qualification, process validation and product validation. When the protocols have been executed successfully they produce documented evidence that the system has been validated.

Validation scope: The scope answers the question: What is to be validated? In the instance of the manufacturing plant, this would include the elements which impact critically on the quality of the product. The elements which require validation are facilities, utilities/systems, process equipment, process and product.

Worst case: A set of conditions encompassing upper and lower processing limits and circumstances, including those within standard operating procedures, which pose the greatest chance of a process or product failure when compared to ideal conditions. Such conditions do not necessarily induce product or process failure.

So, what is required to develop the documentation for validation of the coating process?

11.4   PROCESS DESCRIPTION

Initially we need the process description. This can be divided into two parts: the manufacture of the core and the coating process.

11.4.1   Manufacture of the core
This should detail the following:

● formulation;
● list of ingredients and their specifications;
● equipment required for manufacture, e.g. mixer, granulators, driers, compressing equipment, etc.,

- validated analytical methods for raw materials, in-process testing and finished product testing.

11.4.2 Tablet-coating process

This should detail the following:

- formulation
- list of ingredients and their specifications
- equipment required for the coating process, e.g. coating solution or suspension, preparation vessels, mills, mixers, homogenizers, coating pans, spray-guns
- service requirements such as compressed air, purified water, vacuum, etc.
- computer systems
- process monitoring and control systems
- validated analytical methods for raw material, in-process testing and finished product testing.

The process can be illustrated by using a block flow diagram, Fig. 11.2, Figs 11.3 and 11.4 enable the relevant computer system to be identified.

Table 11.1 shows a total of 37 installation qualification (IQ), operational qualification (OQ) and process/product validation (PV) protocols that will be needed for the various utilities, systems and processes.

Particular attention should be paid to the requirements for computerized systems documentation. Validation of the PCMS system can be handled as part of the OQ and PV protocols for the film- or sugar-coating processes.

11.5 EQUIPMENT HISTORY FILE

The establishment of equipment history files plays a central role in the timing and orderly execution of validation activities. These records are instrumental in providing the validation team with the documentation required to complete the validation protocols and certify utilities, systems and processes.

Equipment history files must be assembled for all items subject to validation for specifications, purchase orders, invoices, receipts, receiving records, certificates, performance curves, manuals, drawings, vendor product information and test results, and any other relevant documentation. The assembly of the equipment history files is an activity that will continue through the start-up and validation phases of the project. Maintenance of these files will continue beyond validation.

11.6 PHYSICAL VALIDATION

The physical validation is ready to commence when:

- The design review has been completed.
- All SOPs relating to the validation effort have been written.
- All appropriate SOP training has been conducted and documented.
- Document, procedure and equipment change control is in place.

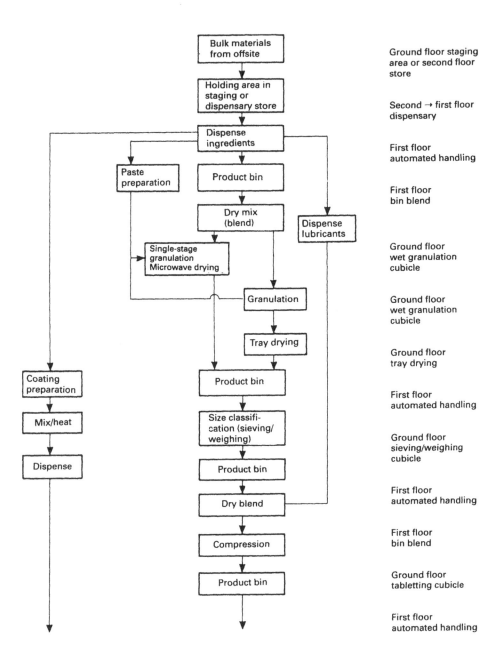

Fig. 11.2 Process plan: preparation and packaging of sugar-coated tablets, using wet granulated methods. From Cole, G.C. (1990) *Pharmaceutical Production Facilities: design and applications*, Ellis Horwood.

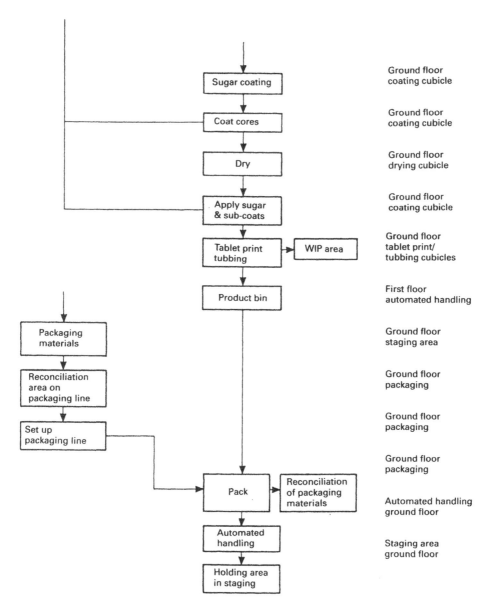

Fig. 11.2 *continued.*

- All passivation, welding and hydrostatic tests have been completed and documented.
- All instruments, gauges, test equipment, etc., have been recently calibrated.
- The protocols have been completed and accepted.
- The descriptive information (equipment identification, SOP numbers, etc.) contained in the protocol has been entered in advance by the validation team.

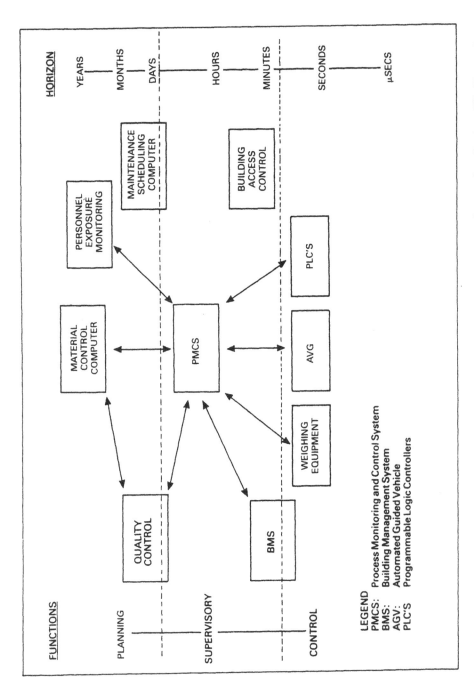

Fig. 11.3   Systems architecture from Cole, G.C. (1990) *Pharmaceutical Production Facilities: design and applications*, Ellis Horwood.

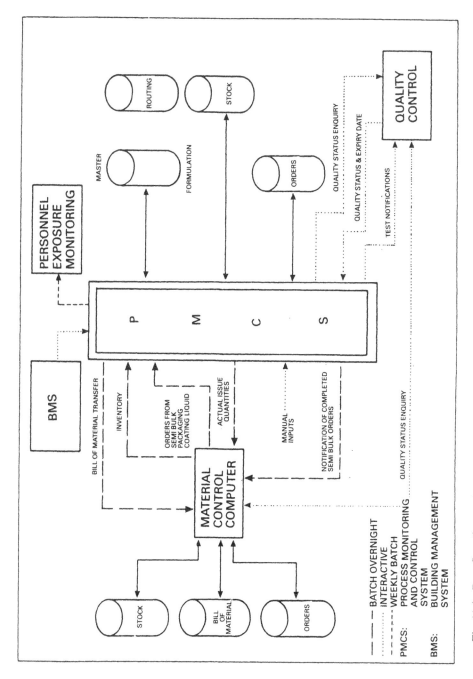

Fig. 11.4   Data flow diagram from Cole, G.C. (1990) *Pharmaceutical Production Facilities: design and applications*, Ellis Horwood.

Table 11.1.   Protocol requirements for utilities, systems and processes

		IQ	OQ	PV
Facility		×	—	—
Utilities	Purified water USP	×	×	×
	Compressed air	×	×	×
	HVAC	×	×	—
	Emergency electrical generator	×	×	—
	Drying air	×	×	×
	Process steam	×	×	×
Systems	Process control and monitoring computer system	×	×	×
	Clean-in-place	×	×	×
Processes	Powder mixers	×	×	—
	Granulators	×	×	—
	Mills/sieving equipment	×	×	—
	Dryers	×	×	—
	Compressing equipment	×	×	—
	Coating pans	×	×	—
	Liquid mixing equipment	×	×	—
	Product process	×	×	×

The physical validation begins with the execution of the installation qualifications for the facility and for those utilities such as HVAC, which support equipment and other utilities. The implementation of the operation qualifications for these same utilities begins as soon as the IQ has been concluded. This same pattern follows all the remaining entities in the order: utilities, systems and processes, as enumerated in Table 11.1.

11.7   STANDARD OPERATING PROCEDURE (SOP) DEVELOPMENT

All pharmaceutical facilities and their operations require SOPs to be in place to comply with the regulations. All new processes require SOPs to be written that cover a number of essential operating areas.

- Documentation system, i.e. batch records.
- Equipment use and cleaning procedures.
- Personnel procedures.
- Operating procedures.

It is necessary that all SOPs should be reviewed prior to the implementation of the validation programme.

11.8 ANALYTICAL SUPPORT

All analytical methods used in support of the validation programme must be validated prior to the physical validation of the facility, its process utilities, its equipment and product process.

11.9 CALIBRATION

All instruments used in measuring parameters in the processes must be divided into two groups: those which are critical to the performance of the equipment and process and those which are strictly convenience instruments. All critical instruments must be calibrated against a traceable national standard.

11.10 TRAINING

Training is an essential part of all cGMP programmes and records must be maintained for all staff responsible for the operation of the processes.

11.11 SUMMARY OF MAIN COMPONENTS OF ANY VALIDATION PROGRAMME

1. Prepare a Master Validation Plan.
2. Prepare complete protocols customized for the facility.
3. Develop SOPs as required.
4. Prepare a training programme.
5. Prepare a schedule of activities.
6. Conduct the physical validation.
7. Review and evaluate all data.
8. Assemble the completed validation packages.
9. Prepare and action the final certification of the facility, utilities, systems and processes.

An example is shown in Table 11.2 of the attributes the IQ, OQ and PV must cover for compressed air, used in a coating pan and for the coating process. Compressed air is the utility service selected as it is a product contact material, i.e. it is used in the spraying operation.

The coating pan listed in Table 11.1 will have several parts:

1. the pan;
2. the spraying equipment;
3. the unit that holds, mixes, and pumps the coating solution to the spray-guns;
4. the autowash system, if fitted;
5. the system used to monitor and record the amount of coating applied;
6. the air-handling system.

The main item is the coating pan and the development of protocols will follow the same pattern as for the compressed air. It is necessary to define the materials of

Table 11.2.   Protocol outline for compressed air

Installation qualification	Operation qualification	Process/product validation
Approval page	Approval page	Approval page
System description	System description	System description
Statement of purpose	Statement of purpose	Statement of purpose
Inspection checklist	Unit operation	Testing procedures
Installation checklist	Production rate	Sampling plan
Drawings	Capacity	Intensive monitoring
Materials of construction	Alarms	Acceptance criteria
Pressure test reports	Point of use filters	Summary, analysis and certification
Cleaning reports	Miscellaneous testing	Appendix reference documents
Manufacturer's certification	Acceptance criteria summary	
Calibration review	Summary, analysis and certification	
Standard operating procedures	Appendix reference documents	
Training		
Supporting utilities		
Expendables/consumables		
Spare parts list		
Punchlists		
Summary, analysis and certification		
Appendix reference documents		
Manuals		
Purpose orders		
Specifications		
Coating pan		

construction for the product contact parts, i.e. the pan and all parts of the auxiliary equipment that is in product contact, i.e. spray-guns, pipework, pumps and containers. Generally, 316L stainless steel will be used wherever possible. It should be remembered that the IQ is basically a check after installation to ensure that it meets the design specification requirements. Where flexible pipes are required then materials such as VITON/EPDM/PTFE may be acceptable.

It is important to emphasize that the manufacturers of equipment, systems and components must supply the necessary certification with their goods and that it meets the specification. The preparation of a comprehensive specification with all the documentation required by the purchaser can eliminate many of the problems associated with validation of the installation of the system. It is true that the major suppliers will provide this information if it is a requirement of supply, but if requested retrospectively then extra payments are usually demanded. These can be considerable.

The smaller equipment supply companies tend to be less aware of the requirements and their response to these requirements is patchy.

Components such as valves, nozzles, flow meters, pumps and pipework are just as critical as the coating pan from the quality viewpoint.

Each product is unique in many of its process requirements, but fundamentally there are many aspects which are common when developing OQs and PVs. It is necessary to determine that the unit operates within the range required by the process, i.e. the pan rotates at a speed which has been optimized for that product. It should be remembered that some tablets are more friable than others and, therefore, the rotation speed must be adjusted to ensure that sufficient coating is applied before serious damage occurs to the surface.

Calibration of the instruments will be required and it is necessary to determine which are critical and which are convenience—a critical instrument being defined as one which will seriously affect the quality of the finished product if it operates out of the defined range due to an inherent fault. Temperature and pressure gauges are good examples.

The OQ coating protocol is checked to ensure that the IQ is completed and approved and that all the moving parts, controls and process utilities operate within their defined ranges. These should be related to the process and product requirements.

To ensure that the process operates within its defined range, placebo or blank tablets can be used initially to develop sampling plans and define the range of process parameters. Two aspects of this part of the validation development programme are critical. Side-vented coating pans can have poor mixing characteristics, and if the coating on a tablet is designed to provide part of a sustained release profile, then all the tablets must have the required amount of coating applied to them. This may well mean experimentation with different types of baffles and speeds to optimize the process.

Validated analytical procedures are also essential to ensure that the quality of the product is maintained. These tests will apply to such services as compressed air, the drying air and the raw materials that will include solvents and purified water where aqueous coatings are applied.

Once all the process parameters have been defined and validated, the next stage is to manufacture three consecutive batches of product without changing the process parameters. Once three batches of coated tablets have been produced, approved, all the data documented (if it's not written down it hasn't been done!) and the product sold, the validation programme will have been completed.

However, this is not the end of validation for this product. If an item of equipment, raw material or set of process parameters is changed, then a proper change control procedure must be enacted to ensure that the quality of the final product is not compromised. It may be that only part of the process needs to be revalidated, but in extreme cases, i.e. where a new plant is built, then the whole programme may have to be repeated. Also a periodic review of validation requirement of a process must be maintained.

Fig. 11.5 shows a bar chart for a typical facility design and build project. This is the programme that would be required in the building of new plants. How much is required will depend on the nature and range of the project. How many of the resources needed to implement the programme from within the company concerned will have to be identified. Many companies use outside resources to enable them to overcome the initial documentation creation programme. The schedule in Fig. 11.1 does give an indication of the length of time required and should be integrated with the schedule in Fig. 11.5. It is never too early to start the validation programme.

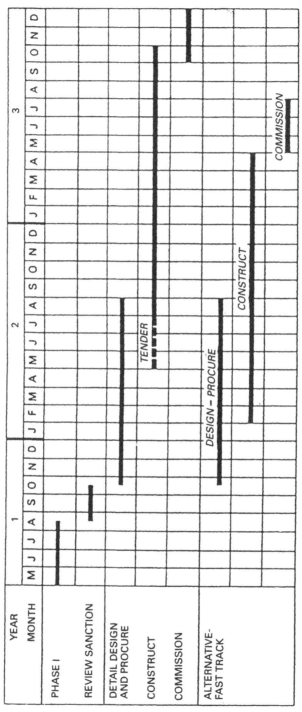

Fig. 11.5   Bar chart for a typical facility design and build project from Cole, G.C. (1990)
Pharmaceutical Production Facilities: design and applications, Ellis Horwood.

12

Mechanical properties of film coats

Michael E. Aulton

SUMMARY

This chapter discusses the need for a film coat to possess the correct mechanical properties. One of the requirements of a film coat is that it should provide adequate protection to the dosage form. The capacity of the film coat to afford physical protection depends to a large extent on its mechanical characteristics. After considering those desirable properties, the chapter explains how to assess such properties. It also explains the need for a standardized approach to film preparation prior to testing.

The main techniques that have been used successfully for the assessment of pharmaceutical film coat properties are indentation hardness and tensile testing. These techniques are described in detail and representative data for polymeric film coat formulations are presented.

The source and consequences of internal stresses within a film coat are explained and the consequences with respect to film-coating defects are discussed.

12.1 INTRODUCTION

12.1.1 Desirable mechanical properties of polymeric film coats

Tablets and pellets are film coated for many reasons. One of the requirements of a film coat is that it should provide adequate physical protection to the dosage form. The capacity of the film coat to afford this protection depends to a large extent on its mechanical characteristics. The coating must remain intact, be durable and be resistant to chipping and cracking during handling. Both the film itself and the composite system (i.e. film plus tablet or pellet substrate) should therefore possess *suitable* mechanical properties.

The mechanical characteristics of polymer film coats are an important parameter in dictating their performance in pharmaceutical dosage forms. A commercial film coat does not consist of polymer alone but contains many other ingredients. Additives are often included for a specific reason, either to assist processing or to improve performance. It should be appreciated that other materials added to a polymer system will almost invariably have an effect on the natural physical properties of that polymer. Often a material is added to a polymer specifically to improve its mechanical properties (plasticizers are a notable example), while on other occasions materials are added to the polymer to achieve one function, yet their addition often inadvertently changes its mechanical properties (here the classic example is the addition of insoluble pigments or opacifiers which tend to make the film much more brittle).

It was mentioned above that in order to provide mechanical protection, film coats should have *suitable* mechanical properties. But how do we define suitable, and, having done so, how can it be quantified? It is advantageous to be able to quantify the mechanical properties of polymer films in order that performance predictions can be made at the development stage and that the effect of additives on these properties can be examined so that the formulator can limit any detrimental effects and enhance any beneficial changes.

Banker (1966) considered that the mechanical strength and bonding ability of polymers arose from forces of cohesion within the material and adhesion between the material and its substrate. The magnitudes of these forces depend on the molecular size and structure of the polymer. *Intra*-molecular forces are generally very much weaker than *inter*-molecular forces, but polymers of sufficiently high molecular weight may give rise to large numbers of *intra*-molecular bonds resulting in high cohesive strength. The observed mechanical properties of polymers are a function of 'free volume' (see section 12.1.3) and thus will be modified by the presence of diluent molecules (e.g. plasticizer or residual solvent) and environmental temperature (Ferry, 1961). Depending on environmental temperature or composition, the mechanical properties of high molecular weight polymers may range between an almost perfect elastic state to an almost Newtonian viscous state. The observed properties will also be dependent on the test methodology, particularly strain rate.

The deformation behaviour of high-molecular weight polymers has been categorized into five distinctly different regions by Tobolsky (1971): glassy, transition, rubbery, rubbery liquid and liquid. The five distinct regions of viscoelastic behaviour may be characterized by the type of stress–strain curve exhibited by the polymer at a particular temperature. While the change between regions is, in some respects, analogous to a phase change in true solids or liquids, it is not sharply defined and is gradual.

1. At low temperature, i.e. below the glass transition region, or at very high strain rates, a polymer behaves as an elastic glass. Tensile strength and elastic modulus are relatively high, but extensibility is low.
2. As the temperature is raised, the polymer enters the transition region. Tensile strength and elastic modulus are decreased, but extensibility is increased.

Polymers in this region may show a ductile type of stress–strain curve, characterized by an elastic portion, a sudden fall-off of stress with increasing strain; then as strain is increased further the stress increases again. This process may be accompanied by the formation of a neck in the sample, and is called cold-drawing.

3.   As the temperature is increased further (or the strain rate is decreased) the polymer enters a region called the rubbery plateau. In this region long segments of the molecular chain are free to move, but they are constrained from slipping relative to each other by cross-links or entanglements. In the rubbery state, the polymer may be capable of undergoing considerable extension but, on removal of stress, it returns to its original state.

4.   In the rubbery transition state, the polymer remains elastic and rubbery, but also has a finite component of plastic flow due to failure of cross-links or disentanglement.

5.   Finally, at the highest temperatures or after long periods of straining, nearly all cross-links and entanglements are uncoupled and the polymer flows as a viscous liquid.

Whereas temperature and pressure are the independent variables for phase change, temperature and strain rate (or duration of strain) are responsible for viscoelastic transitions. True plasticization results in a lowering of the glass transition temperature (T_g, see section 12.1.3) of the polymer–plasticizer blend. The influence of plasticization on the observed viscoelastic behaviour can therefore be interpreted in a manner analogous to the effect of increasing temperature.

Later parts of this chapter will explain in detail how the desirable mechanical properties of a polymer can be defined and quantified, and how formulation variables can influence these properties.

12.1.2 Deformation of materials

Fundamentally, most materials deform either *elastically* (i.e. they return to their original dimensions on removal of the deforming stress) or *plastically* (i.e. their deformation is permanent).

When investigating the physical and mechanical properties of real solids or viscous liquids, it is frequently found that deviations occur from the classical theories of elasticity or viscous flow. Deviations involving stress (applied force divided by area of material over which force is applied), strain (deformation divided by original appropriate dimension of the material) and time are of two kinds. First, stress anomalies arise when the strain in a solid or the rate of strain in a liquid are not directly proportional to the applied stress but instead depend on the stress in a more complex manner. Secondly, time anomalies occur when the resultant stress depends not only on strain but also on the rate of strain: the observed deformation behaviour is both liquid-like and solid-like and is therefore termed *viscoelasticity*. Stress and time anomalies may coexist but in the absence of the former the behaviour is said to exhibit *linear viscoelasticity*. This implies that the ratio of stress to strain is a function of time alone and is independent of the magnitude of the applied stress.

Linear viscoelastic behaviour applies, therefore, to cases where the elastic contribution is Hookean and the viscous contribution is Newtonian. To understand viscoelasticity it is necessary first to consider the extreme examples of deformation behaviour exhibited by an ideal elastic solid and an ideal viscous fluid.

Elastic behaviour
An ideal elastic solid is one which recovers its original strain after removal of an applied stress and thus obeys Hooke's law. This states that the stress (σ) is proportional to the linear strain (ε):

$$\sigma = E.\varepsilon \tag{12.1}$$

where E is a constant of proportionality, effectively a measure of the stiffness or rigidity of the solid, known as the elastic modulus or Young's modulus (thus $E = \sigma/\varepsilon$) or the rigidity modulus G. The implicit conditions of the above equation define elastic behaviour. First, the strain in response to an applied stress has an equilibrium value which is completely recoverable; secondly, deformation is ideally instantaneous, i.e. independent of time; and, thirdly, the relationship of strain to stress is linear.

A simple metal-coiled spring exhibits typical Hookean behaviour. Fig. 12.1 shows stress *versus* time and strain *versus* time relationships.

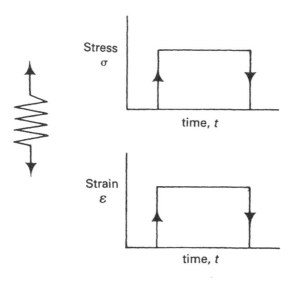

Fig. 12.1   The Hookean spring.

Viscous behaviour

Application of a constant stress to a Newtonian viscous fluid results in a linear increase in strain with time until the stress is removed. The deformation is permanent and the original strain is not recovered. The linear strain–time relationship is characterized by the gradient of the stress *versus* strain-rate plot, i.e.

$$\eta = \sigma/\varepsilon' \tag{12.2}$$

where ε' is the rate of change of strain (the first differential of strain with respect to time, i.e. $\varepsilon' = \varepsilon/t$) and η is the Newtonian viscosity of the fluid.

Newtonian viscous behaviour can be conveniently modelled by a piston and dashpot arrangement in which the dashpot cylinder is filled with a Newtonian fluid. Fig. 12.2 shows the deformation characteristics of such a material.

Real materials

Both stress anomalies and time anomalies result in deviations from the simplest case of Hookean elasticity giving rise to other modes of deformation. Norwick & Berry

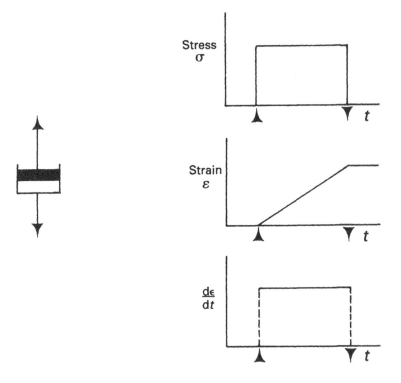

Fig. 12.2   The Newtonian dashpot.

(1972) have classified several types of mechanical behaviour according to the conditions obeyed by the stress–strain relationship (Table 12.1).

Most pharmaceutical materials have combination properties which can only be described by a two-component system in which an ideal elastic phase is combined with an ideal viscous phase. In practice most materials do show, to some extent, both elastic and viscous characteristics (Davis, 1974; Lockett, 1972). Consequently, viscoelastic behaviour covers a wide range of mechanical properties from ideal elastic to ideal Newtonian behaviour.

Mechanical models of linear viscoelasticity
Mechanical models can also be used to represent the properties of a viscoelastic material. The simplest of these use a Hookean spring combined either in series or in parallel with a Newtonian dashpot. These are the Maxwell and Voigt models, respectively. Their properties have been reviewed extensively (see, for example, Castello & Goyan, 1964, and Barry, 1974) and will be be considered briefly here.

The Maxwell model
The Maxwell model is shown in Fig. 12.3. It consists of a Hookean spring in series with a Newtonian viscous dashpot. The strain response with time to an applied stress reflects both the viscous and elastic contributions to the resultant deformation. On application of the stress there is an instantaneous increase in strain associated with the deformation of the spring. This is followed by a time-dependent linear increase in strain due to the movement of the piston of the Newtonian dashpot. On removal of the stress the elastic strain alone is recovered.

Under an applied external force the stress in the spring is equal to that in the dashpot. The total strain (ε_T) in the Maxwell model is the sum of the strains in the spring ε_S and in the dashpot ε_D:

$$\varepsilon_T = \varepsilon_S + \varepsilon_D \tag{12.3}$$

Table 12.1 Types of mechanical behaviour classified according to the conditions obeyed by their stress–strain relationships (after Norwick & Berry, 1972)

Condition	Unique equilibrium relationship (complete recovery)	Complete instant response	Linearity
Ideal elasticity	Yes	Yes	Yes
Non-linear elasticity	Yes	Yes	No
Instantaneous plasticity	No	Yes	No
Anelasticity	Yes	No	Yes
Linear viscoelasticity	No	No	Yes

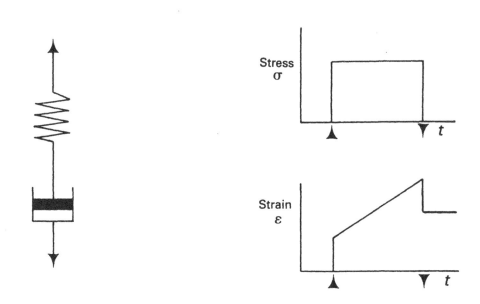

Fig. 12.3   The Maxwell model.

By convention, viscoelastic deformations are studied by calculating compliance (J). Compliance is defined as the strain divided by the applied stress. Its use has the advantage of allowing the comparison of strain data obtained under different stress conditions, or allowing calculation of expected strain for a given applied stress.

If the Maxwell model is maintained under conditions of constant strain, the initial stress in the Hookean spring will be reduced by a viscous deformation in the dashpot until the stress decays to zero. This phenomenon is termed *stress relaxation*. Measurement of stress relaxation in a material, therefore, provides a quantitative measurement of the ability of the material to undergo non-recoverable or plastic deformation.

The Voigt model
The Voigt model is shown in Fig. 12.4. It consists of a Hookean spring in parallel with a Newtonian dashpot. This provides a mechanical analogy for a material in which the response to an applied stress is not instantaneous but is retarded by viscous resistance. Removal of the stress results in a similarly retarded, but total, recovery of the strain. The Voigt model therefore exhibits the properties of creep and creep recovery.

The change in strain with time is exponential, and the greater the apparent viscosity of the Newtonian dashpot the greater will be the retardation. In the Voigt model, on application of an external force, the strain at any time in the spring is equal to that in the dashpot, and the total stress (σ_T) is the sum of the stresses in the spring (σ_S) and in the dashpot (σ_D). Thus:

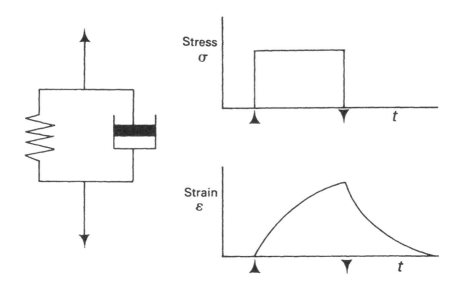

Fig. 12.4   The Voigt model.

$$\text{Total stress } (\sigma_T) = \sigma_S + \sigma_D \tag{12.4}$$

The Voigt model is capable of dissipating energy, a phenomenon known as internal friction. This parameter has the dimensions of viscosity and may be regarded as the apparent viscosity (η) of the Newtonian dashpot. G is the rigidity modulus of the Hookean spring. Unlike the Maxwell model, the Voigt model is incapable of stress relaxation. The quantity η/G is the retardation time (τ) for the unit; that is, the time required for strain to relax to $1/e$ of its initial value on removal of stress. The retardation time is short and strain recovery is rapid where internal friction is small compared with the rigidity modulus. Thus at any time (t):

$$\sigma_T = G.\varepsilon(t) + \eta\varepsilon'(t) \tag{12.5}$$

In real materials there exist a number of molecular interactions resulting in more than one retardation time. The viscoelastic behaviour of such materials can be represented by the generalized Voigt model consisting of n Voigt units in series, where n is the number of discrete retardation times. For a viscoelastic solid exhibiting limited recoverable flow, the generalized Voigt model applies.

If equation (12.5) is rearranged to include the retardation time (τ), then integration without limits for the ith element gives:

$$-\ln\left(\frac{\sigma_i}{G_i} - \varepsilon_i\right) = \frac{t}{\tau_i} + k_i \tag{12.6}$$

When time $t = 0$, strain $\varepsilon_i = 0$ then $k_i = \ln(\sigma_i/J_i)$ and

$$\ln\left[\frac{\sigma_i J_i - \varepsilon_i}{G_i J_i}\right] = -\frac{t}{\tau_i} \tag{12.7}$$

Thus, the strain in the ith element is

$$\varepsilon_i = \sigma_i J_i \left[1 - \exp\left(-\frac{t}{\tau_i}\right)\right] \tag{12.8}$$

or, in terms of compliance,

$$J_i(t) = J_i \left[1 - \exp\left(-\frac{t}{\tau_i}\right)\right] \tag{12.9}$$

The total strain $\varepsilon(t)$ in the generalized Voigt model is the sum of the strains in the individual elements, and thus compliances in series are additive. For the case of n Voigt units in series:

$$J(t) = \sum_{i=1}^{i=n} J_i \left[1 - \exp\left(-\frac{t}{\tau_i}\right)\right] \tag{12.10}$$

Generalized linear viscoelastic model
By combining a Maxwell model in series with one or more Voigt units, a generalized model for linear viscoelastic behaviour is obtained (Fig. 12.5).

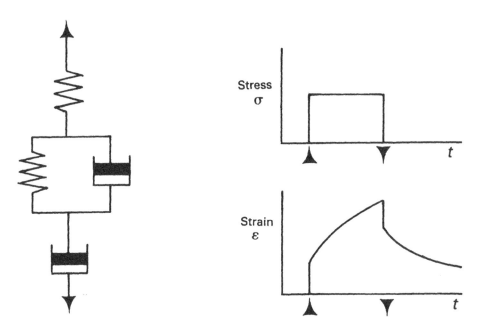

Fig. 12.5   The generalized 'spring and dashpot' model for linear viscoelasticity.

The strain response with time under an applied stress is represented by a plot of compliance $J(t)$ against time t and is termed a creep curve. A typical curve can be rationalized into three distinct regions (see section 12.4.3 for further details). The instantaneous response and the late linear region can be represented, respectively, by the Hookean spring and the Newtonian dashpot of the Maxwell model. The intermediate curved zone can be modelled by one or more retarded elastic Voigt units. An equation for the overall compliance at any time can be derived to include the contribution from each region:

$$J(t) = J_0 + \sum_{i=1}^{i=n} J_i\left[1 - \exp\left(-\frac{t}{\tau_i}\right)\right] + \frac{t}{\eta_0} \qquad (12.11)$$

where J_0 is the instantaneous creep compliance and η_0 is the apparent Newtonian viscosity of the late linear region. Complex viscoelastic behaviour will require more than one Voigt unit to accurately model the observed properties. The middle term of equation (12.11) will then be a summation of the contributions of each discrete Voigt unit.

12.1.3   Thermomechanical properties of polymers

Glass transition temperature
The glass transition temperature (T_g) is a fundamental property of any polymeric system. A good working definition of the glass transition temperature is *that temperature at which a polymer changes (on heating) from a brittle substance (glass) to a rubber solid or vice versa on cooling*. Thus, at the T_g, a polymer undergoes a significant change in mechanical properties which may have implications in coating performance.

The T_g influences many physical properties of coating polymers including: elasticity, adhesion, viscosity, solvent release and permeability.

One theory of what happens at the glass transition temperature is the so-called 'Free Volume Theory'. At the molecular level the total volume occupied by a given number of molecules (V_T) can be pictured as the sum of the 'free volume' (V_F) (the voids) and the 'occupied volume' (V_O) (the volume of the molecules themselves):

$$V_T = V_F + V_O \qquad (12.12)$$

It is assumed that as the temperature increases there is an increase in V_F as thus V_T will increase. This will allow more movement of molecular groups and side chains. As T_g is approached, V_F increases with such magnitude as to bring about changes in measurable mechanical properties.

Determination of glass transition temperature
Most T_g determinations are based either on measurements of bulk temperature coefficients (since these properties undergo marked changes at T_g) or on experiments which are sensitive to the onset of molecular motion in polymer chains. Differential scanning calorimetry (DSC) and thermomechanical analysis (TMA) are the most

commonly used methods to examine pharmaceutical film-coating systems.

Presented below is a very brief introduction to the application of thermal analysis in the study of pharmaceutically relevant polymers. The reader is referred to the book in this series by Ford & Timmins (1989) for a comprehensive explanation with further details and examples.

Differential scanning calorimetry (DSC)

In operation, DSC involves placing a small sample of the material under test in a metal sample holder and raising its temperature at a constant rate. When a transition occurs in the sample material, an endothermic (energy-absorbing) or exothermic (energy-liberating) reaction takes place. With the DSC technique, the change in power required to maintain the sample holder at the same temperature as the reference holder (i.e. at its programmed temperature) during the transition is recorded. The sample and reference holders and their associated heaters and temperature sensors are shown in Fig. 12.6 and a block diagram of the components of a commercial DSC are shown in Fig. 12.7.

The abscissa of the chart output indicates transition temperatures and any peak area indicates the total energy transfer to or from the sample during a phase change. The direct calorimetric measuring principle of the instrument requires that each sample holder has a built-in heater and a temperature sensor. The differential power required to maintain the balance condition is output directly in millijoules per second on the recorder and is always equivalent to the rate of energy absorption or evolution of the sample.

Polymer features, such as T_g, compatibility, moisture interactions and crystallinity, may be determined using this technique. The glass transition is considered to be a second-order transition since it involves a discontinuous change in a secondary thermodynamic quantity, such as specific heat. Since the DSC thermogram is a continuous plot of specific heat as a function of temperature, the glass transition will appear as a discontinuity (step change) in the baseline. The heat capacity change (ΔC_h) at glass transition is the change in heat capacity between onset and the end of transition. T_g is generally taken as either the onset of transition or the intersection or mid-point of the heat capacity change (ΔC_h) with a straight line joining the onset with the end of transition (Fig. 12.8).

Thermomechanical analysis

This technique permits the monitoring of very small changes in sample dimensions as a function of temperature. A typical analysis can be used in a variety of modes, including penetration, expansion, extension and flexure. In the first two modes the sample is under a compressive force while in the latter two the sample is in a state of tension.

In penetration and expansion modes, the sample is placed on the platform of a quartz sample tube. A diagram showing the details of the assembly is given in Fig. 12.9.

The appropriate quartz probe is fitted to the probe assembly which consists of a shaft upon which is the core of a linear variable differential transformer (LVDT).

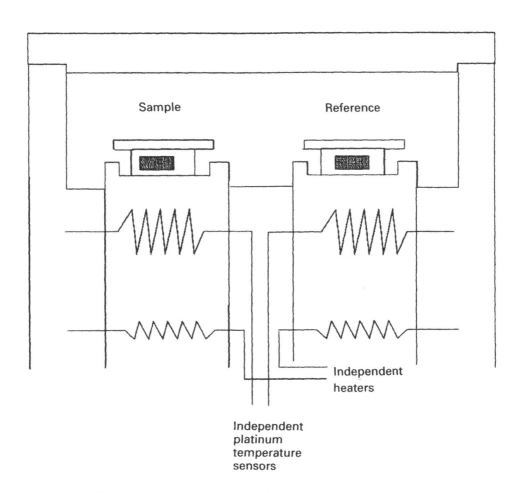

Fig. 12.6   Schematic diagram of the principle of differential scanning calorimetry.

Any change in position of the core in the annular space of the cylindrical transformer results in a change in the voltage output of the transformer. In this way, any motion of the probe caused by penetration or expansion is transmitted with very high sensitivity as an electrical signal to the potentiometric recorder. The entire assembly must be free to move relative to the fixed sample tube and LVDT, yet its weight must be supported in order to permit control of the loading on the sample.

Melting point (T_m), softening point (T_s), T_g and expansion coefficients are a few of the parameters that can be obtained from this test.

In *penetration mode*, below T_g, the polymer exhibits resistance to penetration because there is insufficient thermal energy to allow significant segmental movement of the polymer chains. As the temperature increases, immobilized chain segments are freed, thereby becoming more flexible. Approaching the transition temperature,

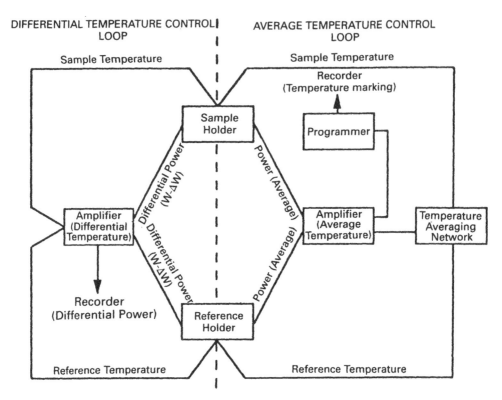

Fig. 12.7   Block diagram of a commercial differential scanning calorimeter.

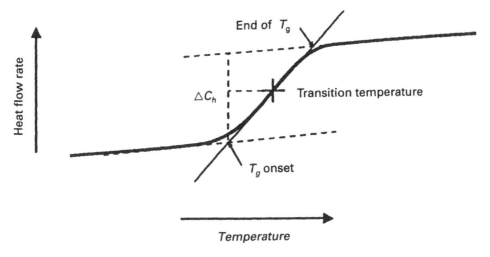

Fig. 12.8   Determination of glass transition temperature from a DSC thermogram.

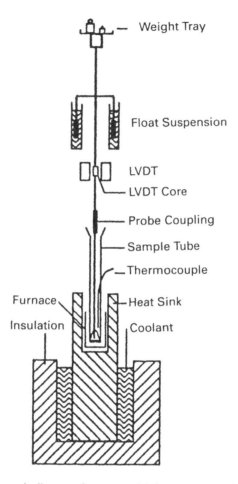

Fig. 12.9 Schematic diagram of a commercial thermomechanical analyser.

there is a corresponding increase in void volume in the polymer, allowing the polymer to become penetrable. The intersection of the extrapolations of the baseline and the penetration line is taken as T_g (Fig. 12.10).

Measurements of T_g by TMA in the *expansion mode* is based on the principle that, at T_g, the rigid polymer chains become mobile, thus increasing the free volume. This is manifest as a thermal expansion of the polymer film which vertically displaces the expansion probe upwards.

In the *tension test*, the material slowly elongates because of creep and thermal expansion. At the transition temperature, the material begins to stretch at a rapid rate over a narrow temperature interval by the same principle involved in the penetration test.

A *dynamic method* of TMA analysis is the torsional braid pendulum, a technique originally used for following rigidity changes during the curing of polymers.

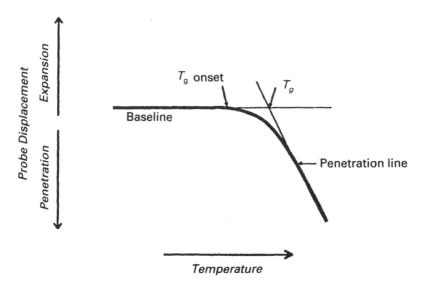

Fig. 12.10   Determination of glass transition temperature from a TMA thermogram.

Sakellariou *et al.* (1985) have examined several pharmaceutical polymer systems. Analysis of plots of relative film rigidity and the logarithmic decrement (a function of the energy loss of the system under test) *versus* temperature enabled glass transition temperatures to be measured with a high degree of precision.

Coefficient of thermal expansion of a material (α) can be determined by using TMA in the expansion mode. These values are calculated from measurement of the linear expansion of the sample material (ΔL) with respect to temperature change (ΔT) using the relationship $\Delta L = L_O \alpha \, \Delta T$ where L_O is the original length/thickness/height of the sample. Expansion coefficient measurements require a 'zero' load on the sample.

Thermomechanical properties of film-coating materials

It is possible to determine the glass transition temperature (T_g) with some precision on a pure polymer sample, but very often coating polymers are mixtures of many ingredients and the addition of these other materials usually leads to a reduction in T_g and a broadening of the transition temperature which makes it more difficult to determine its value accurately.

Some typical DSC thermograms obtained from various HPMC samples are shown in Fig. 12.11. This figure clearly shows how the presence of plasticizer and storage conditions influence the shape of the thermograms.

For the important coating polymer HPMC, using the technique of thermal mechanical analysis (TMA), it has been shown that this polymer possesses three transitions α, β and γ, the α transition being at the higher temperature. The secondary transitions β and γ result from movement of molecular groups and side chains on the polymer.

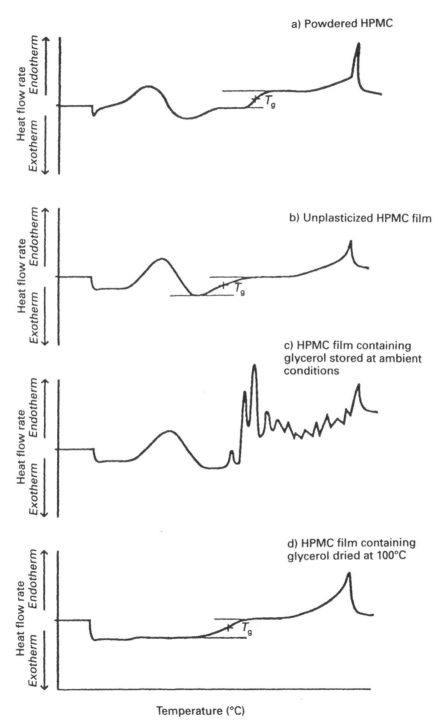

Fig. 12.11   Characteristic DSC thermograms obtained from various HPMC samples.

Various values of T_g have been reported for HPMC; Entwistle & Rowe (1979) stated 177°C; Okhamafe & York (1983a), 155°C; and Abdul-Razzak (1980) reported an exceedingly low value of 56°C but questioned whether this was indeed the primary glass transition.

Porter & Ridgway (1983) demonstrated the characteristic effect of adding a plasticizer—that is, an ability to lower the T_g of a coating polymer. They worked with CAP and PVAP. Fig. 12.12 shows the predicted reduction in T_g of HPMC by the addition of plasticizer (Entwistle and Rowe, 1979).

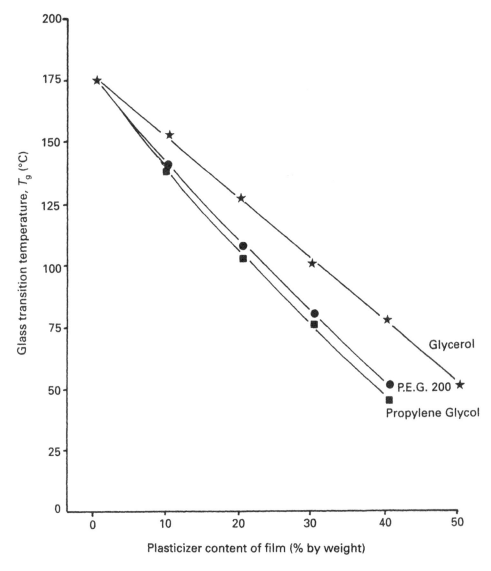

Fig. 12.12   Effect of plasticizers on the glass transition temperature of HPMC.

12.2 TESTS FOR THE ASSESSMENT OF FILM MECHANICAL PROPERTIES

A large number of tests are available for the testing of polymers. An excellent review of the early published literature relating to both official and unofficial tests applicable to polymeric materials can be found in a book by Lever & Rhys (1968). Another useful publication is the *Paint Testing Manual* (Gardner & Sward, 1972) published by the American Society for Testing and Materials (ASTM). In this text, many pieces of apparatus suitable for the testing of films are described, together with a brief description of their use.

In pharmaceutical technology, two tests have proved to be the most useful in the assessment of the mechanical properties of film coats: tensile testing and indentation hardness testing. These two tests are discussed in detail in subsequent sections of this chapter.

12.2.1 Film preparation

Before we can concern ourselves with the testing of film coats, however, we must first consider the various methods of preparing the films prior to testing in order to ensure consistency in the data generated during the tests. Similarly, we must consider if the data so generated are truly representative of the properties of the actual film *in situ* around a substrate tablet core or multiparticulate pellet or bead. Additionally, careful *standardization* of film preparation and test conditions is essential to allow comparisons between potential film coat formulations in a development programme, and also to enable data generated in a number of laboratories to be compared.

Differences in film density, strength, hardness, moisture absorption and surface appearance have been demonstrated between cast and sprayed films (Banker *et al.*, 1966; Zaro & Smith, 1972; Amann *et al.*, 1974; Hawes, 1978; Pickard, 1979). Similarly, films prepared using airless and pneumatic sprays have been shown to possess different properties (Bayer & Speiser, 1971; Spiteal & Kinget, 1977; Pickard, 1979). These papers illustrate the potential importance of the film coat application process in determining the properties of aqueous film-coated products. Characterization of aqueous film-coating process variables and their effect on the properties of the resulting film coat has not been the subject of intensive study, although work has been carried out to try to isolate some of the more fundamental parameters.

Free film or in situ *on substrate?*

A decision must be made whether to test films which have actually been sprayed onto a tablet or pellet, or to test cast or sprayed free films. The use of free films as a means of assessing film coats in practice has been criticized (Rowe, 1977). It is argued that free-film studies should be used only for early predictions and for gross formulation changes. However, there are many benefits in testing free films.

Indentation hardness tests can be performed on films *in situ* on a coated tablet or even a spherical pellet, but for tensile testing the film must be peeled off. This inevitably produces an unsatisfactory film of irregular thickness, since the polymer will have entered the surface voids of the substrate. There will also be damage to the film as a result of the peeling process. This makes accurately quantifiable data impossible to achieve.

Rowe (1976b) found no significant difference between films cast onto a glass substrate and those applied to tablets from dilute organic solutions. Okhamafe & York (1986), however, reported Young's modulus values for cast films to be about two to five times greater than equivalent films applied to aspirin tablets.

Cast or sprayed film?

Similar arguments can be made for the relative merits of testing either cast or sprayed films. A sprayed film is more realistic, but is less easy to control. On the other hand, a cast film is a more perfect specimen, which is better for obtaining fundamental material properties, but is less realistic.

Casting of a film from solution is best achieved by the use of a thin-layer chromatography applicator to apply a uniform layer of solution of known initial thickness on a carefully levelled substrate from which the dried film can easily be peeled. A glass sheet is ideal for many polymers (e.g. HPMC), while other substrate materials may have to be investigated if the adhesion between the film and glass is so great that the film is damaged during removal.

The problem of solids dispersed within the film sedimenting before gelation is complete has been neatly solved by Devereux (1988), who used a horizontally rotating cylinder on which the film was cast on the inside surface. The continual rotation prevented permanent sedimentation up to the point of gelation, at which time the solid particles become trapped in position within the gel matrix.

If the decision is to spray the films, a number of techniques which attempt to mimic a commercial film-coating process have been suggested.

Model systems

The use of a model system which mimics conditions pertaining in commercial coating equipment has obvious advantages for research and development work. Information on the coating process can be obtained without either the considerable capital cost, space or services required for commercial coating equipment or the need for large amounts of tablets or pellets.

In one simple laboratory model system the sample to be coated moves past the spray pattern of a gun for a short time with a fixed interval between successive sprays. This attempts to crudely mimic the fate of tablets in a tumbling bed or multiparticulate pellets in a fluidized bed.

Prater (1982) measured coating conditions experienced in a Model 10 Accela–Cota and used this information to prepare a model system. The apparatus consisted of a timing belt to which the substrate was attached and a timed shutter mechanism which allowed the substrate to be exposed to the spray for a required interval. The apparatus was positioned in a modified fume cupboard and was capable of investigating the effect of the drying air flow rate and temperature, spray rate, atomizing air pressure and nozzle-to-bed distance.

A model system developed by Reiland & Eber (1986), constructed within a specially designed stainless-steel spray box, was also intended to mimic coating in a Model 10 Accela–Cota. The spray gun was mounted on a movable track and the substrate on an assembly rotating at 30 rev/min. The apparatus gave a spray exposure time of 0.12 s with interdispersed drying cycles. Although the apparatus was used for an extensive study on the effect of process variables on the surface gloss and roughness of films prepared from aqueous gloss solutions, no attempt was made to demonstrate that the apparatus was an adequate simulation of practical coating conditions, and no information on drying air volumes or substrate temperatures was given. Neither of the two model systems described above simulated the tumbling action of tablets within the coating pan.

A system for spraying film for testing within an actual coating pan was described by Porter (1980) who placed a vinyl-covered card inside a coating pan during an actual coating run.

Another model system for preparing tablet coatings has been designed and described by van Bommel et al. (1989a). This apparatus consists of a rotating cylinder which has tablet holders attached to its curved surface. The tablets pass in turn in front of a continuously spraying gun and are thus exposed intermittently to the atomized solution. This allows the coated surfaces to partially dry prior to the next application. These authors successfully used this system to generate films of ethylcellulose containing various concentrations of paracetamol and xylitol for their novel Gradient Matrix System. The authors then adapted the apparatus to produce free films in order to study the effect of additives on the physicochemical properties of these films (van Bommel et al., 1989b). Subsequently, these authors adapted a laboratory scale spheronizer to apply the Gradient Matrix System films onto multiparticulate spheres (van Bommel et al., 1990).

Residual solvent
It could be assumed that once the coating solvent has been evaporated from a polymer film during the film-coating process it will have no residual effect on the mechanical properties of the resulting film. Work on ethylcellulose films cast from different organic solvents has shown this not to be the case. Vemba et al. (1980) measured the breaking strength of ethylcellulose films plasticized with 10% ethyl phthalate. They used a range of solvents which were a mixture of 70% Freon 21 with 30% of a range of other solvents. A wide variation in breaking strengths of the resulting 'dried' films (between 7.95 and 28.2 MPa) was observed with this range of solvents under otherwise identical testing conditions.

Other properties which must be very accurately controlled during the testing are the drying time and conditions after casting, the humidity of the air during film storage and testing, and the temperature of storage and testing.

Drying time
It is very important to control the drying time, particularly with aqueous systems when drying times are longer because of slower evaporation rates. Mechanical properties vary considerably with the amount of solvent remaining in the film (see

below). After initial experimentation, drying conditions and times should be accurately standardized.

Storage humidity
Atmospheric humidity during drying, storage and even testing needs to be very carefully controlled, particularly with water-soluble polymers. Water itself can have a very efficient plasticizing effect.

Aulton *et al.* (1981) found that conditioning unplasticized films at high humidity resulted in significant changes in the mechanical properties consistent with a plasticizing action (see Fig. 12.13). This effect was also reported by Masilungan & Lordi (1984) who showed the softening temperature of unplasticized HPMC films to be reduced after storage at 79% r.h. for eight weeks.

Temperature
Obviously this needs careful control during testing. In general terms (i.e. within realistic limits), an increase in temperature will lead to a reduction in film strength and greater elongation prior to fracture, while a reduction in temperature will have the opposite effect, increasing the brittleness of the film.

12.2.2   Tensile and indentation testing
Of the very many tests for the mechanical assessment of polymer films of pharmaceutical interest, the two tests which have proved to be the most successful are

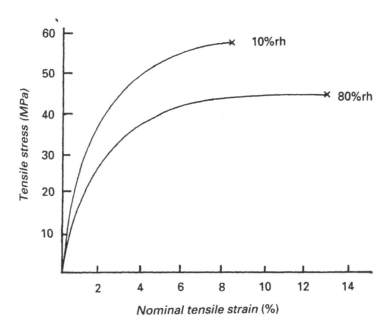

Fig. 12.13   Stress–strain curves for cast HPMC films conditioned at 10% and 80% r.h. atmospheres prior to testing showing the plasticizing effect of water.

tensile testing and indentation testing. The following sections of this chapter consider in detail both of these techniques, which have been used successfully to quantify the mechanical properties of polymer films. Data from pharmaceutical systems are presented.

12.3 TENSILE TESTING

12.3.1 Desirable tensile properties of film coats

Quantification of deformation, for example by measuring the elongation of a material with increasing tensile load, enables information about the fundamental mechanical properties of that material to be derived. An ideal film coat, with respect to retaining its physical continuity, should be hard and tough without being brittle. It is possible to define these properties in terms of yield point, strain at break and elastic modulus data obtained from a tensile deformation test. This information can be interpreted according to the classification of Lever & Rhys (1968) shown in Table 12.2.

Therefore a desirable hard, tough film must have a high tensile strength, a large extension before breaking and a high elastic modulus. It is possible to quantify these properties quite easily in a tensile elongation test in which the film is placed in the jaws or grips of a tensile testing machine which can stretch the film at a carefully controlled strain rate and simultaneously provide a continuous output of force and displacement (or, preferably, stress and strain).

12.3.2 Tensile testing

Sample preparation for tensile testing

Films must be prepared on a substrate from which they can be removed easily without damage to the film. Thus, as mentioned previously, films peeled from a tablet are unsuitable. The subject of sample preparation has been discussed earlier in this chapter. The preferred method for tensile testing is casting or spraying the film into a sheet on a flat substrate (such as a glass plate). The film is cut into strips

Table 12.2 Classification of material properties on the basis of tensile deformations (after Lever & Rhys, 1968)

Film description	Strain at break (elongation)	Yield point (or tensile strength)	Modulus of elasticity
Soft, weak	Low	Low	Low
Soft, tough	Low	High	Low
Hard, brittle	Not defined	Low	Very high
Hard, strong	High	Moderate	High
Hard, tough	High	High	High

or dumb bell-shaped samples (Fig. 12.14) using a sharp scalpel and a metal template
(Fig. 12.15) and then peeled from the substrate.

Care must be taken when cutting to avoid jagged edges. These can produce stress
concentrations leading to rips and tears at that point. These will occur at much
lower force values than the true tensile strength of the material, thus giving misleading data.

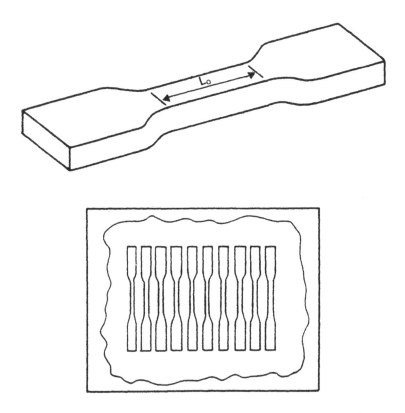

Fig. 12.14   A template for cutting out standard samples for tensile testing. L_O is the gauge
length. Many samples can be cut from the same casting onto a glass plate.

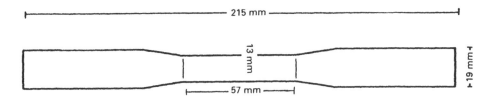

Fig. 12.15   Dimensions of a typical metal dumb-bell template used for cutting samples for
tensile testing from a cast sheet of film-coating polymer.

The tensile test

Test strips are placed in non-slip jaws or grips of a tensile-testing machine, such as an Instron, JJ or Monsanto tester. The grips must be designed and operated so that the film does not slip during testing but they should not be overtightened in order to avoid damage to the film. The machine must pull the sample in tension at a constant speed of grip separation (*speed of testing, v,* mm/min) exactly along the long axis of the sample. It should measure and record the force applied to the sample and its corresponding displacement as the grips move apart until the point of fracture of the film. Some machines convert these data to stress *versus* strain if the dimensions of the test sample are input. Stress is calculated by dividing applied force by the initial cross-sectional area of the film and strain is the ratio of the elongation of the film during the test to the initial length of the test section of the specimen. These definitions are expanded in the following section.

The tests should be performed in a controlled (temperature and humidity) environment if that is deemed to be necessary. With all water-soluble film-coating polymers this is essential. It is recommended that at least five replicates are performed. The results for any samples which slip in the grips or fracture close to the grips should be discarded.

It is common practice, where feasible, to measure the deformation of the test specimen (by means of an extensiometer—a device which measures the extension of the film gauge length either by contact or optically) between two marks on the parallel section of the cut film specimen at pre-determined distance apart (L_0) (see Fig. 12.14). In reality, with polymer films of a composition and thickness equivalent to those used in film coating, this procedure is virtually impossible to perform without damage to the sample. Thus, it is preferable to grip the sample so that only a parallel section is positioned between the jaws of the test apparatus, indeed parallel-sided strips may be used. In this case, the distance between the grips at the start of the test (L) is taken as the gauge length. Slightly different terms are given to data obtained in this way, with the term 'nominal' prefixing the corresponding strain definition—see below.

12.3.3   Interpretation of data from tensile stress-strain curves

The definitions, symbols and explanations which follow are in accordance with the latest ISO specification for the determination of the tensile properties of plastic materials (ISO 570–1, 1993). A number of these terms and definitions differ slightly from previously used conventions. It is recommended that these standard terms and symbols are adopted in all future descriptions of these properties. In this book, where appropriate, previously published data has been re-presented using the correct terms.

Tensile stress (σ)

Tensile stress (or engineering stress) is the tensile force (F in N), carried by the specimen at any given moment, per unit area of the initial cross-sectional area of the specimen (A in mm^2) within the gauge length (L or L_0). It is calculated as $\sigma = F/A$ and the result expressed in megapascals (MPa).

Tensile strain (ε)
Tensile strain is the increase in length of the specimen between the gauge marks (ΔL_O in mm) per unit initial length of the gauge (L_O in mm). It is calculated and expressed either as a dimensionless ratio ($\varepsilon = \Delta L_O/L_O$) or as a percentage ($\varepsilon(\%) = 100 \times \Delta L_O/L_O$). Thus, in general terms:

$$\text{Strain} = \frac{\text{Increase in length}}{\text{Initial length}} (\times\ 100 \text{ if required}) \qquad (12.13)$$

Strictly, this term is used only for strains up to the yield point and only when changes in a marked gauge length are being measured. As explained above, with delicate film coating polymer films, the distance between the grips (grip separation) is often used instead, resulting in nominal tensile strain.

Nominal tensile strain
This is defined as the increase in length of the test specimen (ΔL in mm), measured as the distance between the grips (L in mm). It is expressed as a dimensionless ratio ($\varepsilon_t = \Delta L/L$) or as a percentage ($\varepsilon_t(\%) = 100 \times \Delta L/L$). This term should be used for strains beyond the yield point and when strain measurements are based on grip separation.

Fig. 12.16 shows stress-strain plots for three representative polymeric film materials. Curve (a) represents a polymer film with a yield point which is followed by fracture at the maximum observed stress. Curve (b) represents a material exhibiting a yield point, but this time the maximum stress occurs at that yield point and the film breaks at a lower stress. Curve (c) is a stress-strain curve exhibited by a material not exhibiting a yield point.

Once the stress-strain curve up to the point of fracture has been obtained, the following material properties can be quantified.

Yield point (limit of elasticity)
When a material is stressed beyond its elastic limit, it may fail immediately (in the case of a very brittle material) or it may continue to deform in a non-linear manner. Some materials (certainly not all polymers) show a distinct yield point. This is the first point on the stress-strain curve at which an increase in strain occurs without an increase in stress, i.e. the material has begun to yield (flow, deform plastically).

The yield point is not observable in many polymers and indeed is impossible to determine in the case of hydroxypropyl methylcellulose (Aulton *et al.*, 1980, 1981, 1984), as films of this material show smooth stress–strain curves (see, for example, Figs 12.13, 12.19 and 12.21), but a yield point can be seen clearly in some other polymers, e.g. ethylcellulose (Delporte, 1980a, 1980b).

Tensile stress at yield (or yield stress)
This is the first stress (in MPa) at which an increase in strain occurs without an increase in stress. It may (or may not) be less than the maximum attainable stress see Fig. 12.16, curves a and b. Yield stress (σ_Y) is a measure of a material's resistance to permanent deformation.

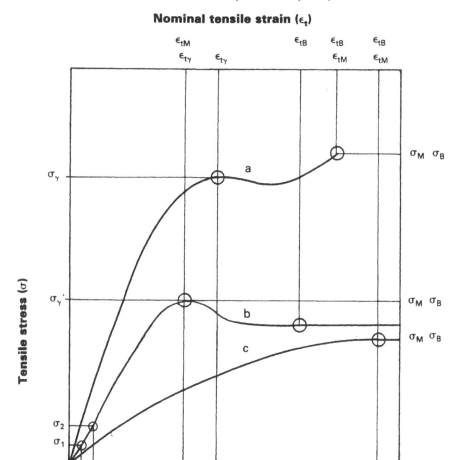

Fig. 12.16 Typical plots of applied stress against strain for polymeric materials being tested to failure in tension. Material properties which can be obtained from the curves are indicated on the axes, the symbols coinciding with the definitions in the text (based on ISO 527–1).

Thus, tensile stress at yield is defined as:

$$\text{Yield stress } (\sigma_Y) = \frac{\text{Force applied at yield point}}{\text{Initial cross-sectional area of test sample}} \quad (12.14)$$

Tensile strength
Tensile strength (σ_M) is the maximum tensile stress (in MPa) sustained by the test specimen during a tensile test. This may or may not be at the point of fracture:

$$\text{Tensile strength } (\sigma_M) = \frac{\text{Maximum force applied during test}}{\text{Initial cross-sectional area of test sample}} \quad (12.15)$$

Tensile stress at break
The tensile stress at break (σ_B) is the tensile stress (in MPa) at which the specimen ruptures. It is the tensile stress applied to a film at its point of fracture. If elongation of the test sample is extensive, the film may 'thin' significantly before fracture. Since tensile strength is generally calculated by dividing applied force by the initial cross-sectional area of the film, this will lead to imprecise values of actual stress at this point. This effect can, however, be compensated for in calculations.

Ultimate tensile strength
This term has been used variably and often incorrectly in the past for either tensile strength or tensile stress at break. Its use is not recommended and should be discontinued.

Tensile strain at yield
Tensile strain at yield (ε_Y) is the tensile strain at the yield stress. It is expressed as a dimensionless ratio $(\varepsilon_Y = \Delta L_{OY}/L_O)$ or a percentage $(\varepsilon_Y(\%) = 100 \times \Delta L_{OY}/L_O)$, where ΔL_{OY} is the elongation in the gauge length at the yield point.

Nominal tensile strain at yield
The equivalent to the above, if grip separation at yield (ΔL_Y) is used rather than change in gauge length, is nominal tensile strain at yield (ε_{tY}). Thus $\varepsilon_{tY} = \Delta L_Y/L$ and $\varepsilon_{tY}(\%) = 100 \times \Delta L_Y/L$.

Tensile strain at tensile strength
Tensile strain at tensile strength $(\varepsilon_M$ or $\varepsilon_M(\%))$ is that tensile strain at the maximum tensile stress observed during the test, if this occurs without yielding and changes in gauge length are measured. It is expressed as a dimensionless ratio $(\varepsilon_M = \Delta L_{OM}/L_O)$ or a percentage $(\varepsilon_M(\%) = 100 \times \Delta L_{OM}/L_O)$, where ΔL_{OM} is the elongation in the gauge length at the tensile strength.

Nominal tensile strain at tensile strength
The equivalent to the above, if grip separation at maximum stress (ΔL_M) is used rather than change in gauge length, is nominal tensile strain at tensile strength. This term must also be used if the material yields before reaching maximum stress (e.g. Fig. 12.16, curve c). Again this may be a dimensionless ratio ($\varepsilon_{tM} = \Delta L_M/L$) or a percentage ($\varepsilon_{tM}(\%) = 100 \times \Delta L_M/L$).

Tensile strain at break
The tensile strain at break (ε_B) is the tensile strain at the tensile stress at break if the sample breaks without yielding (e.g. Fig. 12.16, curve c). It is a measure of the overall extensibility or ductility of a material. This can be expressed as a dimensionless ratio ($\varepsilon_B = \Delta L_{OB}/L_O$) or as a percentage ($\varepsilon_{tB}(\%) = 100 \times \Delta L_{OB}/L$), ΔL_{OB} being the deformation between gauge marks at break.

Nominal tensile strain at break
If the sample yields prior to fracture (e.g. Fig. 12.16, curves a and b) or grip separation is used in measurements, nominal tensile strain at break (ε_{tB}) should be calculated. Again this can be a dimensionless ratio ($\varepsilon_{tB} = \Delta L_B/L$) or a percentage ($\varepsilon_{tB}(\%) = 100 \times \Delta L_B/L$), ΔL_B being the deformation between grips at break.

Elastic modulus
An initial linear portion of the curve indicates that the deformation in this region obeys Hooke's law, i.e. the induced strain is directly proportional to the applied stress. The uniaxial modulus of elasticity in tension, or Young's modulus, (E in MPa) is obtained from the slope of the regression of stress (σ) on strain (ε) in the region of linear elastic deformation, i.e. $E = \Delta\sigma/\Delta\varepsilon$. According to Fig. 12.16 (see curve b as an example); this corresponds to:

$$E = (\sigma_2 - \sigma_1)/(\varepsilon_2 - \varepsilon_1) \tag{12.16}$$

Due to their viscoelastic behaviour, many properties of film coating polymers are time-dependent. With regard to the tensile test, this causes non-linear stress/strain curves (bending towards the strain axis) even within the range of linear viscoelasticity (see section 12.1.2 above). Consequently, values of elastic modulus determined by drawing a tangent to the beginning of this curve (*initial tangent modulus*) are operator-dependent and do not yield reliable values for modulus. ISO 527–1 recommends that this technique is no longer used. Instead, two values for ε_1 and ε_2 are recommended – 0.05 and 0.25% respectively. Note that both these strains are small ensuring that the initial part of the curve is assessed. The lower value is not zero in order to avoid errors in the measured modulus caused by possible onset effects at the beginning of the stress/strain curve. A computational linear regression can be performed between these two points if sufficient data points are available.

The modulus of elasticity is a measure of the stiffness and rigidity of the film.

Poisson's ratio
When a material is stretched it becomes thinner. The ratio of these changes in strain is called Poisson's ratio (μ) (or ν is often used). Poisson's ratio is the negative ratio

of the tensile strain (ε_n) in one of two axes normal to the direction of pull (i.e. the width or thickness of film) to the corresponding strain (ε) in the direction of pull (i.e. length of sample) within the linear portion of the stress-strain curve. It is always expressed as a dimensionless ratio and is calculated as:

$$\mu_n = -\,\varepsilon_n/\varepsilon \tag{12.17}$$

The negative sign in the equation compensates for the negative strain of ε_n (because this dimension is decreasing) and thus Poisson's ratio is always a positive number. The Poisson's ratio of a film influences the generation of internal stresses as the film shrinks around the core during coating. This is discussed in detail in Section 12.5.

Area under stress-strain curve
The area under a force-displacement curve (a non-ISO assessment) is equal to the work (force × elongation, Nm) expanded in straining the sample to failure. The area under a stress-strain curve is the work expended in straining unit volume of the sample to failure and is a measure of the material's toughness. Toughness is not clearly definable but is bound up with impact strength. Toughness is an important property in tablet or pellet film coating since it governs the ability of the coated cores to withstand shock loads – within the factory, at the dispensary and when the product is carried about by the patient – without damaging the integrity of the film.

Overall mechanical considerations
It is important when examining the mechanical properties of a material that all relevant mechanical properties are considered together, not just a single parameter. An illustration of this point can be made by considering the addition of titanium dioxide in increasing concentrations to HPMC films. This is discussed in a later section of this chapter (12.3.4), but for this present discussion reference can be made to Fig. 2.10. If one was to consider the effect of titanium dioxide addition on tensile stress at break only, one could be misled into assuming that its addition has a negligible effect on the mechanical properties of the film. Whereas examination of all the data obtainable from stress-strain plots will show that titanium dioxide produces a marked reduction in the toughness of the film. This is due to its effect on nominal tensile strain at break. The marked reduction in this property produces very brittle films at high titanium dioxide concentrations.

Various shapes of stress–strain curve
Different materials may exhibit different characteristic stress–strain relations. A number of workers (Carswell & Nason, 1944; Lever & Rhys, 1968) have classified material properties on the basis of their characteristic stress–strain curves. Stress–stain curves typical of various types of material are shown in Fig. 12.17. These correspond to the classification of Lever & Rhys (1968) given in Table 12.2.

12.3.4 The tensile testing of film-coating materials
Some of the research work published on the effects of additives on the tensile properties of polymer films is described below. It is interesting when examining the

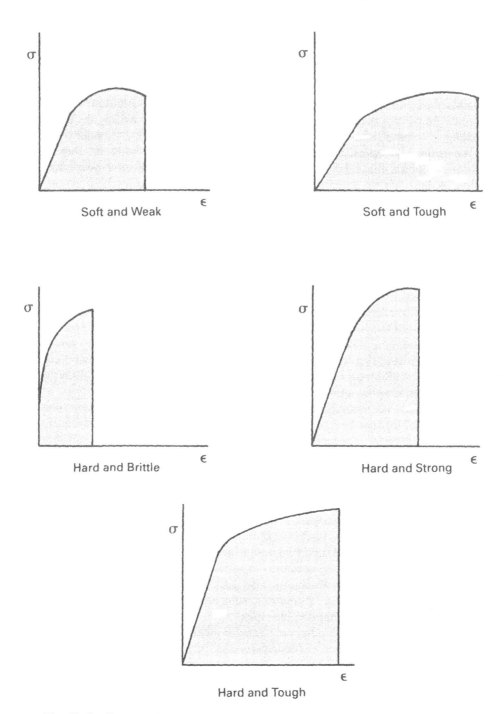

Fig. 12.17 Characteristic stress–strain curves for different types of materials (after Carswell & Nason, 1944).

effects of additives to view the changes in film properties in the light of the scheme of Lever & Rhys (1968) discussed above (Table 12.2).

Plasticizer effects

The addition of plasticizers is often necessary in order to improve the film-forming characteristic, workability and serviceability of a polymer. Their addition will alter the physical properties of the polymer, reducing brittleness by increasing flexibility and ductility. The method by which they impart flexibility to the film is thought to be due to imposition of the plasticizer molecules between the polymer chains and thus disruption of the forces which hold the chains together. The most effective plasticizers are generally those having structures which closely resemble those of the polymer that they are plasticizing. Plasticizers used in aqueous film coating are limited by toxicity and compatibility. For HPMC useable plasticizers include such water-soluble polyols as glycerol or propylene glycol and the series of polyethylene glycols (the PEGs). All of these have hydroxyl groups which enable suitable interactions with HPMC. The compatibility levels of these plasticizers with HPMC have been reported by Aulton *et al.* (1981), Okhamafe & York (1985b and c) and Sakellariou *et al.* (1986).

Interactions between various plasticizers and HPMC, and their effect on the properties of free films, have been investigated by Entwistle & Rowe (1978, 1979), Aulton *et al.* (1981), Okhamafe & York (1983b, 1985b), Masilungan & Lordi (1984) and Sakellariou *et al.* (1986). Since some of the effects caused by adding plasticizers might be detrimental to the properties of the film when applied to substrate cores, Aulton *et al.* (1981) concluded that careful consideration should be given (a) to whether a plasticizer should be included and (b) its concentration.

The volatility of a plasticizer is dependent on both its effective vapour pressure and its rate of diffusion through the polymer matrix. These in turn are dependent on polymer/plasticizer interactions. Pickard (1979) found that a considerable loss of the plasticizer propylene glycol occurred both during the coating process and on storage. This loss resulted in significant changes in film water vapour permeability, strength and elasticity. Loss of propylene glycol during coating has also been reported by Skultety & Sims (1987).

Plasticizers should not be volatile. Thus water, while having a plasticizing effect on many water-soluble polymers (such as HPMC, see Fig. 12.13), is not a true plasticizer and should never be used as such because of its volatility and non-permanence.

Generally, the addition of plasticizer increased the ductility of the film, but this is often accompanied by a reduction in its tensile strength and modulus of elasticity. The addition of plasticizer, therefore, results in a soft, tough film. Increasing the plasticizer concentration enhances this effect.

Porter & Ridgway (1977) observed that the inclusion of increasing amounts of diethyl phthalate resulted in a decrease in the tensile strength of some enteric coating polymers. Hawes (1978) reported the plasticization of HPMC by glycerol and PEG 400. Entwistle & Rowe (1979) studied the influence of chain length of a series of dialkyl phthalates and the molecular weight of a series of ethylene glycol derivatives on the mechanical properties of ethylcellulose and HPMC respectively. A correlation was found between the intrinsic viscosity of polymer/plasticizer solutions and the tensile strength, tensile strain at break and work of failure of cast films. Within a homologous series of plasticizers, the magnitude of the mechanical properties exhibited a minimum when the intrinsic viscosity was at a maximum. No such correlation was found with plasticizers of different structures. A reduction in the tensile strength of ethylcellulose films with increasing content of diethyl phthalate was observed by Vemba *et al.* (1980). In contrast, they found little change with the addition of glycerol, soya oil or PEG 400.

Delporte (1980a and b) observed a reduction both in the elastic modulus and the limit of elastic deformation as the level of PEG 400 or propylene glycol in aqueous HPMC films was increased. Reductions in the strength of sprayed aqueous HPMC films with increasing concentrations of propylene glycol, glycerol, PEG 400 or PEG 4000 were reported by Porter (1980).

The effects of the inclusion of glycerol and a series of polyethylene glycols and moisture sorption on the tensile properties of cast HPMC films has been reported by Aulton *et al.* (1981). Incorporation of glycerol resulted in a reduction in the tensile strength and elastic modulus and an increase in extensibility. The magnitude of the effects increased as the level of glycerol was increased (Figs 2.6 and 12.18).

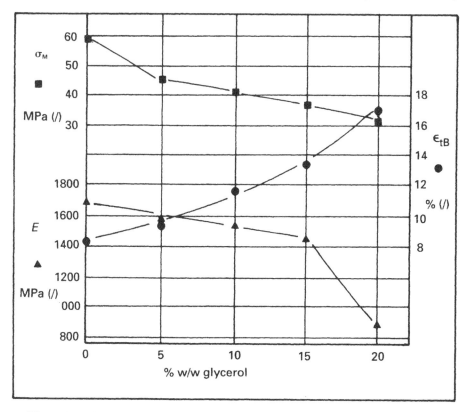

Fig. 12.18 Changes in tensile strength (σ_M), nominal tensile strain at break (ε_{tB}) and modulus of elasticity (E) with change in glycerol content of HPMC films.

Similar effects were observed by Aulton *et al.* (1981) with the inclusion of PEGs. Plasticization efficiency increased with decreasing PEG molecular weight (Figs 2.7 and 12.19), possibly due to the greater number of plasticizer molecules available to interact with the polymer. PEG 600 appears to have optimum plasticization effects.

Okhamafe & York (1983a) observed that increasing concentrations of PEGs 400 and 1000 progressively lowered the tensile strength and Young's modulus of cast HPMC films. The addition of polyvinyl alcohol (PVA) lowered the tensile strength and Young's modulus although to a lesser extent than the PEGs. PEGs generally increased the extensibility of the films while PVA reduced it, implying that, unlike PEGs, PVA inhibited polymer chain mobility. PEG 400 was found to be a more effective plasticizer than PEG 1000, in agreement with the earlier findings of Entwistle & Rowe (1979) and Aulton *et al.* (1981).

The plasticization of acrylic copolymer films, prepared from pseudolatex aqueous dispersions, by inclusion of different glycols was observed by Dittgen (1984). He also concluded that plasticization efficiency increased with decreasing glycol molecular weight.

Reading & Spring (1984b) observed that PEG 600, included as a potential plasticizer, showed no evidence of plasticization in cast films of four polymers used as tablet binders. Cast films containing PEG 600 at concentrations up to 10 % w/w were, without exception, weaker, less extendible and had a higher Young's modulus than the unmodified films.

As mentioned above, water is not a true plasticizer because of its volatility and lack of permanence. Yet its effect on the mechanical properties of polymer films is

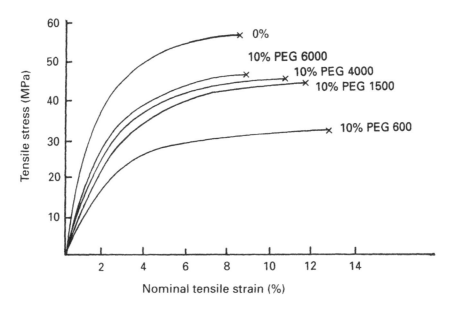

Fig. 12.19 Stress–strain curves for HPMC films containing 10% of different grades of polyethylene glycol.

similar to that observed by the addition of plasticizers. Aulton *et al.* (1981) demonstrated the considerable plasticizing action of water by comparing the properties of unplasticized HPMC films stored at relative humidities of 10 and 80% (as shown in Fig. 12.13). This effect was also reported by Masilungan & Lordi (1984) who showed the softening temperature of unplasticized HPMC films to be reduced after storage at high humidity.

Solid inclusion effects

Colorants and opaquant extenders are often added to coating formulations in order to improve appearance, to facilitate product identification (Rowe, 1983c) and to reduce film tackiness (Lindberg & Jönsson, 1972). Colorants fall into three main categories: synthetic water-soluble organic dyes (e.g. tartrazine, sunset yellow, erythrosine), their insoluble aluminium lakes (these consist of the corresponding water-soluble dyes adsorbed onto small, insoluble particles of alumina) and inorganic pigments (e.g. titanium dioxide, talc, calcium carbonate and the iron oxides). The structures, particle size distribution and properties of these have been reviewed by Patton (1979) and Rowe (1983b, 1985b).

The influence of aluminium lakes and inorganic pigments on the properties of both free and applied films is generally very different to that of plasticizers. Films are usually rendered harder, have an increased modulus of elasticity, are more brittle and exhibit a decreased tensile strain at break and tensile strength (Porter, 1980; Aulton *et al.*, 1984).

A decrease in the tensile strength of cast HPMC films with increasing content of titanium dioxide was noted by Hawes (1978), although the inclusion of a water-soluble dye had no significant effect. Porter (1980) found a significant reduction in the tensile strength of sprayed HPMC films with increasing inclusion of titanium dioxide and also with the inclusion of an aluminium lake. Delporte (1980a and b) found that increasing the titanium dioxide content of HPMC films resulted in an increased modulus of elasticity but little change in the limit of elasticity.

Aulton *et al.* (1984) showed a marked reduction in the work done in breaking the film of HPMC films with increased solids content. This was indicated by a reduction in the strain at break, an increase in elastic modulus but only a slight fall in tensile strength, i.e. there was a general transition towards a more brittle state (see Figs 2.10 and 12.20).

As discussed by Aulton *et al.* (1984), the area beneath a stress–strain curve (AUC) is equal to the work of fracture (MJ/m^3) of the film, as is shown by equation (12.18):

$$AUC = \text{Tensile stress} \times \text{Nominal tensile strain}$$

$$= MPa \times \frac{m}{m} = \frac{MN}{m^2} \times \frac{m}{m} = \frac{MJ}{m^3} \qquad (12.18)$$

The decrease in the value of work of fracture as more solid is added to an HPMC film is illustrated by the data in Table 12.3. The data also illustrate that while the shape of the stress–strain curve is influenced by storage humidity, the toughness of the films stored at widely different humidities is surprisingly similar.

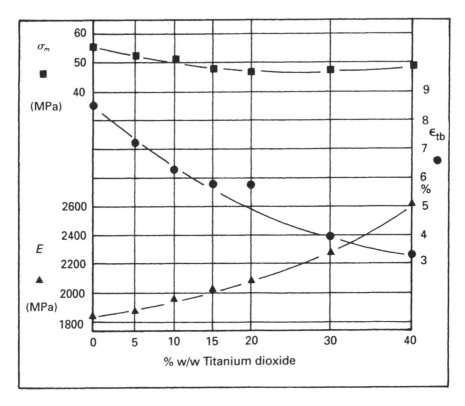

Fig. 12.20 Graphical representation of the effect of titanium dioxide addition on the tensile strength (σ_M), nominal tensile strain at break (ε_{tB}) and modulus of elasticity (E) of cast HPMC films.

Table 12.3 Work of rupture of HPMC E5 films as a function of titanium dioxide concentration and storage humidity (data from Aulton *et al.*, 1984)

Titanium dioxide concentration	Work of rupture (MJ/m³)	
	at 10 %r.h.	at 80 %r.h.
0	3.22	3.20
5	2.26	2.26
10	1.83	1.90
15	1.63	1.61
20	1.53	1.52
30	1.24	1.28
40	1.08	1.00

Aluminium lakes

A similar effect was noted by Aulton *et al.* (1984) for the addition of insoluble aluminium lakes (see Fig. 12.21).

Tobolsky (1971) suggested that filled or pigmented polymer films might be analysed in a manner analogous to suspensions. Rowe (1983c), using this concept, applied a modified Einstein equation to calculate modulus enhancement in pigmented HPMC tablet film-coating formulations. Okhamafe & York (1984b, 1985c) observed that the inclusion of solids (pigments, fillers, talc and titanium dioxide) generally reduced the tensile strength and extensibility while increasing the Young's modulus of HPMC films. The magnitude of this effect was a function both of filler morphology and of filler/polymer interaction.

Dittgen (1984) observed that the inclusion of some drugs to polymer films resulted in a plasticization action on acrylic copolymer films, while others produced films which were significantly more brittle than the parent polymer.

Controlling the particle size of any pigment/opacifier is crucial to efficient film formation. Too large particles not only look unsightly but they also contribute to film weakness by acting as stress loci.

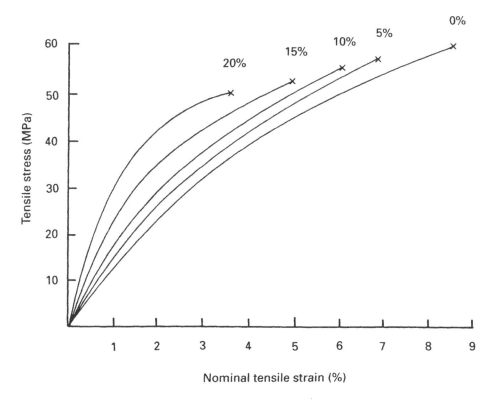

Fig. 12.21 Stress–strain curves for cast HPMC films loaded with a regular grade of Brilliant Blue FCF lake (Colorcon). The figures on the curves refer to the concentration of lake (%w/w) in the dried film.

Other additive effects

The effect of polysorbate 80 (a surfactant) and sodium benzoate (a preservative) on the tensile properties of HPMC films has been examined by Abdul-Razzak (1980). He found that the addition of polysorbate 80 improved the mechanical properties of the films up to a loading of 3 %w/w; above this figure its addition had a detrimental effect. The presence of sodium benzoate was also beneficial up to concentrations of 4 %w/w.

Reading & Spring (1984b) examined the effects of lactose and sodium lauryl sulphate on the tensile properties of films prepared from four polymers. Their inclusion resulted in a reduction of the tensile strength of all the films tested; indeed, some films became too brittle to test.

Processing effects

Allen *et al.* (1972), when spraying solutions of cellulose acetate in acetone in a model system, found that increasing the flow rate could result in films which were stronger and less elastic, as well as being more dense and less permeable to moisture. Also, increasing the spray gun–to–bed distance produced weaker films which were less dense, more permeable and more elastic.

Tensile viscoelastic characteristics of polymer films

Studies of the viscoelastic deformation of film-forming polymers by tensile testing have been limited, probably because of the difficulties in mounting the sample to limit slight slippage at the grips during testing. Castello & Goyan (1964) used the tensile method to investigate the viscoelasticity of glycerogelatin films used in the manufacture of soft gelatin capsules. Thermally aged films showed decreased initial rigidity moduli and decreased equilibrium moduli compared with unaged films, this being associated with a thermally mediated crystalline–amorphous transition in the glycerogelatin melt.

12.3.5   Conclusions on tensile testing

An examination of the tensile deformation of a free film, cut to a suitable shape, can give data on yield point, tensile strength, tensile strain at break and modulus elasticity, as well as the work done in breaking the film. It is possible to define an ideal film in terms of these parameters and, using such a classification, any beneficial or detrimental effects of additives such as plasticizers, opacifiers, colorants, etc., can be quantified.

12.4   INDENTATION TESTING

12.4.1   Quasistatic hardness

In the context of film coating, hardness can be defined as *the quasistatic resistance to local non-homogeneous deformation caused by point or line-shaped force centres* (Braun, 1958). Hardness has also been described as *the ability of the coating, as opposed to its substrate, to resist indentation or penetration by a hard object* (British

Standard, 1992). This latter definition is particularly relevant to the testing of film coats on tablets or pellets as it necessitates careful choice of indenter loads. It is recommended that the depth of indentation should not be greater than one-sixth of the film thickness. Indentation hardness measurements made at depths greater than this may be affected by the substrate, i.e. the tablet core or pellet in this context.

Indentation testing consists of allowing an indenter tip—for example, a hard sphere or square pyramid—to flow under a known load into a film coat and then measuring the penetration of the indenter into the sample. An indenter will travel further into a soft film and less into a harder one.

Reviews of the theory of indentation testing and descriptions of suitable available apparatus have been presented by Aulton (1977, 1982).

The way in which an indentation test can be associated with material properties can be explained as follows. Let us assume that a 'step' load is placed on a spherical indenter (i.e. the load is applied at once, rather than gradually or at a fixed strain rate). At the first point of contact between indenter and sample, the area of contact between the two is infinitely small and thus the stress (load/area) is infinitesimally large. This stress will obviously be greater than the yield strength of the sample and thus the indenter will penetrate into the surface.

As penetration continues, the area of contact between the sphere increases while the applied force remains constant; there is therefore a gradual reduction in the stress beneath the indenter. This continues until the stress is reduced to a level where it no longer exceeds the yield stress of the material. At this point indentation will cease. The resulting shape of the penetration depth *versus* time profile for a non-viscoelastic material is therefore as shown in Fig. 12.22.

Recovery is also shown in the diagram. Here the driving force is the relaxation of the elastic strain within the material as a result of the indentation.

Thus indentation under load is a measure of the yield stress of the material. Hardness (H) and yield stress (σ_y) of a plastic material are interrelated by the following equation:

$$\sigma_y \approx \frac{H}{3} \tag{12.19}$$

The recovery curve can also yield very useful information. Fig. 12.22 illustrates that the recovery will differentiate between the permanent plastic deformation (h_2) and the elastic recovery Δh, i.e. $h_1 - h_2$). The ratio $\Delta h/h_1$ is known as the *elastic quotient* of the material. High values indicate a high resilience of the sample. Thus, a very simple test can help us to differentiate the relative contributions of the elastic and plastic components of a deformation.

12.4.2 Quantification of hardness
Dimensionally, hardness is expressed in terms of the load applied by the indenter divided by the area beneath the indenter which supports that load when penetration ceases. It therefore has the dimensions of pressure and its units are pascals, typically MPa.

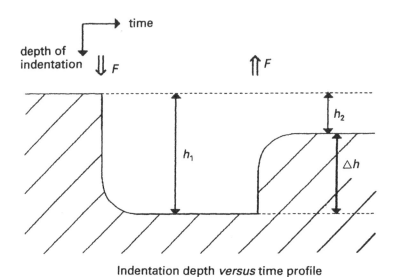

Indentation depth *versus* time profile

Fig. 12.22   Penetration depth versus time profile for the indentation of a material with little time-dependency of deformation.

Hardness values

Brinell and Meyer's hardness

The Brinell and Meyer's tests use a spherical indenter (see Fig. 12.23). Brinell hardness (HB) and Meyer's hardness (HM) values are calculated thus:

$$HB = \frac{\text{Load}}{\text{Curved area of indentation}} \tag{12.20}$$

$$= \frac{2F}{\pi D[D - (D^2 - d^2)^{0.5}]} \tag{12.21}$$

$$= \frac{F}{\pi Dh} \tag{12.22}$$

$$HM = \frac{\text{Load}}{\text{Projected area of indentation}} \tag{12.23}$$

$$= \frac{4F}{\pi d^2} \tag{12.24}$$

In these equations, F is the applied load, D is the diameter of the indenting sphere, h is the depth of indentation and d is the diameter of the indentation in the plane of the film surface.

Meyer's hardness has the advantage that it more closely approximates the mean stress in the material beneath the indenter.

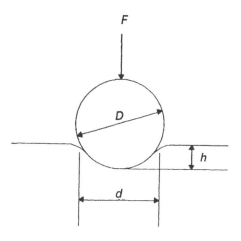

$$\text{Hardness} = \frac{\text{Load}}{\text{Area of indentation}}$$

Fig. 12.23   Geometry of spherical indentation, where F is the load applied, h is the depth of penetration, d is the diameter of the indentation and D is the diameter of the indenter. Hardness is calculated from applied load divided by the area of indentation which supports that load.

Vickers hardness
The Vickers hardness test uses a 136° square-pyramidal diamond indenter (see Fig. 12.24). Vickers hardness (HV), is calculated thus:

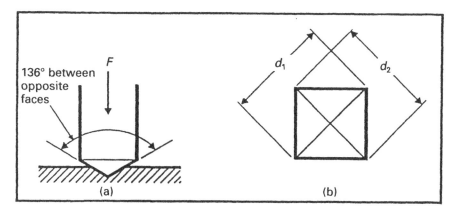

Fig. 12.24   Vickers indentation test: (a) square-pyramidal diamond indenter; (b) form of indentation (plan view). The value d in equations (12.25) and (12.26) is the arithmetic mean of d_1 and d_2.

$$HV = \frac{2F \sin(136°/2)}{d^2}$$ (12.25)

$\sim 1.854F/d^2$ (12.26)

Here d is the arithmetic mean length of the two diagonals of the square impression left by the indenter.

Measurement of hardness

Measurements of hardness are usually performed by lowering an indenter sphere until it just touches the surface to be indented, adding an appropriate weight and monitoring the penetration. The final penetration can be assessed by removing the indenter and examining the impression left in the surface, or by following the vertical movement of the indenter as it penetrates into the test sample.

Indentation testers

Leitz microhardness tester

The Leitz microhardness tester is used to measure Vickers hardness. It is basically a modified microscope with one of the objective lenses being replaced by a pyramidal diamond indenter. It has an adjustable microscope slide sample holder which allows movement of the specimen to be indented in order to allow operator selection of indentation site so that gross defects, etc., can be avoided. The indenter is a square-pyramidal diamond with a point of 136° angle. The indenter is rotated into position above the specimen and brought into contact with the surface at a controlled rate; the indenter load is variable between 5 and 2000 g. On removal of the indenter from the specimen surface, it is rotated away and an optical objective is swung into place. The indentation geometry is measured with the aid of an eyepiece graticule. Illumination is by normal or polarized light shining onto the surface through the objective. Both diagonals of the square impression of the indentation are measured and their mean value inserted into equation (12.25) or (12.26) in order to calculate Vickers hardness.

ICI microindentation tester

Monk & Wright (1965) described the construction and use of a pneumatic microindentation apparatus for measuring the hardness of paint films. The precision of the instrument and its application in characterizing the viscoelastic properties of thin polymer films have been discussed by Morris (1970, 1973). A commercial version of this design was marketed by Research Equipment (London) Ltd. It consists of a spherical indenter, of selectable diameter, which can be lowered gently onto the test surface under a selected load of a few grams (1 to 32 g are available). The indenter is fitted at the end of a beam mounted on cross-flexure bearings which are affixed to a triangular-shaped main chassis of steel plate supported on a base by three adjustable legs. The depth of the indentation and recovery on load removal can both be measured. The timing of the loading–unloading cycle can be controlled automatically. On the original machine the indenter movement is measured by a double pneumatic amplification system of the flapper and nozzle type powered by compressed oxygen-free nitrogen. The outlet pressure from this circuit is displayed on a pneumatic chart recorder, full-scale deflection being equivalent to 6 μm depth of indentation.

The main advantage of this type of machine is that changes in indentation depth with time can be recorded continuously, thus enabling the continuous calculation of creep compliance changes allowing the creep analysis of viscoelastic film-coating materials by following the procedures discussed below in section 12.4.3.

Aulton *et al.* (1986) developed this machine by replacing the pneumatic amplification system used to measure indenter penetration with a LVDT, the output of which is logged, *via* an analogue-to-digital converter, by a microcomputer. The advantages of this type of data gathering *versus* the original chart recorder are at their greatest with respect to accuracy of measurement of indentation depth and time, and speed of data manipulation. The apparatus is now accurate to better than 0.1 μm. These authors have also written a suite of software to perform the mathematical and graphical manipulations necessary to perform both discrete mechanical and continuous spectral analyses of creep compliance (as described in next section).

12.4.3 Time-dependent indentation

Introduction

One major characteristic of the indentation profile of polymer films, particularly if plasticized, is their time-dependent nature. Thus the profile shown in Fig. 12.22 is rarely seen and indentation curves are more likely to appear as those in Fig. 12.25.

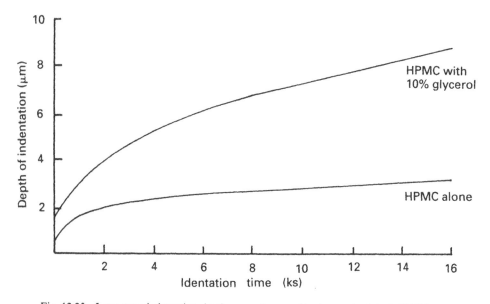

Fig. 12.25   Long-term indentation depth *versus* time profiles for unplasticized HPMC and HPMC plasticized with 10 %w/w glycerol.

The shape of these curves causes difficulty in the interpretation of single-point indentation data. The measured hardness value, using the equations described above, will depend on the duration of the test, since the indentation profile of a polymer may not achieve an equilibrium depth and thus hardness apparently decreases with time. Indeed, Aulton (1982) questioned the validity of using single-point hardness values at all for such polymers. This problem may be overcome by the adoption of a standard indentation duration (as suggested in ISO, ASTM and BS specifications). However, this single-point determination can fail to discriminate between films with quite different deformation characteristics. Indeed, depending on the time of indentation, equivalent hardnesses may be obtained for polymers of vastly differing viscoelastic properties, as is illustrated by Fig. 12.26.

Both qualitative and quantitative indentation assessments have been utilized to investigate time-dependent deformation in polymeric materials of pharmaceutical importance.

Qualitative assessments

Probably the most informative technique for studying time-dependent deformation of polymer films is the creep test, in which a (ideally instantaneous) load is imposed on a sample at zero time and maintained at a constant value while resulting changes in the strain are measured with time. Creep rheological methodology has been applied to a wide range of materials of pharmaceutical interest, including polymers. Micro-indentation techniques have proved to be particularly informative in this context.

A qualitative approach to the interpretation of these data is to compare visually the indentation depth *versus* time profiles for a range of polymers and formulations. Glassy and rubbery polymers show rectangular-shaped curves and viscoelastic materials give characteristically curved traces. The technique can be used, for

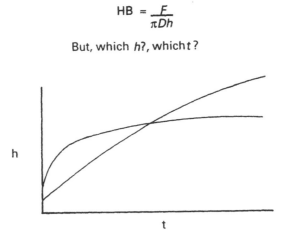

$$HB = \frac{F}{\pi Dh}$$

But, which *h*?, which *t*?

Fig. 12.26 Indentation depth *versus* time profiles of two polymer formulations with different deformation characteristics (after Aulton, 1982).

example, to estimate the efficiency of various plasticizer types and levels in a film coat formulation. This approach is reasonably informative; representative indentation depth *versus* time curves are shown later in this chapter.

Quantitative assessments

The changes in the geometry of the indentation as penetration increases with time, and the consequential change in stress conditions, potentially limit the use of indentation apparatus for fundamental studies. A solution to the problem of the partial penetration of an incompressible semi-infinite plane viscoelastic surface by a smooth rigid sphere has been suggested by Lee & Radok (1960). They derived the following equation:

$$J(t) = \left(\frac{16}{3}\right) \cdot R^{0.5} \cdot \left(\frac{1}{F}\right) \cdot h(t)^{3/2} \tag{12.27}$$

where $J(t)$ is the overall creep compliance at time t, R is the radius of the indenting sphere, F is the indenting force and $h(t)$ is the depth of indentation at time t.

As a test sample is penetrated by an indenter sphere, the geometry of the indentation and hence the stress conditions beneath it are continually changing, but indentation depths can be converted easily to creep compliance using equation (12.27).

Analysis of creep compliance

Data obtained from the ICI microindenter are in the form of a depth of indentation *versus* time profile. In order to yield the most information it is necessary to convert these data to the form of a creep curve.

Indentation profiles are determined only under load and not in recovery. The stress conditions beneath the indenter during loading are given explicitly by the solution of the Lee & Radok equation. On removal of the indenting load, however, the prevailing stress conditions are an unknown. During this phase, the observed strain recovery may be a function of stress transmission from the test sample to the indenter sphere (decreasing with time as the sample recovers) and of the elastic recovery of the crossed flexure bearings of the beam (or other balancing mechanism) of the indenter.

Polymer film indentation depth profiles can be converted to creep compliance and examination shows them to be represented by the idealized creep compliance curve shown in Fig. 12.27.

Figure 12.27 is annotated with the three discrete components of creep under load described below. Analysis of such a curve is carried out using the classical methods reviewed by Barry (1974). This analysis, detailed below, quantifies the instantaneous elastic compliance (J_0), the overall creep compliance of the time-dependent elastic deformations (J_R), the instantaneous elastic modulus ($1/J_0$), creep compliance of non-recoverable viscous deformation (J_N) and the Newtonian viscosity (t/J_N).

Region of instantaneous compliance

The line A–B in Fig. 12.27 is the region of instantaneous elastic deformation. The instantaneous compliance (J_0) is obtained by dividing the strain (ε_0) measured at the onset of applied stress (i.e. at time $t = 0$) by the applied stress (σ). Thus,

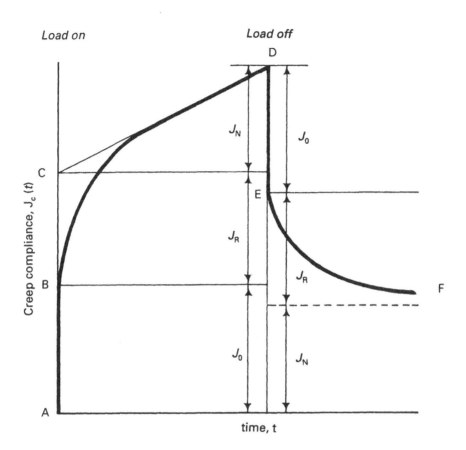

Fig. 12.27   An idealized creep curve (creep compliance *versus* time) for a typical polymer film. J_0 = the compliance of initial instantaneous elastic deformation, recoverable on removal of load, J_R = the overall creep compliance of the time-dependent elastic deformations (also recoverable in time) and J_N = the creep compliance of the non-recoverable viscous deformation.

the instantaneous compliance (J_0) is the reciprocal of the instantaneous elastic modulus (G_0):

$$J_0 = \frac{\varepsilon_0}{\sigma} = \frac{1}{G_0} \tag{12.28}$$

Time-dependent retarded elastic region
The curve B–D in Fig. 12.27 is the retarded elastic region. The region B–D also contains an element of viscous (permanent) deformation. Subtracting the creep compliance of this $(J_N$, see next section) leaves a time-dependent retarded elastic compliance of J_R.
   Using mean values for the parameters:

$$J_R = J_M \cdot \left[1 - \exp\left(-\frac{t}{\tau_M} \right) \right] = \frac{\varepsilon_R(t)}{\sigma} \qquad (12.29)$$

where J_M is the mean compliance of all the bonds involved and τ_M is the mean retardation time (= J_M/η_M). η_M is the mean viscosity associated with the retarded elastic region and $\varepsilon_R(t)$ is the strain in this region at time t. This equation holds where the retarded elastic behaviour can be characterized by a single Voigt unit.

Where more than one Voigt unit is necessary, J_R (the time-dependent retarded elastic compliance) is a summation of the individual compliance (J_i) of all the Voigt units involved, thus:

$$J_R = \sum_i J_i \left[1 - \exp\left(-\frac{t}{\tau_i} \right) \right] \qquad (12.30)$$

τ_i is the retardation time of the ith Voigt unit and is equal to $J_i.\eta_i$ or η_i/G_i.

Linear Newtonian viscous region
The line C–D in Fig. 12.27 is the linear region of non-recoverable (Newtonian viscous) compliance (J_N) where:

$$J_N = \frac{t}{\eta_0} = \frac{\varepsilon_N(t)}{\sigma} \qquad (12.31)$$

η_0 is the apparent Newtonian viscosity of viscous flow and $\varepsilon_N(t)$ is the strain at time t. In this region bonds may rupture so that the time required for them to reform is greater than the test period and the entities flow past each other.

The total creep compliance at any time ($J_C(t)$) for n Voigt units is given by:

$$J_C(t) = J_0 + \sum_{i=1}^{i=n} J_i \left[1 + \exp\left(-\frac{t}{\tau_i} \right) \right] + \frac{t}{\eta_0} \qquad (12.32)$$

Region following load removal
On removal of the indenting stress, there is some strain recovery. This comprises an instantaneous elastic recovery (D–E, Fig. 12.27) of the same magnitude as the initial elastic deformation (A–B) followed by a retarded elastic recovery (E–F), the compliance of which is equivalent to B–C. In the viscous region C–D, bonds are irreversibly broken and the initial structure is not recovered, i.e. the deformation is plastic and permanent.

Discrete mechanical analysis of creep compliance
Characterization of the creep curve in terms of Maxwell and Voigt mechanical models (see section 12.1.2 earlier in this chapter) is termed discrete mechanical analysis. The viscoelastic response can then be quantified and represented visually in terms of mechanical properties of Hookean springs and Newtonian dashpots.

Classical analysis of the creep curve using graphical techniques is illustrated in Figs 12.28a–c.

The instantaneous elastic compliance J_0 is obtained directly from the creep curve as time tends to zero. The rigidity modulus G_0 is given by the reciprocal of J_0. The apparent Newtonian viscosity η_0 associated with the compliance of non-recoverable deformation is obtained from the slope of the late linear portion of the creep curve since:

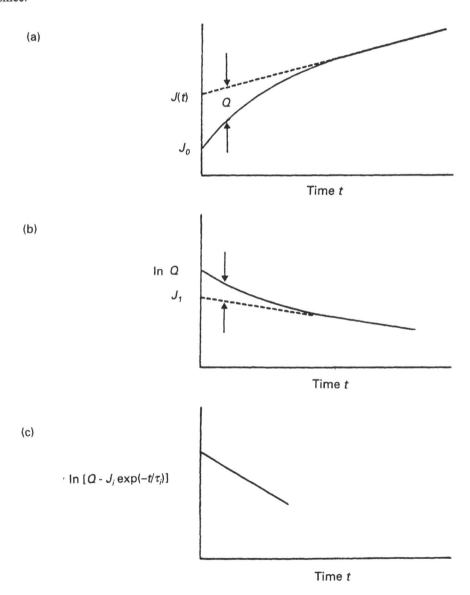

Fig. 12.28   Discrete mechanical analysis of the creep curve using a graphical technique.

$$J_N = \frac{t}{\eta_0} \tag{12.33}$$

Resolution of the discrete Voigt units required to model the retarded elastic region is achieved graphically using an exponential stripping technique. The retarded elastic compliance J_R is the summation of compliances due to the individual Voigt units:

$$J_R = \sum_i J_i \left[1 - \exp\left(-\frac{t}{\tau_i} \right) \right] \tag{12.34}$$

Expanding the expression and defining a function Q such that:

$$Q = \sum_i J_i \exp\left(-\frac{t}{\tau_i} \right) \tag{12.35}$$

Q represents the distance at any time t between the curved portion of the creep curve and the extrapolated late linear region, assuming that linearity is attained (Fig. 12.28a).

Ignoring the summation and expressing the equation logarithmically,

$$\ln Q = \ln J_i \left(-\frac{t}{\tau_i} \right) \tag{12.36}$$

ln Q is then plotted against time (Fig. 12.28b). At late times the plot again tends to linearity. The intercept of the extrapolated linear plot and the reciprocal of the slope gives the compliance J_1 and retardation time τ_1 respectively for the first Voigt unit. The apparent viscosity of the dashpot component of the Voigt unit is given by:

$$\eta_1 = \frac{\tau_1}{J_1} \tag{12.37}$$

Non-linearity at early times indicates the presence of more than one resolvable Voigt unit. The magnitude of the compliance and retardation time of the second Voigt unit is found by plotting $\ln[Q-J_i \exp(-t/\tau_i)]$ against time. This is equivalent to the distance between the curved region at early times and the extrapolated late linear region (Fig. 12.28c). The general process is repeated for subsequent Voigt units until the early time data are linear.

The results of Aulton et al. (1986) for a discrete mechanical analysis of a film-coating polymer (HPMC) alone and with increasing amounts of plasticizer are shown in 'spring and dashpot' form in Fig. 12.29.

Continuous spectral analysis of creep compliance
An alternative to discrete mechanical analysis is the use of continuous spectral analysis. The creep compliance curve can be manipulated so as to construct a continuous spectrum of retardation times. This spectrum represents viscoelasticity in a more generalized manner than functions such as $J_c(t)$ although interpretation of

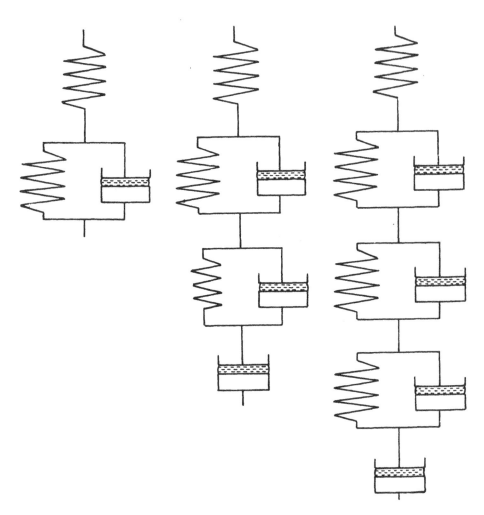

Fig. 12.29   Spring and dashpot models for a typical film-coating polymer; unplasticized
(left) and increasing plasticizer content (centre then right) (Aulton *et al.*, 1986).

the spectra obtained is difficult. The number of Voigt units in the retarded elastic
region of the creep curve is regarded as extending to infinity, and the retardation
spectrum, $\mathscr{L}$, is defined by the continuous analogue of creep compliance:

$$J(t) = J_0 + \int_{-\infty}^{+\infty} \mathscr{L}(\tau)\left[1 - \exp\left(-\frac{t}{\tau}\right)\right] \mathrm{d} \ln \tau + \frac{t}{\eta_0}\right] \qquad \text{(Eqn 12.38)}$$

$\mathscr{L}$ has the properties of a distribution function with the dimensions of compliance.

This treatment accepts that in a complex (real) material there is such a large
number of different molecular interactions that a wide range of retardation times
exist and that differences between adjacent retardation times may be infinitesimal.

The complete spectrum may extend over several orders of magnitude, so, by convention, a logarithmic representation is used. Maxima in the spectrum indicate concentrations of retardation processes (which are time-dependent elastic strain mechanisms at a molecular level) as measured by their contribution to the overall compliance.

Methods for the construction of retardation spectra have been described by Alfrey (1948), Schwarzl & Staverman (1952) and Barry (1974). The value of the distribution function $\mathcal{L}(\tau)$ at any time can be derived from a first-order differential approximation:

$$\mathcal{L}(\tau) \approx \left(\frac{\mathrm{d}}{\mathrm{d}\ln t}\right) \cdot \left[J(t) - \left(\frac{t}{\eta_0}\right)\right] \tag{12.39}$$

The elastic component of creep compliance $(J(t) - t/\eta_0)$ derived from the creep curve is plotted against $\ln(t)$. The gradient of this curve is calculated at selected points in order to provide the data to calculate $\mathcal{L}(t)$. This method has the disadvantage that η_0 must be known, i.e. the steady-state region of viscous flow must be attained. Where the linear viscous region is not reached—for example, in systems where several hours are required to ensure that all Voigt units are fully extended—a second-order approximation (for $t = 2\tau$) may be used:

$$\mathcal{L}(\tau) \approx \left(\frac{\mathrm{d}}{\mathrm{d}\ln t}\right) \cdot \left[J(t) - \left(\frac{\mathrm{d}J(t)}{\mathrm{d}\ln t}\right)\right] \tag{12.40}$$

Application of the second-order approximation (Schwarzl & Staverman, 1952) is illustrated in Fig. 12.30.

Both discrete mechanical and continual spectral analysis can, of course, be performed by computer with suitably written software (e.g. Aulton et al., 1986).

12.4.4 Indentation properties of film-coating materials
The use of microindentation testing in the assessment of the hardness and elastic/viscoelastic properties both of film-coating materials and film-coated tablets has been reported by several authors. The results from these studies have been used to assess such factors as the effect of plasticizers and colorants/fillers (Rowe, 1976a; Aulton et al., 1981, 1984; Okhamafe & York, 1986), stability behaviour (Okhamafe & York, 1986) and the potential for film defects such as edge splitting and intagliation bridging (Rowe, 1982).

Plasticizer effects
Several workers have used microindentation to characterize the mechanical properties of film-coating polymers in order to assess the performance of potential plasticizers. Rowe (1976a) used the ICI microindenter to measure the elastic properties and hardness of HPMC coatings on tablets. Incorporation of glycerol and propylene glycol into HPMC films resulted in films which were softer and more elastic. A similar effect was noted with low molecular weight liquid PEGs. With higher molecular weight solid PEGs, an increase in elastic modulus occurred which, in the case

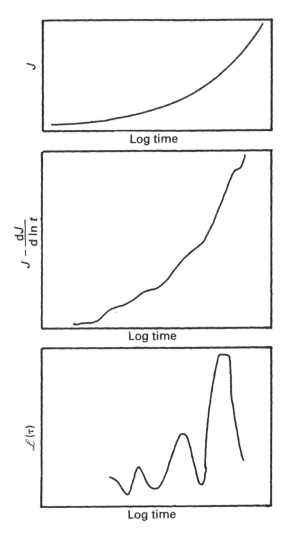

Fig. 12.30 Continuous spectral analysis of the creep curve using a second-order
approximation.

of PEG 20 000, exceeds the modulus of the unplasticized film. The molecular weight
of the PEGs did not appear to have a significant effect on the Brinell hardness of
the film although in all cases the hardness was less than that of the unplasticized
film.

Porter & Ridgway (1977) used an ICI microindenter to evaluate polyvinyl acetate
phthalate (PVAP) and cellulose acetate-phthalate (CAP) films *in situ* on tablet cores.
At low plasticizer concentration, CAP films exhibited much greater hardness than
PVAP films. But an increase in plasticizer level resulted in a decrease in hardness for
both films, with the hardness of CAP approaching that of PVAP.

Aulton *et al.* (1980, 1981), using the vertical displacement indentation tester of
White & Aulton (1980), reported indentation-depth profiles recorded over a 600 s
period for unplasticized and plasticized films of HPMC cast from aqueous solution.
They showed that both sorbed moisture and the presence of a plasticizer increased
time-dependent indentation compared with the unmodified polymer. The viscoelastic nature of HPMC deformation was clearly evident. The results of Aulton *et al.*
(1981) are shown in Figs 12.31 and 12.32.

Rowe (1976b) showed that increasing the molecular weight grade of PEG, at a
fixed plasticizer concentration of 20 %w/w, was found to produce less elastic HPMC
films, a fact that was attributed to the decrease in mole fraction of the hydroxyl
groups. The same conclusions was reached by Aulton *et al.* (1981). Some of their
data are reproduced in Fig. 12.33.

Porter (1980) investigated the mechanical properties of tablets coated with
HPMC films plasticized with glycerol, propylene glycol, PEG 400 and PEG 4000 at
concentrations of up to 40 %w/w. The inclusion of all the plasticizers studied
produced tablets possessing lower diametral crushing strengths, the effect becoming
greater as the plasticizer concentration increased. Little effect on film adhesion was
apparent, however.

Polymer molecular weight effects
The molecular weight of a polymer is important since it determines certain key
attributes of film properties. For instance, Rowe (1976b, 1980) has shown that for
HPMC, an increase in molecular weight provides a film which is harder, has a
greater elastic modulus and is more resistant to abrasion.

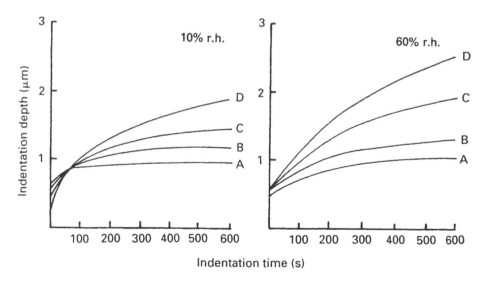

Fig. 12.31 Penetration of a spherical indenter into cast HPMC E5 films stored at two
different humidities showing the effect of the addition of glycerol. Curve A = 0%, B = 10%,
C = 20% and D = 30% (all %w/w in dried film).

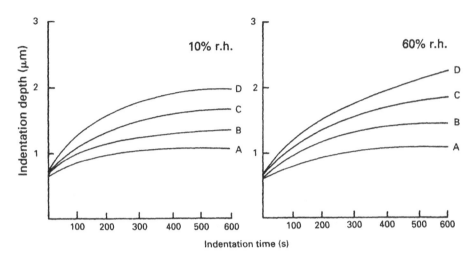

Fig. 12.32   Penetration of a spherical indenter into cast HPMC E5 films stored at two different humidities showing the effect of the addition of polyethylene glycol 600. Curve A = 0%, B = 10%, C = 20% and D = 30% (all %w/w in dried film).

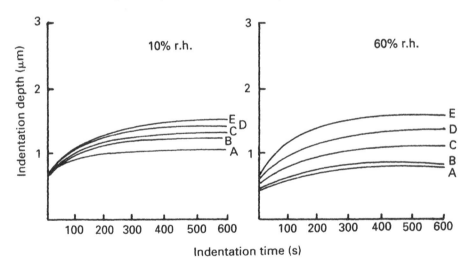

Fig. 12.33   Penetration of a spherical indenter into cast HPMC E5 films stored at two different humidities showing the influence of the grade of polyethylene glycol. A = HPMC alone; B = +10 %w/w PEG 6000; C = +10 %w/w PEG 4000; D = +10 %w/w PEG 1500; and E = +10 %w/w PEG 600.

Further evidence of the influence of HPMC grade on film mechanical properties was shown by Fell *et al.* (1979) when measuring the mechanical strength of film-coated tablets. For grades of nominal viscosity between 3 and 60 mPa s it was found that the maximum breaking strength of the coated tablets themselves progressively increased as the polymer average molecular weight increased.

Water content effects

The microindentation technique has also been applied to evaluate similar polymeric materials, such as those used as tablet binders. Rubinstein & Healey (1973) used the method to investigate moisture effects on gelatin binder films. Reading & Spring (1984a) used an ICI microindenter to study the hardness and creep compliance of a series of hydrophilic polymeric tablet binders. The binders examined were gelatin (Byco C), maize starch, methylcellulose (Methocel A15) and polyvinyl pyrrolidone (40 000 Da). The Brinell hardness of all films was decreased with increasing moisture content. Creep curves determined for films conditioned at 12% r.h. were elastic in nature with no time dependency under load. Conditioning at 81% r.h. (58% r.h. for PVP) resulted in films which deformed both elastically and plastically.

The influence of storage humidity on the indentation profiles of HPMC films have been shown above (Figs 12.31–12.33). At higher humidity storage, the films were softer and more viscoelastic in nature.

Process effects

Increasing the spray gun–to–bed distance, when spraying solutions of cellulose acetate in acetone in a model system, was found by Allen *et al.* (1972) to produce weaker films which were less dense, more permeable and more elastic. They also found that increasing the flow rate could result in films which were stronger and less elastic, as well as being more dense and less permeable to moisture.

Pickard (1979) reported that with organic–based coating formulations, the use of a spray gun resulted in films which were weaker and had a lower modulus of elasticity when compared with poured films. The differences in hardness/elasticity could have arisen potentially from either fundamental differences in the properties of the polymer or from the way in which the film was formed.

Okhamafe & York (1986), when applying an aqueous 10 %w/w HPMC solution (Pharmacoat 606) in a Wurster column, found that the Young's moduli of the sprayed films (determined using indentation testing) were about two to five times lower than those of equivalent cast films (values determined from tensile tests). These authors suggested that the morphology and molecular features (such as crystallinity and glass transition temperature) of a polymeric film formulation can be influenced by the film drying rate. Thus coating conditions which allow a greater time for film formation and molecular orientation would be expected to produce harder, less elastic films. These coating conditions could include: low atomizing air pressures, narrow spray cones, spray guns which tend to concentrate the droplets within the centre of the spray, high spray rates or low drying air temperatures and volume flow rates. Twitchell (1990) found that some of these conditions, e.g. the use of a narrow spray cone and guns with a high density of droplets in the central region, tend to cause harder/more elastic films.

The formation of aqueous film coats is a gradual process which may take several hours to complete. The film is made up from a series of droplets which impinge initially on the uncoated substrate and subsequently on a partly produced film coat. In order for the film hardness to approach a maximum, the film should be continuous with no entrapment of air, as occurs when films are cast from solutions. This is only likely to occur when there is no significant spray drying of the droplets during coating and when each droplet hitting the surface is able to flow and spread sufficiently to exclude air from within the film. In the practical situation the above criteria are unlikely to exist during the aqueous film-coating process, since evaporation may occur from the droplets during their passage to the substrate and the formulation and coating conditions may be such that droplet spreading is restricted. Film coats applied using organic solvent systems are thought more likely to have higher hardness values, since they utilize considerably higher spray rates (typically around five times higher) and lower solution viscosities. This may explain why Rowe (1976a) found little difference in indentation behaviour between films cast onto glass substrates and those coated onto flat-faced tablets when using organic coating solutions.

Application conditions will influence the thickness and density of the film and the spreading behaviour of droplets at the substrate/film surface. Conditions which increase droplet spreading and film density (higher atomizing air pressure, areas of greater droplet density within the spray, low solution viscosity, reduced gun–to–bed distances and in some instances increased spray rate), and thus reduce the amount of entrapped air, were found by Twitchell (1990) to produce harder, less elastic films. This could explain why this author found a significant correlation between the film arithmetic surface roughness and both the film Brinell hardness and modulus of elasticity.

12.5 INTERNAL STRESS WITHIN FILM COATS

12.5.1 Origins and consequences of internal stress

Cracking and edge splitting of the film coat or bridging of the intagliations are problems that film formulators often encounter during tablet film coating. It is well acknowledged that these coating defects are a manifestation of inherent high residual stresses distributed within the plane of the film coat (Rowe, 1981a, 1981b; Rowe & Forse, 1980a, 1981). Coating defects are important, not only because they destroy the integrity and elegance of the film, but also because they affect the shelf-life and durability of the product. Additionally, and more seriously, they may affect the release kinetics of the drug in the case of enterosoluble and/or sustained release films. The effect of defects on film quality is discussed in Chapter 13. This section will concentrate on the origins and quantification of internal stress.

Internal stress within the coating is implicated in some common problems associated with film-coated tablets, such as bridging of logos, cracking of the film, edge splitting and film peeling (Rowe, 1981a, 1982). These visible defects are associated with a means of providing stress relief to the film, since they allow it to contract further.

Bridging will occur if the stresses within the film are such that their reaction at the film–tablet interface exceeds the intrinsic adhesion of the coating, while cracking will occur if these stresses exceed the tensile strength of the coating (Rowe, 1976b).

Cracking, edge splitting and peeling will occur when the total internal stress generated within the plane of the film exceeds the tensile strength of the film (Rowe & Forse, 1982). Similarly, bridging of the intagliations will be observed when this stress is high enough to cause a reaction stress which exceeds the adhesion forces acting at the tablet substrate–film coat interface in the opposite direction (Rowe, 1981b); this is discussed in section 5.5 of this book.

Changes in the dimensions of the tablet or pellet core both during and after film coating is an additional contributor towards internal stress (Okutgen et al., 1991a, 1991c).

The possibility of splitting of sugar coats by high viscoelastic strain relaxation of tablet cores following sugar coating was discussed by Aulton et al. (1973). Tablets undergoing unloading following the application of a maximum pressure, spring back towards their final dimensions resulting in both an expansion in volume and a distortion in shape (Danielson et al., 1983; Çelik & Travers, 1985). Long periods of time may be required for the tablets to attain their final dimensions (Aulton et al., 1973; York & Bailey, 1977). This duration depends on the viscoelastic characteristics of the tabletting materials and on compact size (Okutgen et al., 1988).

Significant volume increases can also occur due to swelling when certain tablets are exposed to humid conditions (Reier & Shangraw, 1966; Sangekar et al., 1972; Wurster et al., 1982). The importance of moisture uptake in high humidity conditions on the dimensional stability of the compacts was discussed by White (1977) who obtained volume changes of up to 21% when tablets made from ibuprofen granules were stored in saturated humidity conditions. Porter (1981, 1982) and Rowe (1983b) have suggested that this kind of dimensional change occurring in tablet cores would affect the build-up of internal stress within the film coats.

Shrinkage effects
When coatings are applied to tablets, it is sometimes assumed that when the coating solution hits the substrate it solidifies instantly to form a film which undergoes very little further change. This, unfortunately, is not always true.

While the film is forming at the tablet surface, it is constantly losing solvent (organic or aqueous). In order to accommodate this loss, the film contracts in volume (i.e. it begins to shrink around the core). No stress is developed during the early stages of solvent evaporation (i.e. before the solidification point) because any resulting stress is relieved by mobility of the polymer molecules. Eventually, however, the film reaches a solidification point beyond which further solvent loss cannot be offset by shrinkage.

According to Croll (1979), the internal stress generated within the film as a result of shrinkage (P_S) is given by the equation:

$$P_S = \left[\frac{E}{3(1-\nu)}\right]\left[\frac{\phi_S - \phi_R}{1 - \phi_R}\right] \tag{12.41}$$

where E and ν are the Young's modulus and the Poisson's ratio of the film, respectively; ϕ_S is the volume fraction of solvent at the solidification point; ϕ_R is the volume fraction of the solvent remaining in the 'dry' film at ambient conditions.

Thermal effects
Another origin of residual internal stress in film coatings is proposed by Sato (1980) and is based on differences between the coefficient of thermal expansion of the coating and substrate. This results in thermal strain during changes in temperature. Above the glass transition temperature of the polymer formulation, the film is flexible enough to absorb these effects without increase in internal stress. Internal stress is generated, therefore, during cooling from the glass transition temperature to the ambient temperature of the film. Its effect decreases, therefore, with increasing ambient temperature, and *vice versa*.

Sato (1980) proposed that the internal stress due to thermal effects (P_T) is given by the equation:

$$P_T = \left[\frac{E}{3(1-\nu)}\right][\Delta\alpha_{cubic} \cdot \Delta T] \tag{12.42}$$

where $\Delta\alpha_{cubic}$ is the temperature difference between the cubic thermal expansion coefficients of the film coat ($\Delta\alpha_C$) and the tablet substrate ($\Delta\alpha_S$); ΔT is the difference between the T_g of the film and the test temperature (T).

Dimensional change effects
In order to estimate the internal stress (P_V) created within the film coat as a result of tablet core expansion effects, Rowe (1983b) suggested:

$$P_V = \left[\frac{E}{3(1-\nu)}\right]\left[\frac{\Delta V}{V}\right] \tag{12.43}$$

where ΔV is the volume change of the tablet core during storage and V is the volume of the core before storage. Employing equation (12.43) and taking the example of a film coating with an elastic modulus of 103 MPa and a Poisson's ratio of 0.35, Rowe (1983b) estimated a P_V value of 5.13 MPa for a 1% volume increase in the tablet core on storage, while a 10% volume increase would produce an internal stress of 51.3 MPa, which is very close to the tensile strength of such a film.

Total internal stress
Rowe (1981a) suggested that the total internal stress (P) in a film coat applied to a tablet substrate is composed of the sum of the stress created by film shrinkage during solvent evaporation (P_S) and the stress caused by thermal strain due to temperature changes during the film-coating process (P_T). Modifying and combining the equations derived by Croll (1979) and Sato (1980), Rowe (1983b) obtained equation (12.44) for the calculation of total stress:

$$P = \left[\frac{E}{3(1-\nu)}\right]\left[\frac{\phi_S - \phi_R}{1-\phi_R} + \Delta\alpha_{cubic} \cdot \Delta T\right] \tag{12.44}$$

It is proposed that the total internal stress created within the film coat applied to a tablet core is the sum of three major stresses, i.e.

$$P = P_S + P_T + P_V \tag{12.45}$$

The total internal stress, P, can be calculated by combining the equations derived by Croll (1979), Sato (1980) and Rowe (1983b) and the resulting equation is shown below:

$$P = \left[\frac{E}{3(1 - \nu)} \right] \left[\frac{\phi_S - \phi_R}{1 - \phi_R} + \Delta\alpha_{\text{cubic}} \cdot \Delta T + \frac{\Delta V}{V} \right] \tag{12.46}$$

12.5.2 Tensile strength/elastic modulus quotient (σ/E)

Film coat cracking will occur if the total internal stress, P, is greater than the tensile strength, σ, of the film, i.e.

$$P > \sigma \tag{12.47}$$

A practical problem in calculating internal stress, using an equation such as equation (12.46), is that many of the parameters are not easily determined. However, by combining and rearranging equations (12.46) and (12.47) we obtain equation (12.48):

$$\frac{\sigma}{E} < \left[\frac{1}{3(1 - \nu)} \right] \left[\frac{\phi_S - \phi_R}{1 - \phi_R} + \Delta\alpha_{\text{cubic}} \cdot \Delta T + \frac{\Delta V}{V} \right] \tag{12.48}$$

For coating conditions using the same polymer, solvent, spray rate, inlet air temperature and inlet air volume flow rate, the variables on the right-hand side of equation (12.48) are likely to remain unchanged. Thus when investigating the influence of changes in formulation, any changes in the value of σ/E for a given polymer film will predict changes in internal stress within the film. This is a useful approach since both σ and E are very easily measured, by tensile testing for example. Changes in this quotient should therefore be a good indicator of the likely incidence of defects occurring in the film (Rowe, 1983c; Franz & Doonan, 1983). The extent of edge splitting would be expected to arise from changes in the ratio σ/E. The larger the value of σ/E, the higher the stress crack resistance of film, edge splitting occurring if the value of the σ/E quotient drops below a certain value.

Rowe (1983c) found a linear relationship between a decrease in the value of the σ/E quotient and an increase in the incidence of film cracking and edge splitting for films prepared from polymers with different molecular weight and containing different pigments. Okhamafe & York (1985c) observed similar results for films containing other additives.

The incidence of bridging of intagliations, on the other hand, has been found to be related mainly to changes in the value of E measured on free films. A linear relationship has been found between a decrease in the measured value of E and a decrease in the incidence of bridging.

12.5.3   Influence of formulation on internal stress
The potential impact of formulation parameters on the performance of films in break lines and in company logos (Rowe, 1992b) can now be considered.

Polymer effects
Polymer type and molecular weight can have an effect on the following:

- Tensile strength, σ
- Elastic modulus, E
- σ/E ratio
- Film adhesion to the tablet substrate.

As an example, an increase in polymer molecular weight usually increases the tensile strength, increases elastic modulus, increases the σ/E ratio, and decreases film adhesion to substrate (Rowe, 1976b).

In all cases, Rowe (1992a) states that the use of a grade of polymer with a molecular weight near or above the critical molecular weight was beneficial. The critical molecular weight for cellulose derivatives is in the order of 8×10^4 Da (Rowe & Forse, 1980a).

Plasticizer effects
The presence of plasticizers in a polymer film coat usually reduces σ, E (Aulton et al., 1981) and T_g (Entwistle & Rowe, 1978). The reduction in E and T_g reduces internal stress (see equation (12.46)). Although σ is reduced, the σ/E ratio is usually increased since the value of E is often reduced to a greater extent. Thus, plasticizers can be used to reduce both cracking and bridging (Rowe & Forse, 1981).

Pigment effects
The effect of the presence of pigments appears to be dependent on the type, shape and concentration of pigments (Rowe, 1982, 1984, 1985a; Gibson et al., 1988). For example, the incidence of edge splitting of HPMC falls with increase in the content of talc but rises with increasing levels of calcium carbonate. Pigments may reduce σ or they may have very little effect, depending on the pigment type, particle size and particle shape. Additionally, pigments significantly increase E (Aulton et al., 1984; Porter, 1985). The magnitude of any effect (particularly on σ) will be dependent on the efficiency of dispersion.

If used to excess pigments can have a detrimental effect on the coating. The presence of poorly dispersed pigment agglomerates in the coating can act as a focus for stress, initiating cracking (Porter, 1982). As far as an effect on bridging is concerned, the tendency to increase E can increase the risk in this area.

Rowe (1986b) has calculated the localized internal stress generated by the difference in thermal expansion between pigment particles and the polymer film and found this to be in the order of 13 MPa for one typical example.

Solvent effects
Solvents generally govern the concentration at which solidification occurs. The

volume fraction of solvent at the solidification point, ϕ_S, tends to increase with the poorer solvents. This can increase the resultant internal stress since there is now potential for a large solvent loss to occur beyond the solidification point. Additionally, the poorer the solvent is, the poorer will be the mechanical properties of the coating (Rowe, 1981a). Thus, there is potential for the incidence of both bridging and cracking to be enhanced.

Film thickness effects
Internal stress increases with increasing film thickness, as does the incidence of bridging of intagliations (Rowe, 1978; Rowe & Forse, 1980b). Thus, this may have a significant impact on bridging (see also Rowe, 1992b).

Tablet core ingredients
The only factor in the internal stress calculations which is directly affected by the tablet or pellet core is $\Delta\alpha_{cubic}$ (the difference between the cubical thermal coefficient of expansion of the core and the film coating). The inclusion of tablet components which have low coefficients of thermal expansion compared to the coating polymer HPMC—for example, magnesium carbonate and calcium carbonate—produce film coats which are particularly prone to defects (Rowe, 1980b, 1986b).

Process condition effects
The processing factor most likely to influence internal stress generation is the processing temperature, which will influence the value of ΔT in equation (12.42) (i.e. the difference in temperature between the T_g of the formulation and the temperature of the film). Data of Rowe & Forse (1982) show that at higher tablet bed temperatures (i.e. a lower ΔT), bridging of intagliations is reduced but edge splitting is increased. This anomaly can be explained by reference to the internal stress equations (see Rowe, 1992b).

12.5.4   Role of dimensional changes in internal stress generation
During a typical film-coating run, tablet cores may undergo significant changes in their dimensions. This can result from thermal expansion or contraction and sorption or desorption of moisture. This section describes the temperature and humidity changes occurring during coating, and describes how these dimensional changes can be measured. It will then explain how these dimensional changes can increase significantly the resulting internal stress within the film coat.

Temperature and humidity variations during film coating
In the manufacture of film-coated tablets, prior to the actual coating process, freshly compressed tablet cores are usually stored at ambient conditions for a few hours or days. A typical aqueous film coating time for 150 kg of cores in a side-vented, perforated drum coater (e.g. Accela–Cota) is up to two hours (Hogan, 1982). Although the tablet bed temperature is influenced by many factors—such as drying air temperature, the duration of the spraying and drying periods, the rate of rotation of coating pan, the temperature of the coating solution and the kind of solvent applied

(Lindberg & Jönsson, 1972) during the aqueous film-coating process itself—it should be maintained at a constant value of approximately 37–40°C (Hogan, 1982). This, as a result of evaporative cooling in the coating chamber, requires an inlet air temperature of between 50 and 80°C. The tablet bed temperature can be reduced to 30–40°C when using organic solvents (Lantz *et al.*, 1970).

A typical aqueous film-coating process in a side-vented, perforated drum coater can be divided into three stages:

1. *Pre-warming stage*, in which the tablet cores are warmed to minimize the penetration of water into the tablet surface during the initial stages of spraying.
2. *Spraying stage*, where the actual tablet film coating takes place, during which the coating solution is sprayed onto the rotating tablet cores.
3. *Post-spraying stage*, where the spraying is stopped and the chamber air continues to flow for 2 or 3 min. In some circumstances this period may be prolonged in order to ensure that (i) the solvent is fully evaporated from the tablets, and (ii) the film-coated tablets are sufficiently dried.

The temperature changes in the outlet duct and/or at several locations in the tablet bed have been measured by many workers and the effects of certain processing variables on these thermal patterns have been evaluated.

Early work on this general area was focused on organic solvent-based film coatings. Lantz *et al.* (1970) used a thermocouple and thermistors placed in the tablet bed to record temperature changes during organic solvent film coating in a conventional pan. They found distinguishable differences in the tablet bed thermal patterns. Lindberg & Jönsson (1972) reported that the bed temperature rose at the beginning of the run but gradually an equilibrium temperature was reached with only periodic cyclic variations. These authors also found that the rotation rate of the pan, the duration of spraying and drying periods, the inlet air temperature and the velocity and temperature of the coating solution had significant influences on the tablet bed temperature. Franz & Doonan (1983) determined the effects of some of these processing variables on the surface temperature of the tablet bed during aqueous film coating in an Accela–Cota. Their equilibrium temperature measurements taken at different locations indicated that only small temperature differences existed over the surface of the bed of rotating tablets.

Little work has been carried out, however, on the relative humidity changes in the tablet bed during film-coating processes.

Typical temperature and relative humidity patterns occurring at various locations of the tablet bed during a complete actual aqueous film coating process have been measured by Okutgen *et al.* (1991b) and the effects of inlet air temperature variations on these patterns have been investigated. A diagram of an Accela–Cota, showing the measurement locations, is shown in Fig. 12.34.

The temperature and relative humidity variations occurring in a tablet bed during a typical film-coating process exhibited a characteristic profile (Fig. 12.35). The pattern of the temperature was found to be very similar to the typical infrared thermal pattern obtained by Franz & Doonan (1983). A good correlation is observed between the temperature and the relative humidity of the tablet bed. The

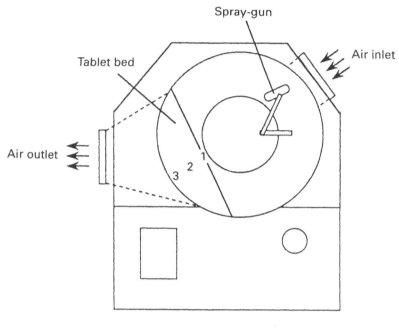

The Manesty Accela–Cota

Fig. 12.34 Diagram of Manesty Accela–Cota Model 10 showing the measurement locations in the tablet bed. Position 1, at the surface of tablet bed; Position 2, at the centre of tablet bed; Position 3, at the base of tablet bed, close to the exhaust air duct.

different stages of the coating process were also easily distinguishable. At the initial warming stage (OA), the relative humidity gradually decreases with increasing temperature of the tablet bed. Initiation of the spraying cycle at point A causes a rapid increase in the relative humidity and a drop in the temperature of the bed until an equilibrium is attained after approximately 10 min. At the end of the spraying cycle, B, the relative humidity in the tablet bed drops rapidly and significantly, whereas the temperature rises only a little until the inlet air flow is shut down (C).

Effect of inlet air temperature
Although the tablet bed temperature and the relative humidity changes during the initial tablet warming stage (OA) depend on the initial ambient values of these parameters, it can be generalized that at the end of this stage (A), the peak tablet bed temperature increased and the final relative humidity decreased with increasing inlet air temperature. During the spraying stage (AB), as the inlet air temperature decreased, the relative humidity of the bed increased (see Table 12.4), also becoming more uneven (Okutgen *et al.*, 1991b).

These results are in good agreement with the findings of other workers who have reported that increasing the drying air temperature increases the tablet bed

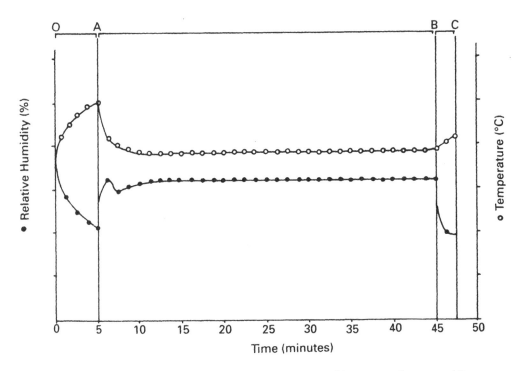

Fig. 12.35   Temperature and r.h. changes at Position 2. OA, pre-warming stage; AB, spraying stage; BC, post-spraying stage.

temperature at a constant spray rate (Lindberg & Jönsson, 1972; Franz & Doonan, 1983; Pickard & Rees, 1974). Wide variations in relative humidity are observed when inlet air temperature is low, probably caused by the inefficient solvent evaporation. It has been noted that the mean values of tablet bed temperatures and outlet air temperatures at the spraying stage are close, as shown in Table 12.4. This confirms the suggestion made by Hogan (1982) that the bed temperature is registered most conveniently by recording the temperature of the exhaust air.

At the end of spraying stage (B), the rapid drop in the relative humidity of the tablet bed is more pronounced at lower inlet air temperatures. This is also a result of the higher value of relative humidity of the tablet bed which is achieved during the spraying stage at these temperatures.

Effect of location within tablet bed

The circulation of heat and the distribution of coating solution in a rotating pan is always of concern. At a constant inlet air temperature, the temperature of the tablet bed during the spraying stage was found (Okutgen *et al.*, 1991b) to be highest at the surface of tablet bed (Position 1 in Fig. 12.34) and lowest at the base of tablet bed (Position 3), whereas the relative humidity of the tablet bed was the lowest at

Table 12.4 Effect of inlet air temperature on mean equilibrium values
of tablet bed temperature and relative humidity during the spraying stage

Average inlet air temperature (°C)	Mean tablet bed[a] temperature (°C)	Mean Tablet bed[a] relative humidity (%)	Average outlet air temperature (°C)
48.7	30.3	42.7	31.6
63.9	39.3	32.5	43.6
68.5	45.2	18.1	46.2

[a] All tablet bed readings are taken at Position 2, which is illustrated in Fig. 12.34.

Position 1 and usually about the same at the centre of the bed (Position 2) and at
Position 3, as shown in Table 12.5.

The tablet bed surface is the location where the product first experiences the
direct exposure to heat and spray. Therefore, evaporation of the solvent and drying
of the tablet cores are rapid at that point. The heat transmission is relatively slow
through the inner parts of the tablet bed due to the distance to the inlet air duct and
the closer arrangement of the tablet cores. This results in a cooler and wetter tablet
bed at these points.

The results of an investigation by Okutgen *et al.* (1991c) of the dimensional
changes occurring in tablet cores exposed to both temperatures and relative humidities which mimic the film coating process are discussed in the next section.

*Exposure of tablet cores to temperatures and relative humidities which mimic the
film-coating process*
It has been observed (Okutgen *et al.*, 1991a) that tablets exposed to temperatures
which mimic the film coating process undergo extensive dimensional changes owing

Table 12.5 Effect of locations within the tablet bed on mean equilibrium values of tablet bed temperature and relative humidity during
spraying stage[a]

Position[a]	Tablet bed[b] temperature (°C)	Tablet bed[b] relative humidity (%)
1 (surface)	43.2	22.4
2 (centre)	39.3	32.5
3 (base)	38.3	32.4

[a] The position number indicating the test locations are illustrated in Fig. 12.34.
[b] All tablet bed readings are taken at an average inlet air temperature of 63.5°C and an average outlet
temperature of 43.1°C.

to temperature and moisture variations. The most significant dimensional changes occur on re-equilibration of the tablets to room temperature—a stage which corresponds to the completion of the film-coating process. This section reports the significance and consequences, with respect to internal stress generation, of the dimensional changes of tablet cores exposed to the influence of changes in both humidity and temperature which simulate the conditions of a tablet bed during and after a typical film-forming process. The experimental conditions used were based upon the results obtained from temperature and humidity measurements carried out within a bed of tablets during an actual aqueous film-coating run in a Manesty Accela–Cota by Okutgen *et al.* (1991b), as described above.

Dimensional changes occurring during *a film-coating process*
The dimensional changes exhibited by tablets of maize starch on exposure to temperatures and relative humidities simulating a film-coating process depend to a great extent on the test conditions (Okutgen *et al.*, 1991c). The tablets exposed to test conditions of 30°C and 45% r.h. (Fig. 12.36), and 40°C and 33% r.h. (Fig. 12.37) for one hour expanded at high rates, being greater in the former case. The expansion in the axial direction was greater than in the radial direction. The tablets exposed to test conditions of 45°C and 20% r.h. (Fig. 12.38), however, underwent a gradual axial contraction during the 1 h exposure after a slight expansion which took place in the first 15 min. Radially, only contraction was observed.

It can be suggested that the moisture absorption and desiccation characteristics of maize starch tablets at different test conditions are responsible for this behaviour. At the test conditions of 30°C and 45% r.h., both the relative humidity and the temperature are higher than the pre-test storage conditions. Thus the expansion observed in Fig. 12.36 over the first hour is a result of two components: (i) due to

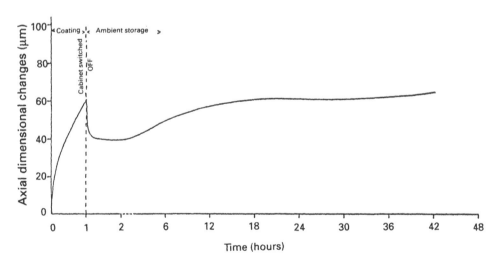

Fig. 12.36 Axial dimensional changes of maize starch tablets during exposure to 30°C, 45% r.h. test conditions for 1 h and re-equilibration to ambient conditions.

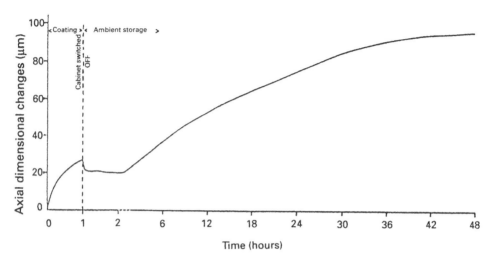

Fig. 12.37   Axial dimensional changes of maize starch tablets during exposure to 40°C,
33% r.h. test conditions for 1 h and re-equilibration to ambient conditions.

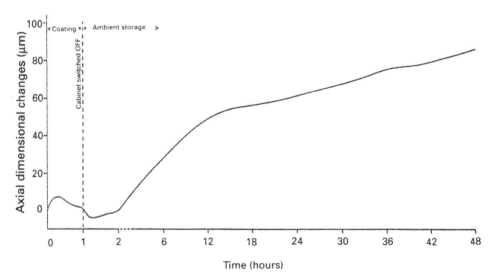

Fig. 12.38   Axial dimensional changes of maize starch tablets during exposure to 45°C,
20% r.h. test conditions for 1 h and re-equilibration to ambient conditions.

thermal expansion and (ii) due to moisture absorption. At the 40°C and 33% r.h.
test conditions, the expansion over this time is lower (Fig. 12.37) because the test
relative humidity is similar to the storage relative humidity, thus only thermal effects
are observed. At the 45°C and 20% r.h. test conditions, the relative humidity is
lower than pre-test storage conditions and therefore there are two contrasting
effects: (i) thermal expansion and (ii) contraction due to water loss. This is reflected
in the data shown over the first hour in Fig. 12.38. The tablets have a nett radial

contraction over the test period, showing that shrinkage due to water loss overcomes any radial thermal expansion.

Dimensional changes occurring after a film-coating process
At the end of the simulated coating process, the tablets were allowed to re-equilibrate to room conditions. The tablets underwent an abrupt contraction in all cases (Figs 12.36, 12.37 and 12.38) due to the rapid drop in the relative humidity and consequent water loss from the compacts. This was followed by expansion of the tablets soon after.

The most pronounced contraction at this point occurred after 30°C and 45% r.h. storage (Fig. 12.36) due to the greatest drop in relative humidity of the environment. It took up to 1 h for the test environment to approach ambient conditions, and at about this time the tablets began to expand. The major part of the tablet expansion took place in the first 5 h of equilibration, but it still continued at a reducing rate for much longer. It was also noted that tablets exposed to the test conditions of higher temperatures and lower relative humidities underwent a higher rate of subsequent expansion. This is again due to a greater amount of water loss taking place during exposure to these conditions than the conditions of lower temperatures and higher relative humidities. Therefore, the tablets are capable of absorbing more moisture at the equilibration stage. It is assumed that the tablets themselves would be re-equilibrated to ambient room conditions before 5 h, thus the continued expansion suggests that the temperature and humidity cycles undergone during this simulated film-coating process have precipitated further viscoelastic strain.

General discussion relating to volumetric changes
Dimensional changes undergone by tablets during the phase of exposure to certain test conditions corresponding to the actual spraying stage of a film-coating process are significant, but they are not as important as the extensive swelling of tablet cores taking place during subsequent ambient storage of the freshly film-coated tablets. At this stage the tablets are fully film coated and large volume increase will create large internal stresses (P_V) within the film coat which, by that time, has dried and has lower flexibility. Additionally, following the spraying cycle, film-coated tablets are sometimes subjected to a short post-spraying stage. At this stage, the relative humidity in the coating chamber will fall. It can be predicted from the results of Okutgen et al. (1991c) reported here that this would cause more moisture loss, more initial contraction of the tablet and, thereby, greater volumetric changes as the tablets return to ambient room conditions.

Aulton et al. (1973) reported that the maximum rate of volumetric expansion occurred at the edges of their compacts on prolonged storage at high humidities. Since Chow (1975) and Hoffman (1981) showed that the largest stresses were also found near the edges of a film when measured along the substrate–film interface, and since the edges of a film-coated tablet are often the thinnest part of the coating, it can be proposed that this would be a preferential region for the beginning of a film failure, leading to edge splitting and subsequent peeling of the film coat.

Table 12.6 shows calculated P_V values (based on the example of film properties used by Rowe, 1983b, for actual core expansions observed by Okutgen et al., 1991c). During the calculations, the change in volume of the tablet (ΔV) is calculated by considering the volume of the compact following ejection from the die, during 24 h ambient storage, during the coating process, during sudden contraction due to moisture loss after the coating process, and finally during the significant post-coating expansion stage. These ΔV values are significant enough to play an important part in the development of the final internal stress within all film coatings.

There is no doubt that the role of P_V would be more capable of creating coating defects in the case of the presence of more hygroscopic excipients or drug in the tablet core formulation, a hydrophilic polymer that forms films with high water permeability (Patel et al., 1964; Banker et al., 1966; Swarbrick et al., 1972; Okhamafe & York, 1985a), and in the circumstances of storing the finished products at higher humidities.

Practical suggestions to reduce P_V

The main control of P_V is to limit volumetric changes (ΔV) and therefore to minimize water loss and gain by the tablet core. Hence, the control of the permeability of a film coat to water is of prime concern. The data of Okutgen et al. (1991c) have shown that the largest expansion of the tablet core occurs on completion of a coating process in which the tablet bed temperature is higher (i.e. higher inlet air temperature and/or lower spray rate) due to the consequent lower tablet bed relative humidity. Allen et al. (1972) reported that films formed at a lower spray rate were more permeable to water vapour. Since this would result in even more subsequent moisture absorption, especially if the drug/excipient core has a great affinity for moisture, it will aggravate the development of the internal stress within the film due to volumetric changes of the core and may eventually cause the film to break.

Patel et al. (1964) reported that plasticizers could enhance or retard moisture permeation through a polymer film, depending upon their concentration and type. The use of hydrophobic plasticizers may result in a decrease in film permeability (Porter, 1980, 1982). Inclusion of pigments may decrease permeability as a consequence of the particles themselves serving as a barrier to the diffusing

Table 12.6 Mean percentage volume increase of maize starch tablets on re-equilibration to ambient conditions and resulting internal stress created within a film coat

Test conditions	Volume increase (%)	P_V (MPa)
30°C, 45% r.h.	0.946	4.853
40°C, 33% r.h.	3.095	15.877
45°C, 20% r.h.	4.520	23.188

moisture. However, there is a level at which the polymer can no longer hold all the pigment particles together and voids are created, leading to increase in moisture permeation (Parker *et al.*, 1974; Porter & Ridgway, 1982). This point is described as the 'critical pigment volume concentration' (CPVC) (Chatfield, 1962).

Film thickness is another important factor influencing the permeability of the films. Patel *et al.* (1964), Banker *et al.* (1966) and Parker *et al.* (1974) reported increasing water vapour transmission rates of films with the decreasing film thickness. Patel *et al.* (1964) pointed out that this effect increased as the hydrophilicity of the film increased.

Amann *et al.* (1974) emphasized the importance of an intimate contact between the film and the tablet. They proposed that the lower the porosity and specific surface area of the tablet, the more intimate will be this contact and the lower will be the extent of moisture uptake.

12.5.5   Conclusions relating to internal stress

Film-coating defects, such as cracking, edge splitting, peeling and bridging of intagliations, are known to be caused by the build-up of stress within a film coat. The total resulting internal stress, P, is the summation of P_S (the stress which develops as a result of film shrinkage following solvent loss by evaporation (Croll, 1979)), P_T (the stress which arises from changes in temperature during the coating process as a result of differences in the thermal expansion coefficients of the film coat and the tablet substrate (Sato, 1980)), and P_V (the stress resulting from volume changes of the tablet core as a result of water sorption (Rowe, 1983b) and/or viscoelastic strain recovery (Okutgen *et al.*, 1991c)). If the stress created in the film by these factors exceeds the tensile strength (σ) of the film, cracks (either microscopic or macroscopic in nature) and edge splitting can occur and destroy the integrity of the film. If the internal stress exceeds the forces of adhesion holding the film to the substrate, local detachments and bridging of intagliations can appear (Porter, 1981; Rowe & Forse, 1982).

Estimations of total internal stress from the contributions of P_S, P_T and P_V have been made by Okutgen (1991) from physicochemical and mechanical data generated on plasticized HPMC coats produced on tablet cores at 30 and 45°C. Insertion of these values into equations (12.42–12.45) resulted in the data shown in Table 12.7.

The right-hand column of Table 12.7 is of particular interest since this indicates the difference in magnitude between the calculated internal stress and the measured mechanical strength of the film. These data indicate that films coated onto tablets at 30°C should perform satisfactorily and retain their integrity, while films coated at the higher temperature (45°C) may crack and detach due to the internal stress generated during coating and on storage exceeding the tensile strength of the film.

In conclusion, processing variables of the coating run, storage conditions of final product, water permeability characteristics of the film coat and hygroscopicity of the tablet cores can be considered as the factors which have major importance in

Table 12.7 Calculation of total internal stress (P) within a film coat around a tablet core, summated from the contribution of P_S, P_T and P_V (from data generated by Okutgen, 1991)

Coating temp. & humidity (°C) (% r.h.)	Storage time at 25°C and 50% r.h. (h)	Calculated internal stress			Total P (MPa) (12.46)	Measured strength of film (σ) (MPa)	Diff. $(P-\sigma)*$ (MPa)
		P_S (MPa) (12.41)	P_T (MPa) (12.42)	P_V (MPa) (12.43)			
30 (45)	0	15.69	5.01	5.95	26.64	27.45	− 0.81
	6-48	7.06	5.61	4.88	17.55	27.39	− 9.84
45 (20)	0	45.44	5.01	− 2.91	47.54	30.35	+ 17.19
	6-48	15.94	5.65	12.09	33.68	26.53	+ 7.15

* Thus positive values indicate an internal stress in excess of the measured tensile strength of the film

controlling the generation of internal stress within a film coat as a result of expansion of the tablet core and subsequent film-coating defects.

12.6 GENERAL CONCLUSIONS ON MECHANICAL PROPERTIES

Mechanical test methods form an important part of material and formulation development. The object is to obtain data on a single property while carefully controlling the test conditions and eliminating extraneous factors. Rarely is it possible to eliminate all the other variables, but they can be reduced significantly by a detailed knowledge of their effects and attention to detail during testing. This chapter has indicated some ways in which these assessments can be accurately achieved for tablet film-coating materials.

There are dangers of using data from free films in order to predict the properties of films sprayed onto tablets or multiparticulates—especially those using aqueous systems, since when producing the free films it is extremely difficult to reproduce adequately those conditions experienced with a film-coating pan. The results also illustrate that care should be taken when investigating the effect of formulation variables on film properties using indentation testing. If changes in the formulation also affect solution viscosity or the atomization process, the results may be a reflection of process changes rather than those of the formulation variable intended.

The scheme of Lever & Rhys (1968; see section 12.3.1) is very useful and it can be used, in conjunction with the tensile test, to quantify changes in mechanical properties caused by formulation and process changes in our search for the ideal hard, tough film that has not yet been achieved.

An understanding of the σ/E concept (section 12.5.2) is invaluable in the prediction of coating defects such as edge splitting and bridging of intagliations. This is pursued further in Chapter 13.

Various studies have used microindentation to investigate the influence of either coating polymer molecular weight grade, or formulation additives such as plasticizers and solid inclusions, on the mechanical properties of films. These have included work carried out both on free films (Aulton *et al.*, 1984; Okhamafe & York, 1984b) and on films in place on the tablet surface (Rowe, 1976a, 1976b; Okhamafe & York, 1986). The potential for the Young's modulus of elasticity of film coats to influence the extent of coat defects, such as edge splitting and bridging of the intagliations, has been illustrated in a series of articles (Rowe, 1981a, 1981b, 1983b, 1986a).

REFERENCES

Abdul-Razzak, M.H. (1980) The mechanical properties of hydroxypropylmethylcellulose films derived from aqueous systems, M.Phil. Thesis, De Montfort University Leicester.

Alfrey, T. Jr (1948) *Mechanical behaviour of high polymers*, Interscience Publishers, New York.

Allen, D.J., de Marco, J.D. & Kwan, K.C. (1972) *J. Pharm. Sci.* **61(1)**, 106–109.

Amann, A.H., Lindstrom, R.E. & Swarbrick, J. (1974) *J. Pharm. Sci.* **63(6)**, 931–933.

Aulton, M.E. (1977) *Manuf. Chem. Aerosol News* **48(5)**, 28–36.

Aulton, M.E. (1982) *Int. J. Pharm. Tech. Prod. Mfr* **3(1)**, 9–16.

Aulton, M.E., Abdul-Razzak, M.H. & Hogan, J.E. (1980) *Proc. 2nd Int. Conf. Pharm. Tech., APGI, Paris, France*, June V, 16–25.

Aulton, M.E., Abdul-Razzak, M.H. & Hogan, J.E. (1981) *Drug. Dev. Ind. Pharm.* **7(6)**, 649–669.

Aulton, M.E., Abdul-Razzak, M.H. & Hogan, J.E. (1984) *Drug. Dev. Ind. Pharm.* **10(4)**, 541–561.

Aulton, M.E., Houghton, R.J. & Wells, J.I. (1986) *Proc. 5th Pharm. Tech. Conf., Solid Dosage Research Unit, Harrogate* **II**, 399.

Aulton, M.E., Travers, D.N. & White, P.J.P. (1973) *J. Pharm. Pharmacol.* **25** Suppl., 79P–86P.

Banker, G.S. (1966) *J. Pharm. Sci.* **55(1)**, 81–89.

Banker, G.S., Gore A.Y. & Swarbrick, J. (1966) *J. Pharm. Pharmacol.* **18**, 457–466.

Barry, B.W. (1974) In *Advances in pharmaceutical sciences*, Vol. 4, Academic Press, London.

Bayer, K. & Speiser, P. (1971) *A.P.V.* **17**, 151–158.

Bommel, E.M.G. van, Fokkens, J.G. & Crommelin, D.J.A. (1989a) *J. Contr.*

Release **10**, 283–292.

Bommel, E.M.G. van, Fokkens, J.G. & Crommelin, D.J.A. (1989b) *Acta Pharm. Technol.* **35(4)**, 232–237.

Bommel, E.M.G. van, Fokkens, J.G. & Crommelin, D.J.A. (1990) *Acta Pharm. Technol.* **36(2)**, 74–78.

Braun, A. (1958) *Schweiz Arch. Angew Wiss. Tech.* **24**, 106.

British Standard (1992) No. 2015, *Glossary of paint terms.*

Carswell, T.S. & Nason, H.K. (1944) *Mod. Plast.* **29**, 121–126.

Castello, R.A. & Goyan, J.E. (1964) *J. Pharm. Sci.* **53**, 777.

Çelik M. & Travers, D.N. (1985) *Drug Dev. Ind. Pharm.* **11(2&3)**, 299.

Chatfield, H.W. (1962) *Science of surface coatings*, Van Nostrand, New York.

Chow, T.S. (1975) In *Adhesion sciences and technology*, Vol. 9B, L.H. Lee (ed.), Plenum Publishing Corp., New York and London, p. 687.

Croll, S.G. (1979) *J. Appl. Polym. Sci.* **23**, 847–858.

Danielson, D.W., Morehead, W.T. & Ripple, E.G. (1983) *J. Pharm. Pharmacol.* **72**, 342–345.

Davis, S.S. (1974) *Pharm. Acta Helv.* **49**, 161.

Delporte, J.P. (1980a) *Proc. 2nd Int. Conf. Pharm. Tech., APGI, Paris, France* **V**, 6–15.

Delporte, J.P. (1980b) *J. Pharm. Belg.* **35(6)**, 417–426.

Devereux, C. (1988) Physicochemical properties of some methacylate polymer films produced from aqueous dispersions. M.Phil. Thesis, University of Bradford.

Dittgen, M. (1984) *Proc. 4th Pharm. Techn. Conf., Edinburgh.*

Entwistle, C.A. & Rowe, R.C. (1978) *J.Pharm. Pharmacol.* **30** Suppl, 27P.

Entwistle, C.A. & Rowe, R.C. (1979) *J. Pharm. Pharmacol.* **31**, 269–272.

Fell, J.T., Rowe, R.C. & Newton, J.M. (1979) *J. Pharm. Pharmacol.* **31**, 69–72.

Ferry, J.D. (1961) *The viscoelastic properties of polymers*, Wiley Interscience, New York.

Fisher, D.G. & Rowe, R.C. (1976) *J.Pharm. Pharmacol.* **28**, 886–889.

Ford, J.L. & Timmins, P. (1989) *Pharmaceutical thermal analysis*, Ellis Horwood, Chichester.

Franz, R.M. & Doonan, G.W. (1983) *Pharm. Technol.* **7(3)**, 54–67.

Gardner, H.A. & Sward, G.G. (eds) (1972) *Paint testing manual. Physical and chemical examination of paints, varnishes, lacquers and colors*, American Society for Testing of Materials (ASTM Ref. STP 500), 13th edn.

Gibson, S.H.M., Rowe, R.C. & White, E.F.T. (1988) *Int. J. Pharmaceut.* **48**, 63–77.

Hawes, M.R. (1978) 'The effect of some commonly used excipients on the physical properties of film formers used in the aqueous coating of pharmaceutical tablets', R.P. Scherer Award, Royal Pharmaceutical Society of Great Britain.

Hoffman, R.W. (1981) *Surf. Int. Analysis* **3(1)**, 62.

Hogan, J.E. (1982) *Int. J. Pharm. Tech. Prod. Mfr* **3(1)**, 17–20.

ISO 527-1 (1993) *Plastics—Determination of tensile properties—Part 1: General principles*, International Organization for Standardization.

Lantz, R.J., Bailey, A. & Robinson, M.J. (1970) *J. Pharm. Sci.* **59(8)**, 1174–1177.

Lee, E.H. & Radok, J.R.M. (1960) *J. appl. Mech.* **27**, 438–444.

Lever, A.E. & Rhys, J.A. (1968) *The properties and testing of plastics materials*, Temple Press Books, UK, 3rd edn.

Lindberg, N.-O. & Jönsson, E. (1972) *Acta Pharm. Suec.* 9, 589–594.

Lockett, F.J. (1972) *Nonlinear viscoelastic solids*, Academic Press, London.

Masilungan, F.C. & Lordi, N.G. (1984) *Int. J. Pharmaceut.* 20, 295–305.

Monk, C.J.H. & Wright, T.A. (1965) *J. Oil Col. Chem. Assoc.* 48, 520–528.

Morris, R.J.L. (1970) *J. Oil Col. Chem. Assoc.* 53, 761–773.

Morris, R.J.L. (1973) *J. Oil Col. Chem. Assoc.* 56, 555–565.

Norwick, A.S. & Berry, B.S. (1972) *Anelastic relaxation in crystalline solids*, Academic Press, New York.

Okhamafe, A.O. & York, P. (1983a) *J. Pharm. Pharmacol.* 35, 409–415.

Okhamafe, A.O. & York, P. (1983b) *Proc. 3rd Int. Conf. Pharm. Tech., APGI, Paris, France* V, 136–144.

Okhamafe, A.O. & York, P. (1984a) *Proc. 4th Pharm. Tech. Conf., Edinburgh.*

Okhamafe, A.O. & York, P. (1984b) *Int. J. Pharmaceut.* 22, 273–281.

Okhamafe, A.O. & York, P. (1985a) *Pharm. Acta Helv.* 60(3), 92–96.

Okhamafe, A.O. & York, P. (1985b) *J. Pharm. Pharmacol.* 37, 385–390.

Okhamafe, A.O. & York, P. (1985c) *Drug Dev. Ind. Pharm.* 11, 131–146.

Okhamafe, A.O. & York, P. (1986) *J. Pharm. Pharmacol.* 38, 414–419.

Okutgen, E. (1991) Dimensional changes and internal stress predictions in film coated tablets. Ph.D. Thesis, De Montfort University Leicester.

Okutgen, E., Travers, D.N., Hogan, J.E. & Aulton, M.E. (1988) *4th Int. Pharm. Technol. Symp., Hacetepe University, Ankara, Turkey.*

Okutgen, E., Hogan, J.E. & Aulton, M.E. (1991a) *Drug Dev. Ind. Pharm.* 17(9), 1177–1189.

Okutgen, E., Jordan. M., Hogan, J.E. & Aulton, M.E. (1991b) *Drug Dev. Ind. Pharm.* 17(9), 1191–1199.

Okutgen, E., Hogan, J.E. & Aulton, M.E. (1991c) *Drug Dev. Ind. Pharm.* 17(14), 2005–2016.

Parker, J.W., Peck, G.E. & Banker, G.S. (1974) *J. Pharm. Sci.* 63(1), 119–125.

Patel, M., Patel, J.M. & Lemberger, A.P. (1964) *J. Pharm. Sci.* 53(3), 286–290.

Patton, T.C. (1979) In: *Paint flow and pigment dispersion*, 2nd edn (ed. Patton, T.C.), Wiley, New York.

Pickard, J.F. (1979) Ph.D. Thesis, CNAA.

Pickard, J.F. & Rees, J.E. (1974) *Manuf. Chem. Aerosol News* 45(4), 19–22 and 45(5), 42–45.

Porter, S.C. (1980) *Pharm. Technol.* 4(3), 66–75.

Porter, S.C. (1981) *Drug Cosm. Ind.* 129(9), 50–58.

Porter, S.C. (1982) *Int. J. Pharm. Tech. Prod. Mfr* 3(1), 21–25.

Porter, S.C. (1985) *Pharm. Tech.* 4(3), 67–75.

Porter, S.C. & Ridgway, K. (1977) *J. Pharm. Pharmacol.* 29 Suppl., 42P.

Porter, S.C. & Ridgway, K. (1982) *J. Pharm. Pharmacol.* 34, 5–8.

Porter, S.C. & Ridgway, K. (1983) *J. Pharm. Pharmacol.* 35, 341–344.

Prater, D.A. (1982) Ph.D. Thesis, University of Bath.

Reading, S.J. & Spring, M.S. (1984a) *J. Pharm. Pharmacol.* 36, 421–426.

Reading, S.J. & Spring, M.S. (1984b) *Proc. 4th Pharm. Tech. Conf., Edinburgh.*
Reier, G.E. & Shangraw, R.F. (1966) *J. Pharm. Sci.* **55**, 510.
Reiland, T.L. & Eber, A.C. (1986) *Drug Dev. Ind. Pharm.* **12(3)**, 231–245.
Rowe, R.C. (1976a) *J. Pharm. Pharmacol.* **28**, 310–311.
Rowe, R.C. (1976b) *Pharm. Acta Helv.* **51(11)**, 330–334.
Rowe, R.C. (1977) *J. Pharm. Pharmacol.* **29**, 723–726.
Rowe, R.C. (1978) *J. Pharm. Pharmacol.* **30**, 343–346.
Rowe, R.C. (1980a) *J. Pharm. Pharmacol.* **32**, 116–119.
Rowe, R.C. (1980b) *J. Pharm. Pharmacol.* **32**, 851.
Rowe, R.C. (1981a) *J. Pharm. Pharmacol.* **33**, 423–426.
Rowe, R.C. (1981b) *J. Pharm. Pharmacol.* **33**, 610–612.
Rowe, R.C. (1982) *Pharm. Acta Helv.* **57(8)**, 221–225.
Rowe, R.C. (1983a) *J. Pharm. Pharmacol.* **35**, 43–44.
Rowe, R.C. (1983b) *J. Pharm. Pharmacol.* **35**, 112–113.
Rowe, R.C. (1983c) *Int. J. Pharmaceut.* **14**, 355–359.
Rowe, R.C. (1984) *Acta Pharm. Technol.* **30(3)**, 235–238.
Rowe, R.C. (1985a) *Pharm. Acta Helv.* **60**, 157–161.
Rowe, R.C. (1985b) *Pharm. Int.* **6**, 225–230.
Rowe, R.C. (1986a) *S.T.P. Pharma* **2(16)**, 416–421.
Rowe, R.C. (1986b) *J. Pharm. Pharmacol.* **38**, 529–530.
Rowe, R.C. (1992a) *Int. J. Pharmaceut.* **86**, 49–58.
Rowe, R.C. (1992b) Defects in film-coated tablets: aetiology and solutions, In
    Ganderton, D. and Jones, T.M. (eds), *Advances in pharmaceutical sciences*,
    Vol. 6, Academic Press, London.
Rowe, R.C. & Forse, S.F. (1980a) *J. Pharm. Pharmacol.* **32**, 583–584.
Rowe, R.C. & Forse, S.F. (1980b) *J. Pharm. Pharmacol.* **32**, 647–648.
Rowe, R.C. & Forse, S.F. (1981) *J. Pharm. Pharmacol.* **33**, 174–175.
Rowe R.C. & Forse, S.F. (1982) *Acta Pharm. Technol.* **28(3)**, 207–210.
Rubenstein, M.H. & Healey, J.N.C. (1973) *J. Pharm. Pharmacol.*, **25** Suppl., 168P.
Sakellariou, P., Rowe, R.C. & White, E.F.T. (1985) *Int. J. Pharmaceut.* **27**, 267–277.
Sakellariou, P., Rowe, R.C. & White, E.F.T. (1986) *Int. J. Pharmaceut.* **31**, 55–64.
Sangekar, S.A., Sarli, M. & Sheth, P.R. (1972) *J. Pharm. Sci.* **61**, 939–944.
Sato, K. (1980) *Prog. Org. Coat.* **8**, 143–160.
Schwarzl, F. & Staverman, A.J. (1952) *Physica* **18**, 791–798.
Skultety, P.F. & Sims, S.M. (1987) *Drug Dev. Ind. Pharm.* **13(12)**, 2209–2219.
Spitael, J. & Kinget, R. (1977) *Acta Pharm. Technol.* **23**, 267–277.
Swarbrick, J., Amann, A.H. & Lindstrom, R.E. (1972) *J. Pharm. Sci.* **61(10)**,
    1645–1647.
Tobolsky, A.V. (1971) In *Polymer science and materials* (eds Tobolsky, A.V. &
    Mark, H.F.), Wiley Interscience, New York.
Twitchell, A. M. (1990) Studies on the role of atomisation in aqueous film coating,
    Ph.D. Thesis, De Montfort University Leicester, UK.
Vemba, T., Gillard, J. & Roland, M. (1980) *Pharm. Acta Helv.* **55(33)**, 65–71.
White, P.J.P. (1977) Studies on the deformation of compacts, Ph.D. Thesis De
    Montfort University, Leicester.

White, P.J.P. & Aulton, M.E. (1980) *J. Phys. E: Scientific Instruments* **13**, 380–381.
Wurster, D.E., Peck, G.E. & Kildsig, D.O. (1982) *Drug Dev. Ind. Pharm.* **8(3)**, 343.
York, P. & Bailey, E.D. (1977) *J. Pharm. Pharmacol.* **29**, 70–74.
Zaro, J.J. & Smith, W.E. (1972) *J.Pharm. Sci.* **61(5)**, 814–815.

13

Film coat quality

Michael E. Aulton and Andrew M. Twitchell

SUMMARY

This chapter discusses the desirable properties of polymer film coats with respect to their end usage. The mechanical properties of films were discussed fully in Chapter 12 and so this chapter concentrates on other aspects of film quality such as gloss and roughness, uniformity of film thickness and defects such as cracking, edge splitting, picking, bridging and foam filling of intagliations, etc.

The methods of assessing film coat quality by visual observation, light section microscopy, surface profilimetry and scanning electron microscopy are discussed. Other techniques such as dissolution, adhesion measurements and permeability measurements are mentioned briefly. The influence of formulation and process variables on the quality of the resulting film coat is then discussed and advice for the production of a smooth coat is provided.

Coating defects are discussed with respect to their cause and suggestions are given for possible methods to reduce their incidence.

13.1 DESIRABLE AND ADVERSE PROPERTIES OF FILM COATS

The required properties of a film coat are numerous. The coating may be added to a dosage form for cosmetic, processing or functional drug delivery reasons. A discussion of the reasons for film coating has been given in Chapter 1, and a further discussion relating to desirable mechanical properties was given in Chapter 12. In the context of this chapter, it is necessary to clarify the definitions of gloss and roughness, and also to be aware of the correct terminology for the many possible coating defects that might occur.

Gloss

Gloss can be defined as the attribute of the polymer surface which causes it to have a shiny or lustrous appearance.

Rowe (1985) determined gloss values of film coats by measuring light reflected at 60° by flat-faced film-coated tablets. He reported that, with organic solutions of HPMC, increased polymer concentration, and thus viscosity, caused a reduction in the gloss of the coat. This was attributed to the increase in the roughness of the coat. It was shown for the coating conditions used in the study that tablet gloss and surface roughness could be related directly by a power-law equation.

Roughness

The surface roughness of film coats can be quantified by determining various characteristic values, the most commonly used being the *arithmetic mean surface roughness* (R_a). This may be defined as the arithmetic mean value of the departure of the roughness profile above and below a central reference line over a measured distance. The principle is illustrated in Fig. 13.1. R_a is calculated according to equation (13.1).

$$R_a = \frac{\text{Sum of areas } (r) + \text{Sum of areas } (s)}{L} \tag{13.1}$$

The appearance of a polymer coat is governed to a large extent by its surface roughness. Coats which have smooth surfaces tend to have a glossy appearance, while those with a rough surface appear more matt and may exhibit a surface like that of an orange skin. The surface properties of a coated tablet may therefore be important for aesthetic reasons. Because of the difficulties in achieving glossy film surfaces, gloss solutions are often added after the main coating process (Reiland & Eber, 1986). This inevitably increases batch process time and expense. Knowledge of the factors which would negate use of gloss solutions while still producing an acceptable product in an acceptable time would therefore be beneficial. The measurement of surface roughness may provide information on the behaviour of

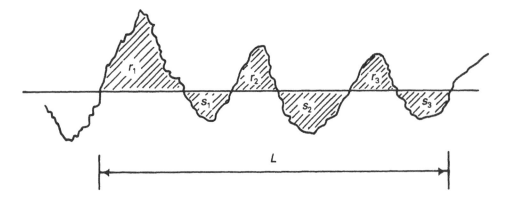

Fig. 13.1 Diagrammatic representation of the calculation of arithmetic mean roughness.

atomized film-coating droplets on the substrate surface and thus aid the optimization of the coating process. It may also be used as a quality control tool to monitor film coating at the production scale (Trudelle *et al.*, 1988).

Coat surface roughness will be dependent upon the roughness of the substrate, the properties of the coating formulation applied and the coat application conditions. Hansen (1972), King & Thomas (1978) and Rowe (1981a) suggested that the inherent roughness of the original substrate is the most important determinant of the roughness of a coated surface.

Film defects

The subject of film-coating defects has been discussed by Rowe (1992) in which thoughts and evidence relating to causes and solutions have been gathered together in a comprehensive summary. As part of this work, Rowe makes the point that the careful use of accurate, standardized definitions and terminology is essential. One can only fully endorse this comment. The following summarizes the definitions used by Down (1991) and Rowe (1992). The reader is referred to these articles for further information.

Blistering is where the film coat becomes detached locally from the substrate, thus resulting in a blister.

Blooming is a dulling of the coating.

Blushing is whitish specks or a haziness, observed generally in non-pigmented films.

Bridging is a defect in which the film pulls out of the intagliation or monograph in the substrate resulting in the film forming a bridge across the indentation. After intagliation bridging a logo may become virtually unreadable.

Bubbling is the occurrence of small air pockets within the film resulting from uncollapsed foam bubbles produced during pneumatic atomization.

Chipping occurs when the film at the edges of a tablet becomes chipped or dented.

Colour variation is self-explanatory.

Cracking is the term used to describe the cracking of the film across the crown of a tablet. Cracking is usually easily observable, although the crack(s) may be microscopic.

Cratering is the occurrence of volcano-like craters on the film surface.

Flaking is the loss of a substantial part of the coating resulting in exposure of the underlying substrate. It usually follows cracking or splitting.

Infilling is the presence of solid material (such as spray-dried droplets) in logos, etc. This differs from bridging although the outward appearance may be the same.

Mottling is an uneven distribution of the colour of a coat.

Orange peel is the phrase used to define a roughened film which has the appearance of the skin of an orange.

Peeling is the peeling back from the substrate of an area of film. It is usually associated with splitting at the edge of a tablet.

Picking occurs as a result of tablets or multiparticulates temporarily sticking together during coating and then pulling apart. It may result in an area of uncoated surface, although this may be partially obscured as coating proceeds.

Pinholing is the occurrence of holes within the film coat formed from collapsed foam bubbles.

Pitting is where pits occur in the surface of the tablet or pellet core without any visible disruption of the film coating itself.

Roughness is due to small vertical irregularities in the surface of the film which affect its smoothness and its visual appearance in terms of glossiness or lustre.

Splitting is the cracking of a film around the edges of a tablet.

13.2 METHODS OF ASSESSING FILM COAT QUALITY

Four techniques have been employed successfully in the assessment of the quality of film coats:

1. Visual examination by naked eye or with a low-power magnifying glass.
2. Light section microscopy to observe surface roughness and variations in coat thickness.
3. Profilimeter measurements of surface roughness.
4. Scanning electron microscopy.

13.2.1 Visual examination

Visual examination will allow a qualitative assessment of the condition of a film coat. Coating defects such as picking, edge splitting, orange peel, bridging of intagliations, etc. (as defined in section 13.1 above) can be recognized.

If sufficient of these observations are made, the incidence of defects can be quantified and quoted, as a percentage, for example.

13.2.2 Light-section microscopy

The thickness of polymer films applied to tablets or pellets is often determined either by using a micrometer to measure the film thickness after its removal from the substrate, or by extrapolation from knowledge of the amount of polymer applied. The former method is destructive and only measures the thickest parts of the applied film. Adhesion of substrate particles to the film may also lead to artificially high thickness values. With the latter method, accurate values for polymer film density and coating efficiency are required before meaningful thickness determination can be made. Both methods yield a single value for film thickness and give no indication of thickness variation.

The light-section microscope

A device known as a light-section microscope (Carl Zeiss, Oberkochen, Germany) is available which non-destructively measures the thickness of transparent coatings, allowing the determination of film coat thickness at selected regions on substrate surfaces. It allows analysis of the variation in film thickness and an estimate of surface roughness without physical contact with the tablet or multiparticulate surface (Twitchell *et al.*, 1994).

The light-section microscope operates on the principle shown diagrammatically in Figs 13.2 and 13.3.

An incandescent lamp of variable brightness illuminates a slit which projects a narrow band of light through an objective (O_1) at an angle of 45° to the plane of the surface being measured. Some of the light is reflected from the surface of the coating; the remainder penetrates the film and is reflected from the surface of the core. In the eyepiece of the microscope at the opposite 45° angle (O_2), the profiles of the coat and core can be seen coincidentally as a series of peaks and troughs after the band of light has been reflected/refracted at the sample, as seen in Fig. 13.4. A cross-line graticule in the eyepiece can be moved within the field of view by means of a graduated measuring drum. The required distance values can then be read off the drum with a sensitivity of 0.1 μm over longitudinal or transversal movements of up to 25 mm.

For the measurement of film thickness, this technique is restricted therefore to transparent films, however, a certain amount of development work could be performed on unpigmented films, and pigments and opacifiers could be added later. Use of the light-section microscope to determine the thickness of polymer film coats applied to granules has been reported by Turkoglu & Sakr (1992).

Analysis of light section microscope images

Thickness
Due to the refraction of the light as it penetrates the transparent layer, the distance between the light bands, as measured through the eyepiece, does not represent the true thickness of the coating (see Fig. 13.3) and this must be calculated.

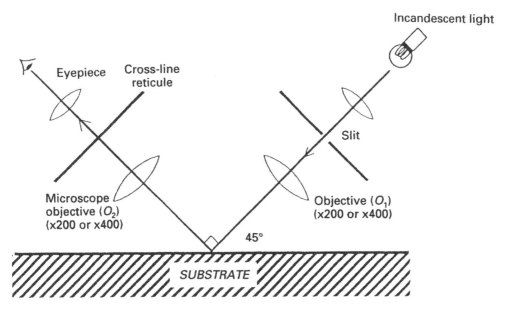

Fig. 13.2 Light-section microscope: schematic representation of principle.

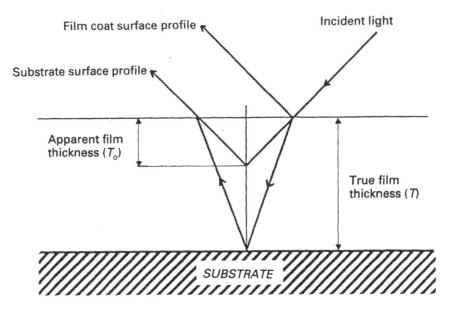

Fig. 13.3   Light path through a transparent film during light-section microscopy.

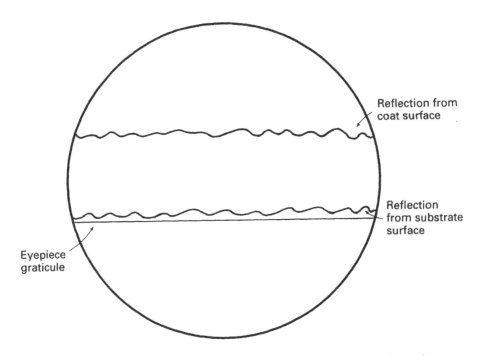

Fig. 13.4   Light section microscopy: impression of light lines and graticule in the eyepiece.

Surface roughness parameters
Surface roughness parameters which can be obtained using the light section micro-scope include:

R_T the distance between the highest peak and deepest valley (μm)
R_{TM} the average of five peak-to-valley distances (μm) and
R_W the average horizontal surface distance between peaks or troughs (μm).

Calculation of R_a (the arithmetic mean roughness, see equation (13.1) above) is diffi-cult in light section microscopy and can only be undertaken after a photographic record has been obtained.

Visualization of light section microscopy images
The diagrams in Fig. 13.5 are representations of light-section microscopy images. They indicate how the roughness of both the coat and the substrate may influence the thickness profile of the coat.

Fig. 13.5(i) indicates that if both the substrate and the coat are smooth, then a film with little variation in thickness will be produced. This combination would represent a desirable situation for film coating since the coat is smooth and of even thickness.

Fig. 13.5(ii) shows how contours of an underlying rough substrate can be over-come if appropriate coating conditions are used. The production of a smooth coat in this case may lead, however, to considerable variation in film thickness, with the thinnest areas of the coat occurring at the peaks of the substrate surface. A similar variation in film thickness may occur if a smooth substrate is coated using condi-tions which produce a rough coat (Fig. 13.5(iii)). In this case the thinnest parts of the coat corresponds to the troughs on the coat surface. In examples (ii) and (iii) the variation in film thickness may be important if the film is intended to confer controlled release properties to the substrate tablet or multiparticulate.

In the case where a rough coat is applied to a rough substrate (Fig. 13.5(iv)), the coat generally tends to follow the contours of the substrate, resulting in a coat of relatively even thickness.

The examples given in Figs 13.5(ii) and (iii) are particularly significant when the coat has been added to the substrate to control the rate of drug release from the core. A wide variation in coat thickness is apparent and since the rate of drug release through a water-insoluble polymer coating is directly proportional to its thickness, the consequences are obvious. The ideal scenario is that depicted by Fig. 13.5(i) where the coat is of very uniform thickness. It cannot be overemphasized here that both a smooth core and a smooth coat are essential requirements.

The role of the substrate in film coating is discussed in section 13.3.2 and the effect of formulation and process conditions on the quality of the coat are discussed in sections 13.3.3 and 13.3.4 respectively.

13.2.3 Surface profilimetry
Surface roughness can be assessed more accurately by *surface profilimetry*. Surface

(i) Smooth substrate and smooth coat

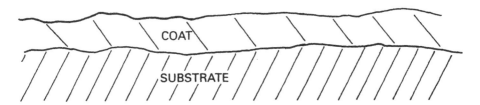

(ii) Rough substrate and smooth coat

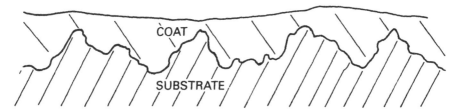

(iii) Smooth substrate and rough coat

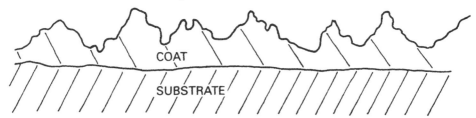

(iv) Rough substrate and rough coat

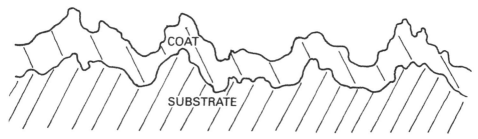

Fig. 13.5   Light section microscopy images for various substrate and coat combinations.

roughness can be quantified, often automatically, in terms of the arithmetic mean surface roughness (R_a), or other surface roughness parameters.

Surface roughness measurements can be made by use of a profilimeter (e.g. a Talysurf 10 surface measuring instrument (Rank Taylor Hobson, Leicester)). This instrument assesses surface roughness from the vertical movement of a stylus traversing the surface of a tablet (see Fig. 13.6). The vertical movement is converted into an electrical signal which is amplified and processed to give an R_a value. Typically, individual coat surface roughness measurements are averaged over a 5 mm traverse length using an 0.8 mm sampling length. R_a values up to 5 μm can be obtained. A hard copy trace is also produced.

It is important to ensure that the skid and stylus do not damage the surface of the film during the test process (therefore generating erroneous readings). It is recommended that five repeat R_a values are determined over the same length of sample. If repeated determinations of R_a values over the same area give identical results, this indicates that the skid and stylus are not damaging the film surface during measurement.

Values of the arithmetic mean surface roughness (R_a) have been calculated for a wide range of formulation and process conditions by Twitchell (1990) and Twitchell *et al.* (1993). The manner in which these conditions influence values of R_a are discussed in detail in section 13.3.

13.2.4 Scanning electron microscopy
Examination of a film coat surface or section by scanning electron microscopy gives a very clear visualization of coat quality. The spreading and coalescence of individual droplets can be clearly seen. These observations can be correlated with solution viscosity, droplet size and process conditions in order to help explain measured roughness values. These correlations for HPMC E5 films are discussed in section 13.3.

13.2.5 Dissolution
Generally, unless it is deliberately intended, the application of a film coating to a tablet or multiparticulate should not have a negative effect on drug release and bioavailability. However, an important application for coating of pharmaceutical systems with polymers is to control drug release, particularly when using multi-particulate pellets. The achievement of the desired release profile must be confirmed by drug dissolution/release testing. This is a complex issue which is dealt with in many other pharmaceutical texts and thus will not be discussed further here.

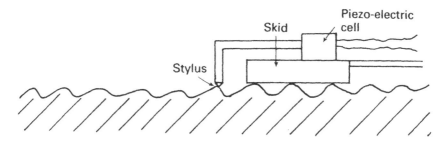

Fig. 13.6 Principle of surface profilimeter.

13.2.6   Adhesion measurements

A strong adhesive bond between the polymer film and the substrate is essential in film-coating practice. The evaluation of the adhesion of a tablet film to the underlying core is important also from the point of view of understanding certain formulation-related film-coating defects. Fisher & Rowe (1976) and later Porter (1980) have provided details of measuring techniques and adhesion values.

The principles, measurement and factors affecting the adhesion between polymer films and substrate have been discussed fully in Chapter 5 and the reader is referred to that chapter for further details.

13.2.7   Permeability measurements

A film coat may be required to act as a permeability barrier to gases and vapours, notably water vapour and in some cases atmospheric oxygen.

Based on Fick's Law of Diffusion and Henry's law relating the quantity of water vapour dissolving in the polymer to the partial pressure of that vapour, the quantity Q (the amount of water vapour permeating the film of thickness d in time t) can be denoted by:

$$Q = \frac{P_T A \Delta p\, t}{d} \tag{13.2}$$

where P_T is the permeability constant, A the cross-sectional area of the film, and Δp the vapour pressure difference across the film.

The evaluation of the permeability of applied films has been studied extensively (see Okhamafe & York, 1983), and the most frequently used apparatus is the 'permeability cup' (Fig. 13.7).

While the permeability cup is very simple to use, it suffers from certain disadvantages in practice, for example the difficulty of obtaining a good seal between the film and the holder. Stagnant layers of water vapour may also act as a permeation barrier. Commercial dynamic methods of measurement are available, and these offer greater accuracy and are much quicker.

The permeability of water vapour through a film is susceptible to alteration by both plasticizers (Okhamafe & York, 1983) and pigments (Prater *et al.*, 1982). Oxygen permeability has been studied by Prater *et al.* (1982).

13.3   THE INFLUENCE OF FORMULATION, ATOMIZATION AND OTHER PROCESS CONDITIONS ON THE QUALITY OF FILM COATS

13.3.1   Introduction

The properties of film coats will depend primarily on four factors: the constituents and properties of the substrate, the coating formulation applied, the process conditions under which that film coating is applied and the environment in which the product is subsequently stored.

The following sections consider the above four factors. The relevance to changes in the mechanical properties of the film has been discussed in Chapter 12.

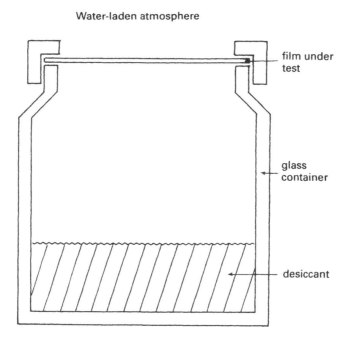

Fig. 13.7 Permeability cup for assessing film permeability to water vapour.

13.3.2 Substrate properties

During the film-coating process, tablets or multiparticulates are subjected to abrasive and mechanical forces while tumbling in the coating pan or fluidized bed. The cores must therefore be sufficiently robust to withstand these forces in order that the product is satisfactory with respect to appearance and performance.

Tablet cores

The problems associated with preparing tablet cores with suitable mechanical properties and their subsequent evaluation have been discussed by Gamlen (1983). Seager *et al.* (1985) concluded that direct compression, precompression, wet massing, fluidized-bed granulation and spray-drying techniques could all be used to prepare tablets for film coating, although the method of preparation could give rise to differences in biopharmaceutical characteristics.

Simpkin *et al.* (1983) illustrated the importance of considering the proportion and solubility of the active ingredient within a tablet core. Tablets in which the active ingredient comprised the majority of the tablet were shown to be particularly susceptible to coat defects, such as poor adhesion and peeling, if the active ingredient was soluble in the coating solvent. This applied whether the solvent was aqueous or organic. It was suggested that this effect was due to the formation of an intermediate surface layer between the tablet core and the film coat which interfered with the adhesive forces through physical or chemical means.

The importance of considering the melting point and purity of the tablet components has been illustrated by Rowe & Forse (1983b) with respect to pitting. Pitting was shown to occur when the tablet bed temperature exceeded the melting point of one or more of the constituents. This phenomenon was illustrated with reference to stearic acid (which has a melting point between 51 and 69°C depending on its quality), PEG 6000 and vegetable stearin (which have melting points of 60 and 62°C respectively).

The initial porosity and surface roughness of tablets intended for film coating will be dependent on both the compaction pressure used in their preparation and their shape (Rowe, 1978a, 1978b, 1979). Fisher & Rowe (1976) showed a direct correlation between the arithmetic mean surface roughness of tablets and their porosity. For tablets with porosities of up to 20%, it was shown that a rise in porosity yielded film coats with a proportionately larger value of measured adhesion to the tablet substrate. These findings were attributed to differences in the rate of penetration of the film-coating solution into the core. Nadkarni et al. (1975) also demonstrated an increase in film adhesion with increasing tablet surface roughness. They suggested, however, that this was due to an increase in interfacial area between the tablet and solution rather than to enhanced tablet-coating solution penetration.

The increase in arithmetic mean roughness with increasing tablet porosity has also been shown to influence the surface roughness of the final coated product (Rowe, 1978b). Generally the higher the initial surface roughness, the greater is the surface roughness after the completion of the coating process. The surfaces of biconvex tablets were demonstrated to be rougher than those of flat tablets of the same diameter, composition and porosity. These differences were still found to be apparent after film coats had been applied.

Zografi & Johnson (1984) suggested that the adhesion of film coats to rough surfaces may be facilitated by the tendency of droplets to exhibit receding contact angles approaching zero on rough substrate surfaces. This would ensure good coverage of the surface on evaporation of the coating solvent.

Rowe & Forse (1974) showed that for 6.5 and 10 mm biconvex tablets coated in a 24 in. (600 mm) Accela–Cota, the proportion of tablets failing a film continuity test increased as the tablet diameter increased. This was attributed to the greater momentum of the larger tablets as they struck the coating pan, resulting in greater attrition forces.

Leaver et al. (1985) showed that when coating in a 24 in. (600 mm) Accela–Cota, the size of the tablet core influenced the duration of the core at the bed surface and the time between surface appearances (circulation time). For tablets between 7.5 and 11 mm diameter, it was found that the larger the tablet the longer was the average surface residence time and circulation time. This was attributed to changes in the balance of forces acting on the tablets, the smaller tablets being lifted further and forming a steeper bed surface angle.

The selection of intagliation shape was shown by Rowe (1981a) to be an important consideration in the preparation of tablets for film coating. It was demonstrated that tablets with larger and/or deeper intagliations were less susceptible to the defect of intagliation bridging. This was thought to be due to enhanced film-to-tablet adhesion arising from the greater intagliation surface area.

Multiparticulate cores
The effect of multiparticulate core properties on the quality of the final coated product has not been researched as extensively as that of tablet cores. It can be envisaged, however, that the substrate properties mentioned in the previous section as affecting the quality of the coat will be equally applicable to multiparticulate systems.

Of particular importance when coating multiparticulates is the geometry (size and shape) of the substrate. For a given substrate formulation, varying the size of the substrate can affect dramatically the surface area to be covered by the coating, resulting in a variation in coating thickness for a fixed weight gain. This is particularly important for controlled drug release preparations since different rates of release will result (Porter, 1989). Ragnarsson & Johansson (1988) demonstrated that the rate of drug release from multiparticulate cores is directly proportional to the surface area of the cores. They emphasized that the particle size (and therefore surface area) of the cores needed to be tightly controlled in order to ensure product quality and production economy.

Surface area variations may also occur as a result of differences in surface roughness, again resulting in variable drug release rates (Mehta, 1986). Areas of high surface rugosity on a pellet surface have been shown by Down (1991) to potentiate the likelihood of pinhole or bubble formation in the coated product.

The choice of binder used to prepare beads with high drug levels has been shown by Funck *et al.* (1991) to influence bead shape, bead friability and the ability of the beads to remain intact during dissolution testing.

Differences between the size, density and disintegration behaviour of spheres prepared either by extrusion/spheronization or by building up in a conventional coating pan have been shown to result in differences in the release behaviour of the coated products (Zhang *et al.*, 1991).

13.3.3 The influence of the formulation of the coating solution/suspension
The physical properties of aqueous film coating solutions have been discussed in section 4.2. Their influence on the atomized droplet size distribution produced during aqueous film coating is detailed in section 4.4. Once droplets of film coating solution have impinged on a tablet or multiparticulate surface, their physical properties may influence the contact angle, degree of spreading and degree of penetration into the substrate surface. The influence of these changes on the quality of the resulting film coats in discussed in detail in the following sections.

Polymer type and molecular weight
Hydroxypropyl methylcellulose (HPMC) is the most commonly used coating polymer for non-modified release coats. HPMC is available in a variety of grades, these being characterized by the apparent viscosity (in cP = mPa s) of a 2% aqueous

solution at 20°C when measured under defined conditions. The viscosity grades used in aqueous film coating are predominantly those with viscosity designations between 3 and 15 mPa s. A particular polymer grade is made up of a wide variation of molecular weight fractions, as demonstrated by Rowe (1980), Tufnell *et al.* (1983) and Davies (1985). These fractions are responsible for the viscosity of the polymer solution and contribute to the resulting film properties. Rowe (1976) showed that, for HPMC grades having a nominal viscosity between 3 and 50 mPa s, the properties of films applied to tablets could be related to the average molecular weight of the polymer. Higher molecular weight polymers were shown to be harder, less elastic, more resistant to abrasion, dissolve more slowly and give rise to an increased tablet crushing strength.

The effect of polymer average molecular weight on the incidence of cracking and edge splitting of HPMC aqueous film coated tablets has been investigated by Rowe & Forse (1980) using a tablet substrate which was known to be prone to these defects. HPMC grades between 5 and 15 mPa s were examined; the films were plasticized with glycerol and pigmented with titanium dioxide. Increasing the molecular weight from 4.8×10^4 Da to 5.8×10^4 Da (equivalent to a change from a 5 mPas grade to a 8 mPa s grade) was shown to produce a marked reduction in the incidence of film splitting, but a further increase to 7.8×10^4 Da (equivalent to a 15 mPa s grade) had little additional effect. These results were compared with data from Rowe (1980) generated from free films and it was demonstrated that there was an inverse relationship between the incidence of edge splitting and free film tensile strength.

It has been postulated by Rowe (1986a) that, in the absence of other changes, if the film modulus of elasticity is decreased, then the incidence of edge splitting and bridging of intagliations should be reduced. Unfortunately with the aqueous filmcoating process one factor can never be changed in isolation. Conditions which influence the modulus of elasticity may also influence the spreading, penetration and adhesion of droplets, film strength, and coat thickness, roughness and density. Hardness and elasticity are therefore only two of the many factors contributing to the nature of film defects.

Polymer solution concentration and viscosity

The influence of polymer solution concentration on film coat surface roughness was investigated by Reiland & Eber (1986) using aqueous gloss solutions prepared from the 5 mPa s grade of HPMC. Coats were applied in a specially designed spray box using solution concentrations of between 1 and 8 %w/v. It was found that when solution concentrations of less than 5 %w/v were applied there was no discernible difference in film surface roughness. Increasing the concentration from 5 to 8 %w/v, however, produced a doubling of the film roughness.

The influence of HPMC solution concentration has also been studied by Rowe (1978b) using organic solutions. He found an increase in coat roughness with increasing solution concentration. With organic solutions the effect was pronounced at concentrations as low as 1 %w/w, whereas with aqueous solutions it only became marked when the concentration rose above 5 %w/w.

The role of the coating formulation in determining the surface characteristics of aqueous film-coated tablets has been studied extensively by Twitchell (1990) and the following results are from his work (unless otherwise credited). Table 13.1 lists the effects of aqueous HPMC E5 concentration on the atomized droplet size and film roughness.

Data from Twitchell (1990) and Twitchell et al. (1993) indicate that the increase in film coat roughness with increasing formulation viscosity is approximately linear over the viscosity range likely to be encountered in practice, with both the HPMC E5 and Opadry coated tablets fitting into the same general pattern. The data appeared to suggest that for pseudoplastic formulations, estimation of the likely surface roughness from minimum likely viscosities may yield values which are too low and estimation from the calculated apparent Newtonian viscosities may give values which are too high.

Scanning electron micrographs (SEMs) of the surface of some film coated tablets are shown below. The main process variable(s) illustrated by the SEMs is/are given with each figure.

The SEMs in Figs 13.8 and 13.10 (magnification ×300) and Figs 13.9 and 13.11 (magnification ×1000) illustrate how the nature of the film surface is influenced by coating solution viscosity. In each case the coat was applied using a Schlick model 930/7-1 spray gun set to produce a flat spray shape. An atomizing air pressure of 414 kPa and a spray rate of 40 g/min were used and the gun-to-bed distance was 180 mm.

Figs 13.8 and 13.9 represent the surface of tablets from a coating run in which a 9 %w/w HPMC E5 solution (viscosity 166 mPa s) was applied. Figs 13.10 and 13.11 are the corresponding SEMs for a 12 %w/w HPMC E5 solution (520 mPa s). The R_a values are 2.53 and 3.51 μm respectively. It can be seen from these figures that

Table 13.1   The influence of HPMC aqueous solution concentration on the mass median droplet diameter and arithmetic mean roughness of the resulting coats

HPMC E5 concentration (%w/w)	Solution viscosity (mPas)	Mass median droplet diam. (μm)	R_a (μm)
6%	45	17.1	1.83
9%	166	20.5	2.53
12%	520	29.0	3.51

Conditions
Schlick gun
414 kPa (60 lb/in²) atomizing air pressure
40 g/min liquid flow rate
Flat spray
180 mm gun-to-bed distance

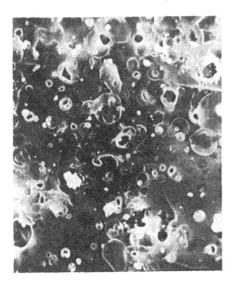

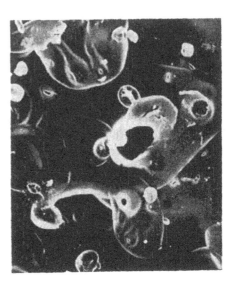

Fig. 13.8 Scanning electron micrograph of the surface of a tablet coated with 9 %w/w aqueous HPMC E5 solution (original = ×300). R_a = 2.53 μm.

Fig 13.9. Scanning electron micrograph of the surface of a tablet coated with 9 %w/w aqueous HPMC E5 solution (original = ×1000). R_a = 2.53 μm.

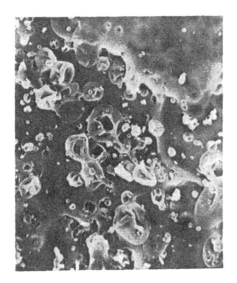

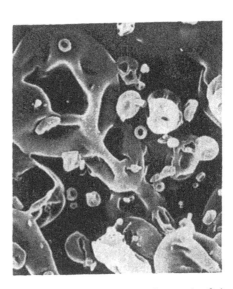

Fig 13.10 Scanning electron micrograph of the surface of a tablet coated with 12 %w/w aqueous HPMC E5 solution (original = ×300). R_a = 3.51 μm.

Fig 13.11 Scanning electron micrograph of the surface of a tablet coated with 12 %w/w aqueous HPMC solution (original = ×1000). R_a = 3.51 μm.

the extent of droplet spreading and coalescence on the tablet surface is dependent on the viscosity of the solution applied. Droplets produced from the 9 %w/w HPMC E5 solution are seen to generally have spread reasonably well. All except the smallest droplets appear to have coalesced to some degree with other droplets on the surface. Droplets produced from the 12 %w/w solution, however, are seen as more discrete units which have a far more rounded appearance, indicating a lack of spreading and droplet coalescence on the surface.

The figures also illustrate the range of droplet sizes produced during the atomization process and the heterogeneous nature of the film. Some of the smaller droplets appear opaque, suggesting that spray drying has occurred in these cases. Generally the smaller droplets are seen to spread less well than the larger droplets. Holes or craters are apparent in the centre of some of the dried droplets. This is particularly noticeable in Figs 13.10 and 13.11 where the 12 %w/w solution was applied. These holes are thought to be due to solvent vapour bursting through the partially dried crust of the droplet surface. The reduction in spreading, coalescence and evaporation on the tablet surface arising as a consequence of increased droplet viscosity are likely to have potentiated this phenomenon.

Thus, the viscosity of the coating formulation has an influence on both the visual appearance of the tablet and their surface roughness parameters. Increases in solution viscosity from 46 to 840 mPa s produced tablets which had progressively rougher and more matt surfaces. Similar behaviour was reported by Rowe (1979) for organic film-coating solutions and Reiland & Eber (1986) for aqueous film-coating gloss solutions in a model system.

Unlike at higher concentrations, the application of 6 %w/w HPMC E5 solutions (viscosity 46 mPa s) using different spray guns produced tablets with very similar R_a values and surfaces, each of which were much smoother than the original uncoated tablet. These results reflect the relatively small amount of kinetic energy necessary to force droplets of low viscosity solutions to spread and coalesce on the substrate surface and illustrate why dilute polymer solutions can be used to impart a gloss finish to coated tablets or multiparticulates. Any initial penetration that may have occurred as a result of the low viscosity would have potentiated the formation of a low contact angle and contributed to low initial surface roughness values.

The ease of droplet spreading of low-viscosity coating solutions would also explain why Reiland & Eber (1986) found HPMC E5 solutions of between 1 and 6 %w/v to produce very similar surface roughness values when applied using their model coating system. As the coating solution viscosity increases, there is a greater resistance to spreading on the substrate surface and a reduced tendency to coalesce, both of which increase surface roughness. This is illustrated by the SEMs shown above. The greater incidence of holes or craters in the centre of the dried droplets, caused by the reduced spreading, coalescence and drying rate, will have contributed to the increased roughness.

Other factors arising from an increase in solution viscosity which may potentiate surface roughness include the larger mean droplet size produced on atomization and the reduced penetration into the uncoated tablet or multiparticulate surface. The rougher nature of the partially coated substrate may itself also contribute to a reduction in spreading, by reducing the advancing contact angle, as discussed by Zografi & Johnson (1984). Any levelling of the droplets on the tablet surface that may occur due to gravitational and surface tension forces (Rowe, 1988) would also be expected to be less significant with higher viscosity solutions.

Variation in solution viscosity may also affect the rate and extent that a coating formulation penetrates into a substrate during application (Alkan & Groves, 1982; Twitchell, 1990). Differences in penetrating behaviour may be important in determining the adhesion of the coat to the substrate. Little or no penetration may lead to poor adhesion; excessive penetration may disrupt interparticulate bonding within the substrate.

Batch variation of polymer
The potential for the coated product surface roughness to be affected by HPMC E5 batch variation may be deduced from the variability in the molecular weight, and thus viscosity, of commercially available polymers. This effect would be expected to be greater with increasing polymer concentration and not to be significant at solution concentrations of around 6 %w/w or below. The effect on surface roughness of any changes in HPMC moisture content that may occur during storage, would be expected to be related to its effect on the coating solution viscosity.

The application of 12 %w/w HPMC E5 solutions prepared from powder batches selected to yield widely varying solution viscosities was shown by Twitchell (1990) to produce film coats exhibiting different roughness values. The solution prepared from a batch giving an apparent Newtonian viscosity of 840 mPa s produced a rougher coat (R_a = 3.99 μm) than that prepared from a batch giving a viscosity of 520 mPa s (R_a = 3.51 μm) which in turn produced a rougher coat than when using a solution prepared from a batch yielding a viscosity of 389 mPa s (R_a = 2.88 μm). The roughness of the applied film coat thus increased as the viscosity of the applied solution increased, and was dependent upon the batch of polymer used.

Plasticizer effects
The effect of plasticizer type and concentration on the incidence of bridging of the intagliations of film-coated tablets was investigated by Rowe & Forse (1981) using PEG 200, propylene glycol and glycerol. At levels of 10 and 20 %w/w the rank order of plasticizing efficiency, as measured by the lowering of the incidence of coat defects, was found to be PEG 200 > propylene glycol > glycerol. These findings were explained in terms of plasticizer volatility and the ability to reduce the residual stresses built up in the film during solvent evaporation.

The inclusion of 1 %w/w PEG 400 in the coating formulation appeared to cause a small increase in the coat surface roughness, the R_a value rising from 2.53 to 2.93 μm, respectively, possibly due to an increase in viscosity (Twitchell, 1990).

Solid inclusion effects
The influence of solid inclusions on the incidence of cracking and edge splitting of HPMC films has been studied extensively by Rowe (1982a, 1982b, 1982c, 1984, 1986a, 1986b) and by Gibson *et al.* (1988, 1989). Iron oxides and titanium dioxide

have been shown to increase the incidence of film defects. This was attributed to the increase in the modulus of elasticity of the film caused by these additives which was thought to increase the build-up of internal stresses within the film during solvent evaporation and film formation. Talc and magnesium carbonate were shown, however, to reduce the incidence of the tablet defects studied. This latter effect was thought to be a consequence of the morphology of the additives, the particles existing as flakes which orientate themselves parallel to the surface resulting in a restraint in volume shrinkage of the film parallel to the plane of coating.

Film permeability to water vapour has been shown to be affected by the nature and concentration of solid inclusions (Parker *et al.*, 1974; Porter, 1980; Okhamafe & York, 1984). Generally, in the presence of low concentrations there is a reduction in permeability, the particles serving as a barrier and thus causing an increased diffusional pathway. As the concentration increases, however, a point known as the *critical pigment volume concentration* (CPVC) is reached where the polymer can no longer bind all the pigment particles together. Pores therefore appear in the film, resulting in an increased permeability to water vapour.

The influence of solid inclusion particle size on film surface roughness was examined by Rowe (1981a) using dolomites of known particle size distribution. The film surface roughness was shown to be dependent on the dolomite concentration and particle size distribution and the inherent roughness of the tablet substrate. For the largest particle size dolomite (mean size 18 μm) there was a marked increase in surface roughness at low concentrations (16 %w/v) and a fall in surface roughness as the concentration increased to 48 %w/v. The opposite effects were noted for the smaller particle size grades used (mean particle sizes below 5 μm).

The importance of the refractive indices of solid inclusions has been discussed by Rowe & Forse (1983a) and Rowe (1983a). It was reported that some solid inclusions possess the property of optical anisotropy—that is, the ability to have different refractive indices depending on the orientation of the particles. Calcium carbonate, for example, was illustrated to possess two refractive indices (1.510 and 1.645) and talc three (between 1.539 and 1.589). HPMC was said to be isotropic, possessing only one refractive index, 1.49. Since the opacity of HPMC film coats is dependent on the refractive indices of all the components, it was postulated that coats could potentially possess differing opacities depending on the nature of the particles and how they were orientated within the film. This phenomenon was proposed by Rowe (1983a) to explain the production of tablets with highlighted intagliations when calcium carbonate was used in the formulation. The pigment was said to orientate equivalent to its lowest refractive index (which is similar to HPMC) on the body of the tablet, thus producing a clear film, and to orientate randomly or to its highest refractive index in the intagliation, thereby producing a degree of opacity. This effect was not found to be substrate dependent.

The mean particle size of the aluminium lakes in the Opadry formulations used by Twitchell (1990) were below 5 μm (manufacturer's data) and their concentration was approximately 50 %w/w (based on HPMC content). The data of Rowe (1981a) indicate that the effect on surface roughness of dispersed solids of this particle size and concentration is likely to be small. The viscosity of the Opadry formulations is therefore likely to have been the main determinant of the surface roughness.

Other additive effects
Reiland & Eber (1986) found that the addition of a surfactant (Brij 30) did not have a significant effect on surface roughness.

13.3.4   The influence of process conditions on film coat quality
The coating process is complex, involving many interacting variables. Although much research has been carried out into how the tablet or multiparticulate formulation and constituents of the coating solution influence the film properties, there have been few extensive studies of the role of process conditions in determining the appearance and behaviour of the coated product.

Although, in film coating, a whole host of problems can occur which may be attributed in some way to the process, many of these may be more closely associated with other factors such as the substrate core and the coating formulation (discussed in previous sections of this chapter). There are, however, two significant coating defects that can be attributed to the process, namely *picking* and *orange peel*, both of which are closely related to problems in controlling the atomization and drying processes.

Picking (see section 13.4.1) will occur if the droplets on the substrate surface are not sufficiently dry when the substrate re-enters the bulk. This may occur, for example, when the rate of addition of coating solution exceeds the drying capacity of the process, resulting in overwetting. Additionally, a condition of *localized overwetting* can occur when the liquid addition is concentrated in one area (for example, when too few spray guns or a narrow spray cone angle are used).

Orange peel, a visualization of excessive roughness, is caused by poor spreading of the coating droplets on the substrate surface. This may be a consequence of premature and excessive evaporation of the solvent from the droplets of coating liquid. This effect may be noticed when:

- the spray rate is too low;
- excessive volumes or temperatures of the drying air are utilized, particularly when the air flow is so high that significant turbulence occurs;
- atomizing air pressures/volumes are excessive.

In extreme cases, these parameters can lead to spray drying.

The use of atomizing air pressures/volumes which are insufficient to cause spreading of the droplets may also cause orange peel, this being more likely to occur as the droplet viscosity increases. Other factors derived from the substrate surface and the nature and formulation of the coating system also affect this property.

Coating equipment design
A variety of coating pans are commercially available for aqueous film coating. These have been reviewed by Pickard & Rees (1974) and Porter (1982). They range from those adapted from traditional sugar-coating pans to those specially

designed for aqueous film coating (see Chapter 8 for more detail on coating equipment).

Tablets have also been coated in various types of fluidized bed equipment. These, although offering excellent drying efficiency, tend to subject the tablets to greater attrition forces. Their use appears to be mainly restricted to small-scale development work where batch sizes as low as 1 kg can be coated satisfactorily. A better use of the fluidized bed is the coating of powders, granules and spherical pellets.

The Accela-Cota is the coating pan most widely used presently within the pharmaceutical industry for aqueous tablet film coating of tablets. It has been the subject of the majority of research work investigating the coating process. It is available in a range of different sizes, from the Model 10 (24 in. (600 mm) pan diameter) which is capable of coating up to about 15 kg of tablet cores and is used for development and small-scale manufacture, up to models capable of coating around 700 kg of tablet cores.

It is envisaged that differences in coating pan design and, consequently, the way in which the films are formed, could lead to the production of coats which exhibit different properties. Little reference to this is available in the literature. Stafford & Lenkeit (1984) demonstrated that some coating formulations based on HPMC which could be coated in an Accela-Cota, could also be coated successfully in a Pellegrini sugar-coating pan with a dip sword, or in a modified conventional sugar-coating pan. Other formulations needed further modification to produce a suitable product in the alternative coating pans.

The design and setting of the spray gun, which are also extremely important, are discussed separately in later sections of this chapter.

The effect of core movement within the tablet bed on film coat surface roughness

It has been suggested that the shear forces generated from mutual rubbing between tablets during the coating process are sufficient to smooth out even the most viscous partially gelled coating formulations (Rowe, 1988). However, large differences in surface roughness of tablets coated with different solution viscosities suggests that mutual rubbing is not enough to completely obliterate other effects. This is probably due to the fact that, in general, the droplets may have dried sufficiently to form part of the thickening viscoelastic film before the tablets enter the circulating bulk where mutual surface rubbing effects mainly occur. There is evidence, however, of surface rubbing when a narrow cone-shaped spray is used to apply the coating solution (see later in this section). In this latter case, the concentration of the spray over a small area tends to cause localized overwetting of the tablets. A proportion of the tablet may therefore subsequently enter the tablet bulk within the coater before the coat has dried and thus the potential exists for the shear forces generated from mutual rubbing between tablets to smooth the partially dried droplets/film.

Any smoothing of the dry film surface arising from attrition forces between the tablets as they tumble in the coating pan would be expected to be greater when applying lower viscosity solutions and when using lower spray rates, since the total coating time will be proportionately longer.

Application conditions
There are several aspects of the coating process which may be subject to variation and may therefore potentially influence film characteristics. These include the properties of the drying air, the setting of the spray gun(s) used and its (their) distance from the tablet bed, the atomizing air pressure and the liquid feed rate (spray rate), etc. Each of these is discussed below.

The effect of atomizing air pressure on film coat surface roughness
The air pressure used to atomize coating solutions has been shown in Chapter 4 to influence not only the distribution of droplet sizes but also the volume and velocity of the atomizing air. Yet, increasing the atomizing air pressure from 20 lb/in^2 (138 kPa) to 50 lb/in^2 (345 kPa), when using a Spraying Systems $\frac{1}{4}$J series spray-gun fitted with a 2850 liquid nozzle and 67228-45 and 134255-45 air caps, was shown to have no significant influence on the coat surface roughness when examined by Reiland & Eber (1986) in their model system for low-viscosity solutions.

The effect of changes in the atomizing air pressure used to apply aqueous HPMC solutions on the roughness of the resultant film coat is demonstrated in Table 13.2 (Twitchell, 1990).

It can be seen that an increase in atomizing air pressure resulted in a decrease in film surface roughness. This was found to occur at a wide range of different solution concentrations, spray rates, spray shapes, spray gun-to-tablet-bed distances and for each spray gun type studied. The extent of the reduction in roughness with increasing air pressure, although varying depending on the other coating conditions, was generally of the same order.

Several factors may be responsible for these observations. Increasing the air pressure will, in some cases, increase the exit velocity of the atomizing air as it leaves the annulus surrounding the liquid nozzle and in all cases increase the mass of the atomizing and spray shaping air. In turn these will increase the velocity and energy of the atomizing air. Since the droplets are propelled by and carried with the atomizing air, their momentum and kinetic energy would increase. Droplets which possess greater momentum are more likely to undergo greater forced spreading at a tablet or multiparticulate surface. Increased atomizing air pressures also produced droplets of smaller mean diameter and reduced the incidence of large droplets. This, coupled with the shorter time to travel to the substrate, may also have contributed to the reduction in surface roughness, especially with the more viscous formulations.

The work of Reiland & Eber (1986) indicates that this dependence is not important at low solution concentrations, since atomizing air pressure was not found to exert a significant effect on surface roughness when applying low-viscosity gloss solutions in a model system.

With the Schlick, Walther Pilot, Binks Bullows and Spraying Systems 45° spray guns, the general spray shape characteristics were similar at all atomizing air pressures. With the Spraying Systems 60° spray gun, however, the spray dimensions were found to be reduced on increasing the atomizing air pressure. This reduction in spray dimensions may have contributed to the lower surface roughness.

Table 13.2 The influence of atomizing air pressure on mass median droplet diameter and the arithmetic mean roughness of the resulting coats

Gun type (spray shape)	Atomizing air pressure (kPa)	Mass median droplet size (μm)	R_a (μm)
Schlick	276	25.1*	1.68
(cone)	414	23.6	1.44
	552	22.9*	1.29
Schlick	276	21.9	2.72
(flat)	414	20.5	2.53
	552	20.2*	2.26
Binks Bullows	276	34.9*	2.41
(flat)	414	27.6*	2.10
	552	—	2.03
Walther Pilot	276	26.8*	2.54
(flat)	414	24.0*	2.05
	552	—	1.90
Spraying	138	—	4.08
Systems 60°	276	—	3.75
(flat)	414	—	3.40
	552	—	3.09

Conditions
40 g/min liquid flow rate
9% aq. HPMC E5
180 mm gun-to-bed distance
See Table 4.6 for details of the guns.

* Estimated by interpolation

The effect of liquid spray rate on film coat quality and surface roughness
When applying aqueous film coats in a Model 10 Accela-Cota, increasing the spray rate between 40 and 60 g/min was found to decrease the exhaust air temperature, reduce the incidence of film edge splitting and increase the incidence of intagliation bridging (Rowe & Forse, 1982). The latter two findings were postulated to be due to an increase in Young's modulus and tensile strength of the film.

Kim *et al.* (1986), using a Model 10 Accela-Cota, found that by reducing the application rate of aqueous coating solutions from 60 to 20 g/min, both the incidence of film bridging and the weight gain required for uniform and complete coating could be reduced. Nagai *et al.* (1989) suggested that for 5 and 6 mPa s grades of HPMC, the spray rate that can be used before coat 'picking' occurs diminishes as the solution concentration is increased.

The effect of changes in coating solution application rate of aqueous HPMC solutions and on film coat surface roughness is shown in Table 13.3 (Twitchell, 1990).

The results do not indicate a clear relationship between spray rate and surface roughness. The effect of changes in spray rate appears to be dependent on the nature of the coating solution applied and possibly the design of spray gun used. For the 9 %w/w HPMC E5 solutions applied with the Schlick and Walther Pilot guns, it would appear that increases in spray rate produce smoother films. When 12 %w/w HPMC E5 solutions and 15 %w/w Opadry suspensions were applied with the Schlick gun, it appeared that an increase in spray rate from 30 to 40 g/min resulted in a rougher surface, but further spray rate increases to 50 g/min caused little further effect.

It is probable that with the 9 %w/w HPMC E5 solution, spreading is enhanced by the increased density of droplets within the spray, the accompanying reduction in spray drying and the lower tablet bed temperature. However, with higher viscosity formulations, where there is a reduced tendency for the droplets to spread and coalesce on the tablet or multiparticulate surface, any effects arising from the increased density of droplets and reduced substrate temperature are likely to be

Table 13.3 The influence of liquid flow rate on mass median droplet diameter and arithmetic mean roughness of the resulting coats

Gun type	HPMC E5 concentration (%w/w)	Liquid flow rate (g/min)	Mass median droplet diam. (μm)	R_a (μm)
Walther Pilot	9%	40	24.0*	2.05
		50	26.4	1.94
Schlick	9%	30	19.2	3.90
		40	20.5	2.53
		50	24.0	1.95
Schlick	12%	30	26.6	2.54
		40	29.0	3.51
		50	31.3	3.56
Schlick	15 %w/w Opadry-OY	30	—	2.61
		40	—	3.11
		50	26.3	2.98

Conditions
414 kPa atomizing air pressure
Flat spray
180 mm gun-to-bed distance

*Estimated by interpolation

much smaller. The increase in roughness with increasing flow rate seen when the 12 %w/w HPMC E5 solution and 15 %w/w Opadry formulation were applied may have arisen from the production of larger droplets which, if they did not spread well or coalesce with other droplets, would produce a rougher surface.

The effect of spray-gun design on film coat surface roughness
The design of spray gun used to atomize film-coating solutions has been shown in Chapter 4 to have a profound effect on the resultant droplet size distribution. In addition, it has been shown to influence the droplet velocity and the volume of atomizing air accompanying the droplets to the tablet surface. The importance of the spray gun and its influence on the process of film formation has tended, however, to be ignored, with many papers failing to define fully the exact nature of spray gun used.

Reiland & Eber (1986) indicated that the type of air cap used with a Spraying Systems spray-gun ($\frac{1}{4}$J series) fitted with a No. 2850 liquid nozzle could exert a significant effect on tablet film coat surface roughness. This was postulated to arise from differences in the atomized droplet size and the atomizing air volume and velocity. No measurement of these parameters was undertaken, however.

The design of spray gun used to apply an aqueous HPMC film-coating solution was shown to have a potentially significant effect on the roughness and appearance of the coated product (Twitchell, 1990). This could have arisen from differences in droplet size distribution, spray shape and droplet distribution within the spray, or the volume and velocity of the atomizing and spray-shaping air. A list of the gun designs used was shown in Table 4.6 and examples of droplet size and roughness data on using different guns are shown in Table 13.4.

The choice of spray gun used to apply the low-viscosity 6 %w/w HPMC E5 solution has a relatively small influence on the resultant film coat roughness. With other coating formulations, however, there are significant differences in roughness when different spray guns are used. The smoothest coats were produced by the Walther Pilot and Binks Bullows guns, the roughness values for these coats being for all practical purposes identical. The next smoothest coats were produced by the Spraying Systems 45° gun followed by the Schlick gun. The roughest coat surfaces were found on tablets coated with the Spraying Systems 60° gun, which generally produced coats which were far rougher than from any of the other guns.

The formation of relatively smooth surfaces when using the Binks Bullows and Walther Pilot guns is considered to be due to the greater total air consumption (especially through the face of the air cap), the high proportion of droplets within the central section of the spray and the low incidence of spray drying. The Schlick gun, although having a higher annulus atomizing air velocity, has a lower total atomizing air mass flow rate and a more evenly distributed spray than either the Walther Pilot or Binks Bullows gun. This, and the increased incidence of spray drying would explain why the Schlick gun produced rougher films than either the Walther Pilot or Binks Bullows gun. The Spraying Systems 45° spray gun produced films with similar surface roughness values to those of the Schlick gun despite its low atomizing air mass (approximately one-third of the Walther Pilot and Binks

Table 13.4   The influence of the design of the spray gun on the mass
median droplet diameter and arithmetic mean roughness of the resulting
coats

HPMC E5 concentration (%w/w)	Gun type (see key below)	Mass median droplet diameter (μm)	R_a (μm)
6%	WP	—	1.75
	SCH	17.1	1.83
	SS 45°	—	1.90
	SS 60°	—	2.00
9%	WP	24.0*	2.05
	BB	27.6*	2.10
	SCH	20.5	2.53
	SS 45°	—	2.30
	SS 60°	18.7*	3.40
12%	WP	29.7*	2.86
	BB	42.5*	2.86
	SCH	29.0	3.51
	SS 45°	—	3.26
	SS 60°	28.2*	> 5.00

Conditions
414 kPa (60 lb/in^2) atomizing air pressure
40 g/min liquid flow rate
Flat spray
180 mm gun-to-bed distance

*Estimated by interpolation

Gun type codes (see Table 4.6 for details)
BB: Binks Bullows 540
SCH: Schlick 930/7-1
SS: Spraying Systems $\frac{1}{4}$J series (45° or 60° air cap and 2850 liquid nozzle)
WP: Walther Pilot WA/WX

Bullows guns and half of the Schlick gun). It is likely that this effect was due to both the smaller surface area covered by the spray, which led to the droplets and atomizing air being concentrated over a smaller area, and the low incidence of spray drying. The Spraying Systems 60° spray gun produced sprays covering the largest surface area, had the lowest atomizing air mass flow rate and produced the smallest droplets. These three factors led to an increase in spray drying and reduced the average droplet momentum. This, in turn, would have reduced the extent of spreading of the droplets on the substrate surfaces (as evidenced by Fig 13.13) and hence led to high roughness values.

Figs 13.12 and 13.13 illustrate the surface appearance of film-coated tablets prepared using two different guns at a magnification of ×100. These coats were applied using a spray rate of 40 g/min, an atomizing air pressure of 414 kPa and a gun-to-bed distance of 180 mm. The film in Fig. 13.12 was prepared using a Walther Pilot gun and a 9 %w/w HPMC E5 solution, and that in Fig. 13.13 a Spraying Systems 60° gun and a 12 %w/w HPMC E5 solution.

The SEM shown in Fig. 13.12 indicates that comparatively good spreading occurs when the Walther Pilot gun is used to apply a 9 %w/w solution. Coalescence between droplets appears to be particularly good and the occurrence of spray dried droplets was comparatively low. Fig. 13.13 shows the very rough surfaces with the Spraying Systems gun. There are many 'craters' present, a lack of spreading and a greater extent of spray drying.

It is considered that the predominant cause of the differences in surface roughness apparent when using different spray guns arose from differences in the average droplet kinetic energy on hitting the tablet surface and the associated degree of spreading. Smoother surfaces are likely to be formed by spray guns which tend to produce sprays which have a high density of droplets in the central region and high atomizing air mass flow rates.

The effect of liquid nozzle diameter on film coat surface roughness
Data in Table 13.5 are from the coating runs using different liquid nozzle orifice diameters. Changes in the liquid nozzle diameter were found to have a minimal effect on film surface roughness values. This is perhaps not surprising, since the atomizing air characteristics and droplet size distributions were essentially unchanged. Any effects arising from differences in the speed of liquid exit from the nozzle or the diameter of the jet of liquid emitting from the nozzle prior to atomization would appear not to have influenced the droplet properties. It should be noted, however, that if changing the liquid nozzle diameter also changes the area of the annulus surrounding the liquid nozzle, differences in the atomizing air characteristics and film surface roughness may result.

The effect of spray shape on film coat surface roughness
A change in spray shape from the standard flat spray shape to a narrow angle cone produced a marked reduction in surface roughness for the conditions studied. Using a spray shape with dimensions approximately midway between a flat and cone shape (see Fig. 4.22) produced a coat exhibiting an intermediate roughness value (see Table 13.6).

Figs 13.14 and 13.15 show SEMs of the surface of a 15 mm diameter 'flat-faced tablets' faced coated with a 9 %w/w aqueous HPMC solution produced by a Schlick gun set to produce a narrow (10°) conical spray. Tablets from this run had a very low mean R_a value of 1.44 μm.

Changing the shape of the spray pattern generated by the Schlick gun, from the commonly used flat shape to a narrow angle solid cone, was found to produce

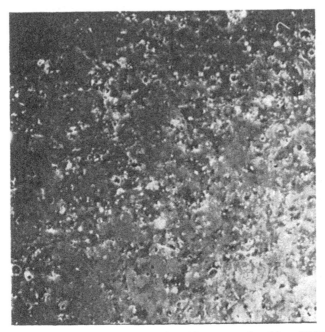

Fig. 13.12   Scanning electron micrograph of a tablet coat produced by a Walther Pilot
spray gun (original = ×100). R_a = 2.05 μm.

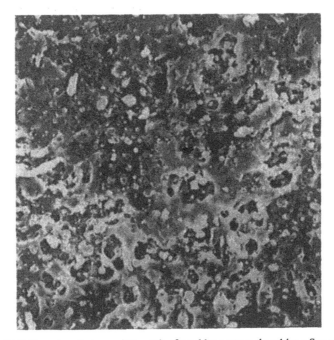

Fig. 13.13 Scanning electron micrograph of a tablet coat produced by a Spraying
Systems spray gun (original = ×100). R_a > 5 μm.

Table 13.5 The influence of liquid nozzle diameter on the mass median droplet diameter and the arithmetic mean roughness of the resulting coats

Schlick gun			Spraying Systems 60° gun		
Liquid nozzle diameter	Mass median droplet diameter	R_a	Liquid nozzle diameter	Mass median droplet diameter	R_a
(mm)	(μm)	(μm)	(mm)	(μm)	(μm)
0.8	20.5	2.53	0.51	—	2.15
1.2	21.6	2.31	0.71	18.7*	2.30
1.8	20.3	2.38			

Conditions
9 %w/w aqueous HPMC E5
414 kPa atomizing air pressure
40 g/min liquid flow rate
Flat spray
180 mm gun-to-bed distance

*Estimated by interpolation

Table 13.6 The influence of spray shape on the mass median droplet diameter and the arithmetic mean roughness of the resulting coats

Spray shape	HPMC E5 concentration (%w/w)	Mass median droplet size (μm)	R_a (μm)
Flat	9%	20.5	2.53
	12%	—	3.51
Elliptical	9%	20.9	2.19
10° Cone	9%	23.6	1.44
	12%	—	2.07

Conditions
Schlick gun
0.8 mm nozzle diameter
414 kPa (60 lb/in²) atomizing air pressure
40 g/min liquid flow rate

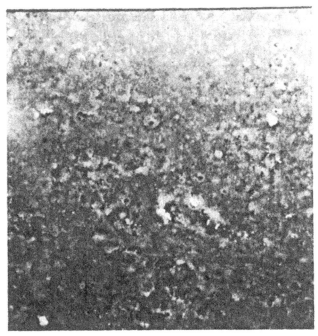

Fig. 13.14   Scanning electron micrograph of an HPMC film produced with a 10° solid
cone spray (original = ×100). R_a = 1.44 μm.

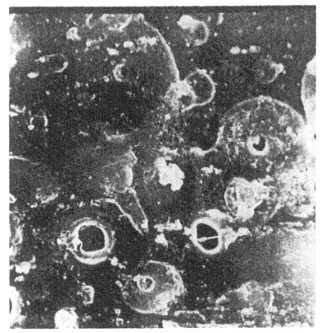

Fig. 13.15   Scanning electron micrograph of an HPMC film produced with a 10° solid
cone spray (original = ×1000). R_a = 1.44 μm.

smoother more glossy surfaces (see Fig. 13.14). Even the 12 %w/w HPMC E5 solutions applied using a cone-shaped spray produced relatively smooth surfaces, these being less rough than those produced by a 9 %w/w solution applied using a typical flat spray shape. These effects are thought to be due partially to differences in average droplet velocity and the extent of spray drying. With the narrow spray cone, because the droplets are concentrated in the centre of the spray, the average distance of droplet travel is reduced and the droplets are propelled by the faster moving central airstream. Both these factors serve to increase the kinetic energy of the droplet on impingement on the tablet or multiparticulate surface, and this, coupled with the reduced incidence of spray drying in the centre of the spray, will increase the extent of droplet spreading.

The increased density of droplets in the central region of the narrow cone spray may also lead to an increase in both the coalescence of droplets on the tablet or multiparticulate surface and the likelihood of droplets hitting partially dried droplets and causing further spreading. Smoothing of the surface due to mutual rubbing between substrates within the coater may also have been a contributing factor, as previously described. This is evidenced by the 'scratched' appearance of the high-magnification SEM shown in Fig. 13.15. Any factors which increase the proportion of droplets with the central region of the spray are therefore likely to reduce coat surface roughness.

These results also illustrate a danger of using model systems such as those described by Prater (1982) and Reiland & Eber (1986) to investigate the coating process, since these systems tend to expose the stationary test tablets only to the central area of the spray.

The effect of spray-gun-to-bed distance on film coat surface roughness
Reiland & Eber (1986) showed that increasing the distance of the spray gun from the tablet surface from 152 to 255 mm resulted in significantly rougher surfaces when coating in their model system. This was attributed to increased spray drying.

The effect on film coat surface roughness of changing the distance between the spray gun and the tablet bed has also been studied by Twitchell (1990) and Twitchell et al. (1993). Some of their data for the Schlick gun are illustrated in Table 13.7. They found that with both the Schlick and Spraying Systems guns, an increase in the gun-to-bed distance resulted in coats exhibiting rougher surfaces. This occurred irrespective of the other coating conditions used. The design and size of the Binks Bullows and Walther Pilot spray guns dictated that it was not possible to perform coating runs where the gun-to-bed distance exceeded approximately 180 mm in the Model 10 Accela-Cota.

Increasing the distance of the spray gun from the point of coating results in a reduced droplet momentum at the point of impingement on the substrate surface, a more even distribution of droplets within the spray and an increase in spray drying. These three factors will tend to reduce spreading and coalescence on the surface and therefore contribute to the consistent increase in surface roughness values which accompanied increasing the distance of the spray gun from the bed.

Table 13.7 The influence of gun-to-bed distance on mass median droplet diameter and arithmetic mean roughness on the resulting coats

HPMC E5 concentration (%w/w)	Gun-to-bed distance (mm)	Mass median droplet size (μm)	R_a (μm)
9%	180	24.0	1.95
	250	33.1	2.27
12%	180	31.3	3.56
	250	40.5	4.06
	300	49.1	4.24

Conditions
Schlick gun
0.8 mm liquid nozzle diameter
50 g/min liquid flow rate
Flat spray
414 kPa (60 lb/in^2) atomizing air pressure

The effect of drying air temperature and volumetric air flow rate on film coat quality and surface roughness

Rowe & Forse (1982) assessed the influence of inlet air temperature on the incidence of intagliation bridging and film edge splitting for aqueous film coats applied in a Model 10 Accela-Cota. Increasing the temperature was found to be beneficial in the case of reducing intagliation bridging but detrimental in the case of film edge splitting. This was thought to arise from an increase in evaporation rate at higher inlet air temperatures and a consequent reduction in the Young's modulus and tensile strength of the film.

Cole *et al.* (1983) when examining the influence of process variables on the appearance of aqueous film-coated tablets prepared in a Model 10 Accela-Cota, concluded that inlet temperature was not an important parameter as long as it was above 50°C for liquid flow rates of 20 to 30 g/min, and 60°C for flow rates of 30 to 50 g/min. They found successful coats could be obtained with inlet air volume flow rates as low as 0.014 m^3/s (equivalent to 30 ft^3/min), although this was not reproducible. Unless the coating pan was sealed, the negative air pressure created inside the pan when using air volume flow rates of 0.014 m^3/s tended to draw cold air in from the room and to displace the spray.

Changing the drying air temperature from 40 to 60°C was found by Reiland & Eber (1986) to cause a significant increase in film surface roughness when aqueous coating solutions were applied in their model system.

Results of Twitchell (1990) in Table 13.8 indicate that a reduction in the drying air volume flow rate from 0.129 to 0.088 m^3/hr or a reduction in its temperature

Table 13.8 Influence on inlet air temperature and volumetric flow rate
on the arithmetic mean roughness of the resulting coats

Drying air temperature (°C)	Drying air volumetric flow rate (m³/s)	Film coat surface roughness (R_a) (μm)
58	0.129	2.43
59	0.129	2.47
65	0.129	2.53
67	0.088	2.39

from 65 to 58°C has only a small effect on coat surface roughness when coating in a Model 10 Accela-Cota. The reduction in both parameters produced coats which were slightly smoother. This may have been due to the overall reduction in heat input into the system, which reduced the tablet bed temperature and evaporation from the droplets during travel to the tablet bed, both of which aid the spreading process.

Film coat thickness and surface roughness at different areas of the tablet surface

Rowe (1988) reported that when applying coats from both aqueous and organic systems, the film coat surface roughness within a tablet intagliation could be 2–3 times higher than on the tablet body. He suggested that on the exposed surface of the tablet the shear stresses induced by mutual rubbing were high enough to partially smooth out even viscous partially gelled coating formulations and to cause alignment of pigment particles if present. Within the intagliations, however, only small surface forces exist and little levelling, smoothing or particle alignment will occur.

Roughness values determined over the outer 0.5 mm edge of coated flat-faced tablets have been found to be considerably lower than on the main body of the tablet (Twitchell et al., 1994). This arises since the predominant point of contact between tablets during the coating process is at the tablet edge and thus the attrition forces at the tablet edge are greater. The effect was more noticeable with 15 mm flat tablets than with 10 mm flat tablets due to their increased weight, and would have been potentiated by any enhanced droplet spreading that may have occurred at the tablet edge due to increased shear forces experienced by the heavier tablet cores. With 10 mm convex tablets, coat and substrate roughness values appeared greater on the crown of the tablet than on the main tablet body, and were lowest within the breakline.

For any particular tablet type, it has been demonstrated by Twitchell et al. (1994) that the film thickness could vary markedly at different points on the tablet surface. This was particularly apparent with tablets coated using conditions which produced smoother, more dense (and thus thinner) films. Since these conditions enhance droplet spreading, the droplets may preferentially 'fill in' irregularities in the substrate surface, as suggested by Prater (1982). This was supported by the image seen though the light-section microscope, which showed the thinnest areas of coat to exist at the peaks of the uncoated tablet surface and the thickest areas at troughs of the uncoated tablet surface (see Fig. 13.5(ii)). Application conditions which tended to produce rougher, less dense, thicker coats tended to form films with a much more even thickness, the film contours tending to follow more closely the contours of the uncoated tablet surface (see Fig. 13.5(iv)).

The variations in film thickness at different points on the tablet surface may have important implications if the coat is to be used to confer controlled release or enteric properties. In these cases, the properties of the coat may depend not upon the average film thickness, but on the thinnest parts of the film coat. In these circumstances it may be possible to reduce the coat level required to achieve the desired effect by producing a coat of even thickness. This may be done by ensuring that the substrate has a low surface roughness and the application conditions produce a smooth coat. The widest variation in film thickness is likely to occur with rough substrates and coating conditions which produce a low surface roughness.

The occurrence of variations in film thickness across the tablet face also highlights the potential inaccuracy of determining film thickness values using a micrometer, since this instrument is likely to measure only the thickest part of the film. Similarly, calculation of theoretical thickness values from cast film density measurements may only be applicable if the coating conditions produce films with a density similar to that of the cast film.

Tablet storage

Rowe (1983b) reported that direct compression tablet formulations coated with HPMC could be susceptible to coating defects, such as intagliation bridging, when stored at high humidities. This was proposed to be due to the build-up of internal stresses within the film, as the tablets swell upon absorbing moisture (see section 12.5.4).

Saarnivaara and Kahela (1985) investigated the stability of aspirin tablets coated with HPMC films and stored at room temperature (25°C) or 40°C. Glycerol or PEG 6000 was used as the coat plasticizer and titanium dioxide as the pigment. Tablets stored at room temperature were shown to exhibit little change in disintegration or dissolution behaviour over a period of 48 months. Storage at 40°C, however, produced tablets with considerably increased disintegration times and slower dissolution rates, this effect being particularly noticeable when glycerol was the coat plasticizer.

Okhamafe & York (1986) showed that little or no change occurred in the Brinell hardness or Young's modulus of some film coatings based on HPMC, when applied to aspirin tablets and stored at 20°C for five months in sealed containers. However at 37°C/75% r.h., unplasticized HPMC (only) films and unplasticized HPMC films with talc or titanium dioxide exhibited a reduced hardness and

Young's modulus. Films plasticized with PEG 400 remained virtually unchanged. The authors attributed these findings to a reduction in crystallinity levels in the unplasticized films arising from the enhanced polymer chain mobility at 37°C/75% r.h. Salicylic acid sublimation into the film was also mentioned as a possible contributing factor. This latter point has been studied extensively by Abdul-Razzak (1983).

The effect of storage at various temperatures and relative humidities on the release properties of theophylline mini-tablets coated with either Eudragit RL or combinations of ethylcellulose with PEG 1500 or Eudragit L was investigated by Munday & Fassihi (1991). They found that coat integrity was maintained at all the storage conditions investigated, but that increasing the storage temperature between 28 and 45°C impeded theophylline release, the extent of which was proportional to the increase in temperature.

13.3.5 Summary of findings for the production of a smooth coat

These can best be expressed by describing the ways in which film coats with low surface roughness and high gloss can be produced. The following factors may be considered:

1. *Reduce solution concentration.* This allows easier spreading of the atomized droplets on the substrate surface. With HPMC E5 solutions, viscosity increases markedly above about 9 %w/w. Consideration should be given to increases in viscosity caused by added plasticizers and colouring agents, and the possible detrimental effects of increased processing times and core overwetting if dilute solutions are used.

2. *Increase atomizing air pressure.* This effect appears to be due to an increase in droplet velocity which may reduce spray drying and increase the forced spreading of droplets on the substrate surface.

3. *Decrease the distance of the spray gun from the substrate.* As with increased air pressure, this serves to reduce droplet spray drying and gives the droplets greater kinetic energy when they hit the substrate surface.

4. *Decrease the width of the spray.* On most guns this can be achieved by reducing the amount of air entering the side-ports of the air cap of the nozzle. This will cause a concentration of the spray over a smaller area and also reduce the average distance over which the droplets have to travel before hitting the tablet or multiparticulate. Care should be taken to avoid overwetting, which may result in the cores sticking together, leading to film picking.

5. *Change the spray gun.* Different guns produce different quality coats. This effect is more pronounced at higher polymer concentrations. The effect appears to depend on the size of the droplets produced by the spray gun, the volume flow rate of the atomizing air, the air velocity at the nozzle exit and the geometry of the liquid and air caps used. A spray gun which has a relatively high atomizing air mass flow rate and tends to produce sprays where the droplets are concentrated in the central region is recommended.

13.4   COATING DEFECTS

13.4.1   The influence of formulation and process conditions on the incidence of film coat defects

This section will describe the cause, consequences and possible cures for a number of film defects that can be related to formulation and process conditions. Those defects resulting from a build-up of internal stress, and therefore strongly dependent on the mechanical properties of the film, have been discussed in Chapter 12.

Tablet and multiparticulate sticking and film picking

Sticking will occur during coating when the cohesive and adhesive forces acting at tablet–tablet interfaces are greater than the forces tending to separate the tablets, i.e. forces arising from the tumbling action in the coating pan. Sticking is also observed between multiparticulates if they are overwetted while being coated in a fluidized bed. The related defect of *picking* arises when tablets or pellets that have become stuck together break apart on subsequent tumbling and film fragments are removed from one core and remain stuck to another. Film picking is obviously unacceptable, but can be detected easily in tablets and they can be rejected. A small degree of picking may be acceptable if the coat is applied for taste masking or reducing dust during packaging, etc. However, since film picking will cause an area of reduced coat thickness on one core and increased thickness on another, enteric or controlled released coats will be compromised.

Flat surfaces are extremely susceptible to sticking with even very small amounts of liquid between the flat faces. Indeed the increased tendency for flat tablets to stick together in this manner is the main reason they are rarely coated in practice; a certain degree of convexity is essential. The sphericity of multiparticulates helps in this respect, but their separation is less efficient due to their lower mass.

The extent and incidence of this defect are dependent upon the coating process conditions; conditions which reduced sticking also reduced picking.

Twitchell (1990) found that the three spray-guns which produced the greatest incidence of sticking and picking were those which produced sprays with either areas of greater droplet density in the centre of their spray pattern (Walther Pilot and Binks Bullows guns) or a reduced area of spray coverage (Spraying Systems 45° gun). Use of these guns can lead to tablets or multiparticulates passing through certain areas of the spray where they are hit by a relatively larger number of droplets. In these areas there would be an increase in the surface area and time over which the cohesive and adhesive forces between partially dried droplets and the film/core could act. The increase in drying time will also lead to a greater likelihood of tablets entering the tablet bulk within a coater in a wetter state. Once in the tablet bulk, the increased proximity of other tablets and the reduction in forces tending to separate the tablets, coupled with the greater area over which the adhesive and cohesive forces can act, will increase the tendency for picking. In the case of the Binks Bullows gun, the larger mean atomized droplet size produced and the presence of some very large droplets may have exacerbated the situation.

A similar argument to that described above can be used to explain the increased sticking and picking which occurred with increasing spray rates and on changing from a flat spray to a narrow cone shape. In the former case the effect is likely to be potentiated by the accompanying reduction in tablet bed temperature and corresponding increase in drying time.

Increasing the spray-gun-to-tablet-bed distance may increase the overall spray dimensions or produce a more evenly distributed spray with a less dense central region. These factors, coupled with the increased potential for evaporation from the droplets before hitting the tablet surface and the reduction in spreading, would explain the reduced incidence of picking observed by Twitchell (1990) when the gun-to-bed distance was increased.

The influence of atomizing air pressure and droplet viscosity on the incidence of sticking and picking is more complex. Decreasing the atomizing air pressure and increasing the solution viscosity will cause larger droplets to be formed and will decrease the tendency of the droplets to spread on the core surface. The production of larger droplets is likely to increase the potential for sticking and picking due to an increase in drying time and to a greater area over which the adhesive and cohesive forces can act. A decreased spreading could either reduce picking and sticking by virtue of the decrease in droplet surface area on the substrate, or increase it by decreasing the drying rate.

As the atomizing air pressure decreased, Twitchell (1990) found that there was a greater tendency for picking and sticking to occur. In this case it was thought that the larger droplets and the reduced evaporation rate had a greater effect than the reduction in cohesive and adhesive forces arising from reduced droplet spreading.

Increasing the solution viscosity was shown, however, to have little influence on the incidence of picking and sticking. It is thought that the main effect of the reduction in spreading is to reduce the cohesive and adhesive forces between the tablets or multiparticulates and that this effect was roughly cancelled by the increase in droplet size. Evidence from the SEMs and surface roughness data in section 13.3.3 suggest that the spreading of droplets produced from the 12 %w/w (520 mPa s) HPMC E5 solution is small. There is therefore little potential for further decreases in cohesive and adhesive forces due to further reduced spreading when the solution viscosity is increased above that of a 12 %w/w solution. The droplet size increases, however, with increasing solution viscosity above 12 %w/w (520 mPa s). This would explain why there was a greater extent of picking and sticking when the 12 %w/w high-viscosity (840 mPa s) HPMC E5 solution was applied. It might also account for the results reported by Nagai et al. (1989) which suggested that the maximum spray rate which could be used before picking occurred decreased with increasing solution viscosity.

The presence of titanium dioxide and an aluminium lake in Opadry formulations reduces the extent to which sticking and picking occurs. This is thought to arise from a reduction in the cohesive forces between droplets on the tablet surface. Chopra & Tawashi (1985) reported that both titanium dioxide and FD&C Blue No.2 aluminium lake reduced tack values.

Film edge splitting and intagliation bridging

Edge splitting/peeling and intagliation/breakline bridging are two defects which may result in the rejection of a batch of film-coated tablets. Bridging, where the film pulls out from an intagliation or breakline, although not necessarily influencing the drug release characteristics of the dosage form, may be aesthetically unacceptable since the identifying monogram may be partially or even fully obscured. Edge splitting and peeling, where the film cracks or splits at the edges and subsequently peels back, as well as being unsightly, may also cause dose dumping if it occurs on controlled-release or enteric-coated tablets. Splitting of controlled-release coatings on multi-particulates is obviously detrimental too.

These two film defects arise from the build up of stresses within the film due to film shrinkage on evaporation of the solvent, to differences in thermal expansion of the coating and the substrate and to volumetric changes in the core during and after coating. These have been fully discussed in the chapter on the mechanical properties of film coats (Chapter 12) and the reader is referred there for further details.

The theoretical aspects of the stress build up and the effect of core and coating formulations on the defects of bridging and edge splitting have been extensively covered, but data indicating the effect of process conditions is more limited (Rowe & Forse, 1982; Kim *et al.*, 1986). In the former study it was shown that decreases in spray rate and increases in inlet air temperature could increase the incidence of edge splitting and reduce bridging. In the latter study the authors also reported that the incidence of bridging could be reduced by decreasing the spray rate. Data generated by Twitchell (1990) indicate that the incidence of edge splitting, as well as being dependent on coat and core formulation, could also be affected markedly by the process conditions. No bridging of the breakline was seen, however, on any of the 10 mm convex tablets coated. This latter finding suggests that the inherent adhesion between the coat and substrate was high. This is supported by data generated by Rowe (1977) which indicated that both microcrystalline cellulose and stearic acid (two components of the direct compression placebo test tablets used by Twitchell, 1990) tended to produce high adhesion values due to the presence of hydroxyl groups which formed hydrogen bonds with corresponding groups of the HPMC. It would be expected that the presence of pregelatinized starch in the formulation would have similarly acted to enhance film adhesion. The relatively rough, porous surfaces would also have been expected to aid adhesion properties, due to the tendency to allow an increased rate and depth of polymer solution penetration (Fisher & Rowe, 1976).

Twitchell (1990) found that edge splitting occurred to a greater extent when the atomizing air pressure was increased, the solution viscosity was decreased and spray shapes which produced a greater concentration of droplets in the centre of the spray were used. These were the same conditions that were shown to cause a decrease in surface roughness and an increase in film density. There is also an increase in film hardness and instantaneous elastic modulus of the applied film. It would appear, however, from the edge splitting data that the relative effect of increasing the elastic modulus was greater than any effect of increasing film strength and thus an increase in incidence of edge splitting occurred.

In each case where edge splitting was prevalent, the films had low surface roughness values indicating that the droplets had spread well on the surface. Work by Zografi & Johnson (1984) on receding contact angles on solids of various roughness suggested that, after the initial droplet spreading has occurred, the droplet base in contact with a tablet surface does not recede on evaporation of the solvent but remains stationary, so that the contact angle gradually approaches zero. The SEMs and surface roughness values indicate that a similar effect is likely to have occurred during the coating studies of Twitchell (1990). Droplets which had spread to a greater extent would therefore cover a larger surface area as the solvent evaporates. This would, in turn, produce a greater internal stress as the film resists the tendency to shrink with solvent loss. The film is in effect being 'stretched' to a greater extent on the tablet surface. Factors which increase the tendency for droplets to coalesce may also increase internal stress since each evaporating unit on the tablet surface is larger. Similarly, any surface spreading arising from mutual rubbing of the tablets would be expected to increase film internal stress and thus potentiate edge splitting.

The lack of edge splitting accompanying the application of a 12 %w/w HPMC E5 solution is likely to have arisen from the lack of droplet spreading and coalescence (the droplets tending to act more as individual units on the tablet surface) and a reduced film elastic modulus. If edge splitting is a problem on a particular substrate, increasing the solution viscosity may be a simple method of overcoming the problem.

Increasing the spray rate was shown to decrease the incidence of edge splitting despite, in some instances, the surface roughness being decreased (Twitchell, 1990). This finding is similar to that of Rowe & Forse (1982). The accompanying reduction in tablet bed temperature may have served to reduce the internal stress by reducing the evaporation rate and film temperature.

The application of 15 %w/w Opadry suspensions was found by Twitchell (1990) to give rise to a greater incidence of edge splitting than when 9 %w/w HPMC E5 solutions were applied, despite the higher viscosity of Opadry suspensions. This is likely to have been due to the inclusion of titanium dioxide and aluminium lakes in the Opadry formulation, these decreasing the σ/E ratio (see Chapter 12).

Foam infilling of intagliations

Down (1982) reported the phenomenon of foam infilling of tablet intagliations experienced during aqueous film coating with a HPMC-based suspension in an air suspension column. He stated that one method of overcoming this defect was by the addition of alcohol to the formulation. This was said to improve the situation by simultaneously reducing the surface tension and viscosity of the formulation.

Droplet spray drying

The occurrence of droplet spray drying during the aqueous film-coating process may cause infilling of a tablet intaglation or breakline. Although unlikely to lead to the rejection of the coated tablet batch, this may be detrimental to the tablet appearance. The occurrence of spray drying may also result in an inefficient coating process, since spray-dried material may either not adhere to the tablet or multiparticulate surface or may be easily abraded off during tumbling in the coating pan or fluidized bed. Incorporation of air within the film due to the presence of spray-dried droplets may also influence the mechanical properties of the film.

The results described in section 4.4 indicated that evaporation from droplets during travel to the tablet bed is unlikely to occur at the centre of the spray due to their greater speed, shorter distance of travel and the local high relative humidity. Data of Twitchell (1990) on the incidence of spray dried material in the breakline of the 10 mm convex tablets supports this, since little or no spray drying was apparent when the majority of the droplets were concentrated in the centre of the spray, i.e. when the Binks Bullows and Walther Pilot guns were used or with the Schlick gun when producing a narrow cone spray. A small amount of spray drying generally occurred when the Schlick gun was used to produce a typical flat spray shape or the Spraying Systems 45°C gun was used. In the former case this is thought to be due to the relatively greater number of droplets towards the spray periphery. These move at slower speed, have further to travel before hitting the tablet bed and are probably exposed to air which is not saturated with water vapour. In the latter case, although the spray dimensions are relatively small, the droplets are thought to be travelling at a relatively slow speed compared to the other guns, allowing an increased time for evaporation to occur. The significantly greater extent of spray drying which accompanied the use of the Spraying Systems 60° gun was likely to have arisen from the greater spray dimensions, the more even distribution of droplets throughout the spray, and the relatively small size and low velocity of the droplets produced.

The lack of any significant effect of atomizing air pressure on the extent of droplet spray drying, indicates that any increased spray drying which might accompany the production of smaller droplets on increasing the air pressure, is compensated by the reduction in evaporation due to the increased droplet velocity.

A factor which is likely to have a significant effect on increasing the extent of spray drying is an increase in the distance of the spray-gun from the tablet bed surface or point of contact with multiparticulates in a fluidized bed. This was demonstrated by Twitchell (1990) and attributed to the greater proportion of droplet towards the spray periphery, the reduced average droplet velocity and the greater distance of droplet travel, all of which led to a greater average time before the droplets hit the surface and thus an increase in the time for evaporation to occur.

The reduction in spray drying which accompanied an increase in the spray rate was likely to have been due to the increased average droplet size and increased concentration of droplets within the spray. The latter factor would have increased the local relative humidity and, therefore, reduced the driving force for evaporation.

13.5   SUMMARY OF THE INFLUENCE OF THE ATOMIZATION AND FILM FORMATION PROCESSES ON THE PROPERTIES AND QUALITY OF FILM COATS

13.5.1   The film coating process
The first stage of the aqueous film-coating process is the preparation of the coating solution or suspension, the components of which will determine its physical proper-

ties. Only the rheological properties of the coating solution are likely to vary to any great extent between different coating formulations based on HPMC. Provided that the components are weighed accurately, the coating formulation properties should be the same irrespective of the preparation method used. There is, however, the potential for the rheological properties to vary when different batches of raw materials are used, especially with respect to the coating polymers. Similarly, incorrect storage may give rise to differences in rheological behaviour. As the coating formulation is fed to the spray-gun, it may be heated as it passes through the feed tubing in the coating pan. The extent to which this occurs will be dependent on the tubing material, tubing length, spray rate, inlet drying air temperature and volumetric air flow rate. On entering the spray gun, the liquid may be cooled by the high-velocity atomizing air in the chamber surrounding the liquid nozzle. Pseudoplastic formulations may undergo changes in viscosity as they pass through the liquid nozzle, the extent of which will depend on the shear rates encountered. On leaving the liquid nozzle, the coating formulation is immediately surrounded by high-velocity atomizing air. This accelerates the liquid stream above a speed at which it is stable and supplies energy to overcome the viscous and surface tension forces, thereby producing droplets. Pseudoplastic formulations may undergo further changes in viscosity at the atomization stage due to the shear forces exerted by the atomizing air.

The droplet size distribution produced will depend on the viscosity and surface tension of the formulation, atomizing air pressure, spray rate and the spray gun used. In the latter case it is the design of the spray-gun air cap which is most important since this determines the velocity of the air as it exits the annulus around the liquid nozzle. The air cap design will also determine the spray shape and the mass flow rate of the atomizing air which accompanies the droplets to the tablet or multiparticulate surface. The latter factor is important in governing the droplet velocity. On leaving the spray gun, the droplets rapidly decelerate but still travel at a velocity which is considerably faster than the accompanying drying air. The droplet velocity will vary at different points within the spray. There may be insufficient HPMC molecules within the small atomized droplets to reduce the surface tension to that of the bulk solution and there may be insufficient time for those molecules that are present in the droplet to reach the droplet surface before the droplet contacts the substrate. Droplets of different surface tension may therefore result.

During passage to the tablet or multiparticulate bed, a certain amount of water will evaporate from the droplets. This is most likely to be significant towards the spray periphery where the density of droplets is less, the droplet velocity is lower and the time taken to reach the surface is greater. Any evaporation which does occur will increase the viscosity of those droplets.

At the centre of the spray, droplet coalescence may occur, the extent of which will depend on the spray shape, spray gun used and spray rate. Droplets hitting the substrate surface will therefore exist in a wide range of sizes which are travelling at different velocities and may have different surface tension and viscosity values.

The formation of a film coat on a pharmaceutical dosage form by the application of an atomized coating formulation is a gradual and intermittent process. As the substrate passes the spray zone, it will be hit by coating formulation droplets possessing different properties, as described above. The number of droplets hitting the substrate during one pass through the spray will depend on the substrate velocity through the spray zone, the position of the substrate in relation to the spray-gun and the spray shape and droplet distribution throughout the spray. The film properties and the way in which the film is formed will depend on the behaviour of the droplets on hitting the substrate surface. In order to form a continuous, smooth film of maximum density and hardness, each droplet hitting the substrate surface should wet, spread, adhere and interact with the substrate or underlying film in such a way that the droplet layers coalesce completely to form a continuous film with no entrapped air. This is unlikely to occur in practice.

The extent to which droplets spread on a substrate surface may depend on the substrate properties and the droplet physical properties and kinetic energy. With droplets of low viscosity, the droplet kinetic energy or momentum is generally sufficient to force the droplet to spread on the surface. With high-viscosity droplets the extent of spreading due to the droplet kinetic energy is considerably reduced and the spreading behaviour will become dependent upon the droplet surface tension, interactions with the substrate and the drying time.

Droplets may dry on the substrate either as separate entities or as part of a collection of coalesced droplets. The extent to which droplet coalescence occurs will depend primarily on the distribution of droplets within the spray, the position at which the tablet or multiparticulate passes through the spray, and the droplet viscosity. Droplets are less likely to coalesce as their viscosity increases.

On the uncoated substrate, droplets may penetrate into the surface, this being governed by the properties of the substrate (porosity and surface composition), the viscosity of the droplets and the drying rate. The extent of penetration may be important in determining the degree of film adhesion and coated tablet mechanical strength. As soon as the droplets hit the substrate, water will start to evaporate and the droplet concentration and viscosity will increase until a gel of the water in an open polymer network is formed. This gel then contracts with further water loss until a viscoelastic film is produced. The extent of interaction and adhesion with the underlying film layers will be dependent on the substrate components, the degree of spreading and penetration, the droplet viscosity and the drying rate. As the water is evaporated and the polymer gel contracts to form a viscoelastic film, stresses are built up within the film. These are dependent on the extent of spreading on the tablet or multiparticulate surface, the speed of drying and the components of the formulation. If these internal stresses are sufficiently high, film edge splitting or intagliation bridging may occur.

13.5.2   The role of coating process variables
Changing any individual coating process parameter will generally have multiple effects on the coating process. Some of these effects may be beneficial for certain aspects of the process or product properties, while others may be detrimental.

The following paragraphs summarize the effect on the coating process of changes in various coating process parameters. It should be borne in mind that the relative effect of any single variable may depend on the other coating conditions used.

Coating solution viscosity

Increasing the viscosity of the coating formulation will lead to the formation of larger droplets and an increased likelihood of problems with spray-gun nozzle blockage. On impingement on the substrate, the more viscous droplets will exhibit a reduced tendency to spread and coalesce. They will penetrate less well into the substrate surface which may lead to problems associated with coat adhesion. The surfaces produced by more viscous droplets will be rougher and more matt in appearance and the films less dense with a greater degree of air entrapment. Mechanically, the films will tend to have a lower elastic modulus and lower Brinell hardness. The effect on coated tablet mechanical strength will depend on the degree of penetration of the coating solution into the tablet surface and, therefore, the relative effects of changes in adhesion and in the disruption of bonds at the tablet surface. The use of coating formulations of increased viscosity will tend to reduce the internal stresses generated within the film during its formation and, therefore, reduce the tendency for edge splitting to occur. There is unlikely to be any significant effect on the incidence of picking and spray drying with changes in formulation viscosity.

Atomizing air pressure

If the atomizing air pressure is insufficient, spray-gun nozzle blockage may occur, especially with more viscous solutions. Increasing the atomizing air pressure will decrease the mean droplet size and the droplets formed will travel to the substrate surface with a greater velocity. These droplets will therefore tend to spread to a greater extent, causing a reduction in surface roughness and a more glossy appearance. The enhanced spreading will also increase the drying rate of the droplets on the surface and therefore decrease the incidence of film picking. Film density and hardness are likely to increase with increasing atomizing air pressure due to a reduction in air entrapped within the film. Coated tablet mechanical strength may be reduced. The enhanced spreading caused by increasing the atomizing air pressure may lead to an increased film internal stress and therefore a greater incidence of film edge splitting. The incidence of spray drying is unlikely to be markedly affected by changes in air pressure.

Spray-gun design

The design of the spray gun and, most importantly, the design of the air cap will affect the droplet size distribution, spray shape and distribution of droplets within the spray, and the momentum of the droplets hitting the surface of the tablets or multiparticulates. Smaller droplets will tend to be produced by spray guns where the air velocity exiting the annulus is higher. Spray guns exhibiting higher total atomizing air mass flow rates will tend to impart more kinetic energy to the droplets and thus produce the effects described earlier. Spray guns in which there are extra holes (angular converging holes and/or containing holes) in the face of the air cap, exhibit higher atomizing air mass flow rates and tend to concentrate the droplets within the central region of the spray. This, in turn, leads to the production of smoother, more glossy film coat surfaces. The films also tend to be harder and more dense. Film defects such as picking and edge splitting may be increased, but spray drying is reduced.

The maximum spray rate which can be successfully applied with a particular spray gun is limited essentially by the area of greatest droplet density within the spray. Thus spray guns which produce sprays of reduced dimensions or where there are areas where the droplets are concentrated will tend to have reduced maximum application rates. In these cases the use of a greater number of guns within the coater, each utilizing a reduced spray rate, may give a more even distribution of droplets and allow an increase in the overall total spray rate.

Gun-to-bed distance
Increasing the gun-to-bed distance results in a greater degree of solvent evaporation from the droplets before they reach the substrate and a reduction in the areas of high droplet density within the spray. The increased distance also results in a reduction in the kinetic energy of the droplets on reaching the substrate. These factors all lead to the production of softer, rougher films which have a greater tendency to exhibit spray drying. Film picking should be reduced.

Spray rate
Increasing the spray rate will increase the mean atomized droplet size and reduce the incidence of spray drying. There will, however, be an increased tendency for picking to occur. The effect on film surface roughness appears to depend on the viscosity of the solution applied. The maximum spray rate that can be successfully applied is generally limited by the design of spray gun used and the temperature and volume flow rate of the drying air.

13.6   CONCLUDING COMMENTS

This chapter has highlighted how the complexity of the film coating process can lead to wide variations in the quality of film coats. There are numerous types of defects which can manifest themselves during coating, but luckily these are relatively rare in practice.

The incidence of these defects and the roughness of the resulting film coat, are dependent on many parameters associated with core and coat formulations and with the process itself. By gaining a knowledge of these influences it is possible to minimize the incidence of defects and to improve the overall quality of the coating with respect to thickness and smoothness, and thus the functional usefulness of the coat.

REFERENCES

Abdul-Razzak, M.H. (1983) Studies on the migration of drugs between polymeric film coats and tablet cores, Ph.D. Thesis, De Montfort University Leicester, U.K.
Alkan, M.H. & Groves, M.J. (1982) *Pharm. Tech.* **6**, 56–67.
Chopra, S.K. & Tawashi, R. (1985) *J.Pharm. Sci.* **74(7)**, 746–749.

Cole, G.C., May, G., Neale, P.J., Olver, M.C. & Ridgway, K. (1983) *Drug Dev. Ind. Pharm.* **9(6)**, 909–944.

Davies, M.C. (1985) Ph.D. Thesis, University of London.

Down, G.R.B (1982) *J. Pharm. Pharmacol.* **34**, 281–282.

Down, G.R.B. (1991) *Drug Dev. Ind. Pharm.* **17(2)**, 309–315.

Fisher, D.G. & Rowe, R.C. (1976) *J. Pharm. Pharmacol.* **28**, 886–889.

Funck, J.A.B., Schwartz, J.B., Reilly, W.J. & Ghali, E.S. (1991) *Drug Dev. Ind. Pharm.* **17**, 1143–1156.

Gamlen, M.J. (1983) *Manuf. Chem. Aerosol News* **54(4)**, 38–41.

Gibson, S.H.M., Rowe, R.C. & White, E.F.T. (1988) *Int. J. Pharmaceut.* **48**, 113–117.

Gibson, S.H.M. Rowe, R.C. & White, E.F.T. (1989) *Int. J. Pharmaceut.* **50**, 163–173.

Hansen, C.M. (1972) *J. Paint Technol.* **44**, 61–66.

Kim, S., Mankad, A. & Sheen, P. (1986) *Drug Dev. Ind. Pharm.* **12**, 801–809.

King, M.J. & Thomas, T.R. (1978) *J. Coating Technol.* **50**, 56–61.

Leaver, T.M., Shannon, H.D. & Rowe, R.C. (1985) *J. Pharm. Pharmacol.* **37**, 17–21.

Mehta, A.H., Valazza, M.J. & Abele, S.E. (1986) *Pharm. Tech.* **10**, 46–56.

Munday, D.L. & Fassihi, A.R. (1991) *Drug Dev. Ind. Pharm.* **17(15)**, 2135–2143.

Nadkarni, P.D., Kildsig, D.A., Kramer, P.A. & Banker, G.S. (1975) *J. Pharm. Sci.* **64(9)**, 1554–1557.

Nagai, T., Sekigawa, F. & Hoshi, N. (1989) In: *Aqueous polymeric coatings for pharmaceutical dosage forms* (ed. McGinity, J.W.), Marcel Dekker, New York.

Okhamafe, A.O. & York, P. (1983) *J. Pharm. Pharmacol.* **35**, 409–415.

Okhamafe, A.O. & York, P. (1984) *Int. J. Pharmaceut.* **22**, 265–272.

Okhamafe, A.O. & York, P. (1986) *J. Pharm. Pharmacol.* **38**, 414–419.

Parker, J.W., Peck, G.E. & Banker, G.S. (1974) *J. Pharm. Sci.* **63(1)**, 119–125.

Pickard, J.F. & Rees, J.F. (1974) *Manuf. Chem. Aerosol News* **45(4)**, 19–22.

Porter, S.C. (1980) *Pharm Tech.* **4(3)**, 66–75.

Porter, S.C. (1982) *Int. J. Pharm. Tech. Prod. Mfr* **3(1)**, 27–32.

Porter, S.C. (1989) *Drug Dev. Ind. Pharm.* **15(10)**, 1495–1521.

Prater, D.A. (1982) Ph.D. Thesis, University of Bath.

Prater, D.A., Meakin, B.J. & Wilde, J.S. (1982) *Int. J. Pharm. Tech. Prod. Mfr* **3(2)**, 33–41.

Ragnarsson, G. & Johansson, M.O. (1988) *Drug Dev. Ind. Pharm.* **14(15–17)**, 2285–2297.

Reiland, T.L. & Eber, A.C. (1986) *Drug Dev. Ind. Pharm.* **12(3)**, 231–245.

Rowe, R.C. (1976) *Pharm. Acta Helv.* **51(11)**, 330–334.

Rowe, R.C. (1977) *J. Pharm. Pharmacol.* **29**, 723–726.

Rowe, R.C. (1978a) *J. Pharm. Pharmacol.* **30**, 343–346.

Rowe, R.C. (1978b) *J. Pharm. Pharmacol.* **30**, 669–672.

Rowe, R.C. (1979) *J. Pharm. Pharmacol.* **31**, 473–474.

Rowe, R.C. (1980) *J. Pharm. Pharmacol.* **32**, 116–119.

Rowe, R.C. (1981a) *J. Pharm. Pharmacol.* **33**, 1–4.

Rowe, R.C. (1981b) *J. Pharm. Pharmacol.* **33**, 423–426.

Rowe, R.C. (1982a) *Pharm. Acta Helv.* **57(8)**, 221–225.

Rowe, R.C. (1982b) *Int. J. Pharm. Tech. Prod. Mfr* **3(2)**, 67–68.

Rowe, R.C. (1982c) *Int. J. Pharmaceut.* **12**, 175–179.

Rowe, R.C. (1982d) *Int. J. Pharm. Tech. Prod. Mfr* **3(1)**, 3–8.

Rowe, R.C. (1983a) *J. Pharm. Pharmacol.* **35**, 43–44.

Rowe, R.C. (1983b) *J. Pharm. Pharmacol.* **35**, 112–113.

Rowe, R.C. (1983c) *Acta Pharm. Technol.* **29(3)**, 205–207.

Rowe, R.C. (1984) *Acta Pharm. Technol.* **30(3)**, 235–238.

Rowe, R.C. (1985) *J. Pharm. Pharmacol.* **37**, 761–765.

Rowe, R.C. (1986a) *S.T.P. Pharma* **2(16)**, 416–421.

Rowe, R.C. (1986b) *J. Pharm. Pharmacol.* **38**, 529–530.

Rowe, R.C. (1988) *Int. J. Pharmaceut.* **43**, 155–159.

Rowe, R.C. (1992) Defects in film-coated tablets: aetiology and solutions, in *Advances in Pharmaceutical Sciences* (eds Ganderton, D. & Jones, T.M.), Academic Press, London, Vol. 6.

Rowe, R.C. & Forse, S.F. (1974) *J. Pharm. Pharmacol.* **26** Suppl., 61P–62P.

Rowe, R.C. & Forse, S.F. (1980) *J. Pharm. Pharmacol.* **32**, 538–584.

Rowe, R.C. & Forse, S.F. (1981) *J. Pharm. Pharmacol.* **33**, 174–175.

Rowe, R.C. & Forse, S.F. (1982) *Acta Pharm. Tech.* **28(3)**, 207–210.

Rowe, R.C. & Forse, S.F. (1983a) *J. Pharm. Pharmacol.* **35**, 205–207.

Rowe, R.C. & Forse, S.F. (1983b) *Int. J. Pharmaceut.* **17**, 347–349.

Saarnivaara, K. & Kahela, P. (1985) *Drug Dev. Ind. Pharm.* **11(2&3)**, 481–492.

Seager, H., Rue, P.J., Burt, I., Ryder, J., Warrack, J.K. & Gamlen, M.J. (1985) *Int. J. Pharm. Tech. Prod, Mfr* **6(1)**, 1–20.

Simpkin, G.T., Johnson, M.C.R. & Bell, J.H. (1983) *Proc. 3rd Int. Conf. Pharm. Tech., AGPI, Paris, France* **III**, 163–169.

Stafford, J.W. & Lenkeit, D. (1984) *Pharm. Ind.* **46(10)**, 1062–1067.

Trudelle, F., Rowe, R.C. & Witkowski, A.R. (1988) *S.T.P. Pharma* **4(1)**, 28–30.

Tufnell, K.J., May, G. & Meakin, B.J. (1983) *Proc. 3rd Int. Conf. Pharm. Tech., AGPI, Paris, France* **V**, 111–118.

Turkoglu, M. and Sakr, A. (1992) *Int. J. Pharmaceut.* **88**, 75–87.

Twitchell, A.M. (1990) Studies on the role of atomisation in aqueous tablet film coating, Ph.D. Thesis, De Montfort University Leicester.

Twitchell, A.M., Hogan, J.E. and Aulton, M.E. (1993) *Proc. 12th Pharm. Technol. Conf., Helsingør, Denmark* **1**, 246–257.

Twitchell, A.M., Hogan, J.E. and Aulton, M.E. (1994) *Proc. 13th Pharm. Technol. Conf., Strasbourg, France* **1**, 660–671.

Zhang, G., Schwartz, J.B., Schnaare, R.L., Wigent, R.J. & Sugita, E.T. (1991) *Drug Dev. Ind. Pharm.* **17(6)**, 817–830.

Zografi, G. & Johnson, B.A. (1984) *Int. J. Pharmaceut.* **22**, 159–176.

14

Modified release coatings

John E. Hogan

SUMMARY

Relevant aspects of the composition and performance of modified release coatings are considered in this chapter. Initially, the basic characteristics of multiparticulate systems are described and comparisons are made with the performance of whole tablets intended for modified release. The properties and effects of the polymers and plasticizers which are used in modified release coatings are illustrated with examples from the literature. This further develops the basic treatment of these materials provided in Chapter 2. Additional ingredients peculiar to modified release coatings, such as pore-forming agents, are also described. A section on the structure and function of modified release films and the mechanism of drug release from the coated particle or tablet is also included.

Enteric coatings as a special form of delayed release coating are dealt with in a separate section due to their importance to the industry. The use of enteric coating is described in terms of gastrointestinal pH and the properties of an ideal enteric coating are suggested.

The following factors as they affect enteric performance are described in some detail: the enteric polymer, the film formulation, the stability of the film coat and the coating process itself.

14.1 INTRODUCTION

In this section we will be concerned with the coating of tablets and multiparticulate systems with the objective of conferring on the dosage form a release characteristic that it would not otherwise possess. The USP has defined a modified release dosage form as 'one for which the drug release characteristics of time course and/or location are chosen to accomplish therapeutic or convenience objectives not offered by conventional dosage forms'.

One particular variant of a modified release dosage form—that is, the enteric or delayed release form—will be dealt with in the subsequent section.

As the coating is designed to perform a function critical to the performance of the product, it is essential that during the development of the dosage form there is an understanding of the nature and properties of the film-coating polymers; the influence of various additives and also the nature of the film-forming process. Equally important is that our manufacturing process be well understood and validated in terms of what we expect from the product.

14.1.1   Possible types of dosage form
These can be tablets or multiparticulates. While tablets coated with a rate-controlling membrane may offer advantages of simplicity from the point of view of production the use of intact tablets has received critical comment in recent years. Much of this criticism has revolved around issues related to gastrointestinal transit time and possibilities of irritancy caused by accidental lodging of the tablet in some location in the gastrointestinal system.

The multiparticulate systems which have been demonstrated to be of use in this technology include

- Drug crystals and powders.
- Extruded and spheronized drug granulates.
- Sugar seeds or nonpareils.
- Ion-exchange resin particles.
- Small compressed tablets.

14.1.2   Characteristics of multiparticulate systems
From the historical origins of multiparticulate systems, techniques have been available for loading drugs onto sugar seeds and then overcoating with a rate-controlling membrane. Traditionally the drug can be applied in a 'lamination' process in which powdered active material is directly loaded onto the sugar seeds in a coating pan. Adhesion to the surface of the particle is greatly assisted by the application of an adhesive or gummy solution. While having the merit of simplicity, the technique can leave a lot to be desired in terms of drug uniformity and drug loss via the exhaust. Alternatively, a process whereby the drug is loaded onto the sugar seeds by a suspension or a solution has a lot to recommend it in terms of comparison.

It is generally accepted that high dose drugs are better treated by using a granulation approach. The physical and chemical characteristics of the uncoated multiparticulates have a part to play in the overall consideration of drug release from these dosage forms. Contributing factors include size and size distribution of the particle, surface characteristics including porosity, friability, drug solubility and the constitution of the other excipients used in the particle.

14.1.3   Presentation possibilities of multiparticulates

In order to constitute a finished dosage form, coated multiparticulates are commonly filled into hard-shell gelatin capsules although they may be compressed into tablets in such a way as to preserve the integrity of the rate-controlling membrane around the individual particles.

The technology of using modified release coatings in combination with multiparticulates is not a particularly new technique and has in fact been practised since the early days of film coating in the 1950s. Nowadays an ever-increasing interest in the subject has been greatly facilitated by developments in suitable coating materials, especially those utilizing application from aqueous systems. Developments in coating equipment and granule production have further facilitated interest in the subject.

14.1.4   Some features of the performance of multiparticulates

Multiparticulate dosage forms have a number of useful features which can be used to advantage in modified release forms. Foremost is their ability to overcome the variation in performance which may arise through variation in gastrointestinal transit time and, in particular, variation occasioned by erratic gastric emptying. The size of most multiparticulates enables them to pass through the constricted pyloric sphincter so that they are able to distribute themselves along the entire gastrointestinal tract. Bechgaard & Hegermann-Nielsen (1978) have produced an extensive review of this particular topic. As the dose of drug is spread out over a large number of particles, then the consequences of failure of a few units has nothing like the potential consequences of failure through dose dumping of a single coated tablet used as a modified release dosage form. Additionally, as the drug is not all concentrated in one single unit, considerations of an irritant effect to the mucosal lining of the gastrointestinal tract are very much reduced.

14.1.5   Mechanisms of action for modified release coated dosage forms

Rowe (1985) has classified potential mechanisms for modified release using film coating into three groups:

- Diffusion
- Polymer erosion
- Osmotic effect.

Diffusion

In this mechanism the applied film permits the entry of aqueous fluids from the gastrointestinal tract. Once dissolution of the drug has taken place it then diffuses through the polymeric membrane at a rate which is determined by the physicochemical properties of the drug and the membrane itself, the latter can, of course, be altered to take into account the desired release profile. Suitable formulation techniques such as optimizing choice of polymer, use of correct plasticizer and concentration of plasticizer will be considered subsequently, as will the use of dissolution rate modifiers. By using these techniques, the structure of the film can be altered so that, for instance, instead of diffusing through the polymer, the drug can be made to diffuse through a network of pores and channels within the membrane, thus facilitating the release process.

In the diffusion process, the membrane is intended to stay intact during the passage of the coated particle down the gastrointestinal tract.

Polymer erosion

This technique has been used in some rather elderly technology where multiparticulate systems were coated with a simple wax or fatty material such as beeswax or glyceryl monostearate, the intention being that during passage down the gastrointestinal tract, at some point the characteristics of the coating would permit the complete erosion of the coating by a softening mechanism. This would, in turn, permit the complete breakup of the drug particle. While this in itself is not modified release, a functioning system can be made by blending together sub-batches of particles coated with varying quantities of retarding material.

Another variant with a different application is that of enteric release where the controlling membrane is designed to dissolve at a predetermined pH and make available the entire drug substance with no delay. This will be dealt with subsequently in section 14.6.

Osmotic effects

This effect is utilized in a group of well-known delivery systems using coated tablets, e.g. 'Oros' from the Alza Corporation. Here a polymer with semi-permeable film characteristics is used to coat the tablet. Upon immersion in aqueous fluids the hydrostatic pressure inside the tablet will build up due to the selective ingress of water across the semi-permeable membrane. Very often these systems are formulated with a tablet core containing additional osmotically active materials as the drug substance may not always be soluble in water to the extent of being able to exert adequate osmotic pressure to drive the device. The sequence is completed by the internal osmotic pressure rising sufficiently to expel drug solution at a predetermined rate through a precision laser-drilled hole in the tablet coating.

These systems are capable of delivering drug solution in a zero-order fashion at a rate determined by the formulation of the core constituents, the nature of the coating and the diameter of the drilled orifice.

Osmotic effects also have a general part to play in release of active materials from many coated particulate systems. This is because pressure will be built up inside the coated particle as a result of the entry of water, which can be relieved by drug solution being forced through pores, channels or other imperfections in the particle coat.

It can, of course, be appreciated that, while formulation design has one predetermined release mechanism, a mixture of all three will be functioning to a certain extent in any modified release coated system.

14.2   THE INGREDIENTS OF MODIFIED RELEASE COATINGS

14.2.1   Polymers
These have a primary part to play in the modified release process and the general characteristics of coating polymers can be found in Chapter 2, together with a description of individual polymers suitable for modified release applications.

The use of polymer blends in modified release coatings
It has been indicated that in order to obtain the optimized film for a particular application, attention should not be solely confined to a single polymer. In an early publication, Coletta & Rubin (1964) described the coating of aspirin crystals with a Wurster technique using a mixed coating of ethylcellulose N10 and methylcellulose 50 mPas grades. They confirmed that the release of aspirin was inversely proportional to the content of ethylcellulose in the coating. Another early publication by Shah & Sheth (1972) examined mixed films of ethylcellulose and HPMC concerning their ability to modify the passage of FD&C Red No. 2 dye. In thin films, a sharp increase in release rate was evident where the content of HPMC was in excess of 10% of the film. At greater than 25% content, film rupture occurred which the authors attributed to mechanical weakness and/or pore formation as a result of the content of water-soluble polymer.

Miller & Vadas (1984) have studied an unusual phenomenon concerning the coating of aspirin tablets with mixed films of ethylcellulose aqueous dispersion (Aquacoat) and HPMC. The authors found that these coated tablets at elevated temperature and humidity suffered a greatly extended disintegration time. These results appeared to be specific to aspirin and the polymer system used. Further investigation using scanning electron microscopy revealed that the coatings in question on storage possessed an atypical structure in which the original outline of the ethylcellulose particles was obliterated and could not be made out. In this connection, Porter (1989) has cautioned that in the incorporation of water-soluble polymers into aqueous ethylcellulose dispersions the introduced polymer will distribute itself mainly in the aqueous phase, so that when the film dries the second polymer will be positioned at the interfaces of the latex particles where they may have the opportunity of interfering with film coalescence.

Other authors have also pointed out that ethylcellulose and HPMC, while a very commonly used combination, are only partially compatible (Sakellariou *et al.*, 1987). Lehmann (1984) has described how mixtures of the acrylic Eudragit RL and RS types of aqueous dispersions can be used to provide modified release coatings. Two different acrylics have been used by Li *et al.* (1991) in the formulation of beads of pseudoephedrine HCl. Eudragit S100 was utilized in the drug-loading process and Eudragit RS, a low water permeable type, was used in the coating stage.

14.2.2   Plasticisers
From what has been described previously in Chapter 2, plasticizers have a crucial role to play in the formation of a film coating and its ultimate structure. It is not surprising, therefore, that several authors have demonstrated that plasticizers can

have a marked effect both quantitatively and qualitatively on the release of active materials from modified release dosage forms where they are incorporated into the rate-controlling membrane.

Rowe (1986) has investigated the release of a model drug from mixed films of ethylcellulose and HPMC under several conditions including variation in plasticizer type and level. On the addition of diethyl phthalate, drug release was decreased with lower molecular weight grades of ethylcellulose (Fig. 14.1a), but with the higher molecular weight grades there was no effect (Fig. 14.1b). The relative decrease in dissolution rate found with increasing plasticizer concentration was greatest with the lower molecular weight grade but gradually decreases with increasing molecular weight of ethylcellulose polymer. Rowe further describes how diethyl phthalate is a good plasticizer for ethylcellulose but is a poor plasticizer for HPMC. When added to mixed films it will preferentially partition into the ethylcellulose component and exert a plasticizer effect by lowering of residual internal stress. For a low molecular weight ethylcellulose where drug release is primarily through cracks and imperfections in the film coat, the addition of diethyl phthalate will be beneficial in controlling release rate. Where drug release is not controlled by this mechanism, as is the

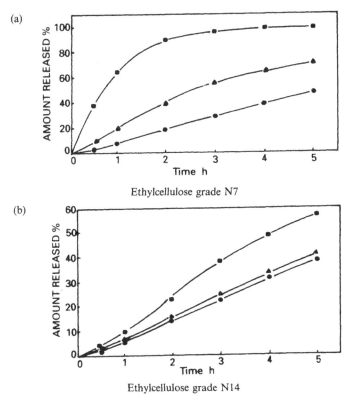

Ethylcellulose grade N7

Ethylcellulose grade N14

Fig. 14.1 The effect of plasticizer concentration on the release of the model drug substance through films prepared with ethylcellulose ■ no plasticizer ▲ 10% diethyl phthalate ● 20% diethyl phthalate

case with the higher molecular ethylcelluloses, the addition of plasticizer will have little effect.

The aqueously dispersed forms of acrylate-based polymers have their own particular characterstics in terms of plasticizer requirements. Thus Eudragit NE30D, which produces essentially water-insoluble films, needs no plasticizer and is capable of forming a film spontaneously. However, the Eudragit RS/RL30D types possess a minimum film-forming temperature of approximately 50 and 40°C respectively and require the addition of between 10 and 20 %w/w of plasticizer to bring the minimum film-forming temperature down to a usable value (Lehmann, 1989).

Li *et al.* (1991) have examined the effect of plasticizer type and concentration on the release of pseudoephedrine from drug-loaded nonpariels. They showed that beads coated with Eudragit RL in combination with lower levels of diethyl phthalate showed slower release profiles than when higher levels of plasticizer were used. They attributed this to the fact that at higher plasticizer levels they experienced higher frequencies of bead agglomeration, sticking and other problems related to the resulting softer film. These effects, it is postulated, would lead to the deposition of an imperfect film. Interestingly Li *et al.* (1991) could find no significant difference in dissolution when the two plasticizers PEG and diethyl phthalate were used in similar concentrations, despite the fact that PEG is more water soluble and therefore might have been expected to release drug faster. Superior film integrity and lack of adhesion of the beads is probably a compensating mechanism allowing the two plasticizers to appear equivalent in action.

Two types of aqueous ethylcellulose dispersion can be distinguished: first, that type which needs the addition of separate plasticizer by the user and, secondly, that type in which the plasticizer has been incorporated within the individual ethylcellulose particles by virtue of the manufacturing process. In a comprehensive study, Iyer *et al.* (1990) contrasted the performance of ethylcellulose dispersions of the two varieties with that of ethylcellulose from an organic solvent solution. The dispersion requiring separate addition of plasticizer, in this case dibutyl sebacate, needed at least 30 min for the plasticizer to be taken up by the ethylcellulose particles. Even then, further differences were noted between the two systems regarding actual performance. The authors stated that for acetaminophen and guaiphenesin beads the combined plasticizer–ethylcellulose aqueous dispersion and the true solution of ethylcellulose in organic solvent were to all intents and purposes identical in performance. This is perhaps not surprising when one considers the high degree of polymer–plasticizer interaction possible with this type of ethylcellulose presentation.

Furthermore, Lippold *et al.* (1990) found that, when adding plasticizers to aqueous ethylcellulose dispersions, periods of between 5 and 10 h were needed for proper interaction between polymer and plasticizer. The two groups of authors did, however, use different methods of assessing plasticizer interaction, Iyer *et al.* (1990) used an analytical technique to determine unused plasticizer while Lippold *et al.* (1990) followed the action of the plasticizer on the minimum film-forming temperature of the polymer. Goodhart *et al.* (1984) have also commented upon the importance of plasticizers in aqueously dispersed ethylcellulose systems.

14.2.3 Dissolution rate modifiers

This is very diverse group of materials providing a variety of means to assist the formulator to produce the desired release profile. Under this heading, of course, can be considered secondary polymers in polymer blends, as described in section 14.3.1, as they may be considered to function under this heading.

Dissolution enhancers and pore-forming agents

Within this group can be considered all manner of usually low molecular weight materials such as sucrose, sodium chloride, surfactants and even some materials more usually encountered as plasticizers, for example, the polyethylene glycols. Some early work in this area was performed by Kallstrand & Ekman (1983) who coated potassium chloride tablets with a 13% PVC solution in acetone which contained microcrystals of sucrose with a particle size of less than 10 μm. The principle involved is that once the coating is exposed to the action of aqueous fluids, the water-soluble pore former is rapidly dissolved leaving a porous membrane which acts as the diffusional barrier.

Lindholm & Juslin (1982) have studied the action of a variety of these materials on the dissolution of salicylic acid from ethylcellulose-coated tablets. As the authors state, very little salicylic acid was released from unmodified coated tablets due to the water insolubility of ethylcellulose. That which did dissolve was due to the solubility of the salicylic acid in the ethylcellulose film (see also Abdul-Razzak, 1983). Altogether, three different types of film additive were used, a surfactant, a fine particle size water-soluble powder and a counter-ion. Depending upon the nature of the surfactant the release of salicylic acid was increased by varying amounts, the greatest increases were seen with the more hydrophobic surfactants such as Span 20 rather than the hydrophilic surfactants such as Tween 20. The authors supposed that the hydrophobic surfactants acted as better carriers of the salicylic acid than did the hydrophilic ones, and that this mechanism prevailed over one where the hydrophilic types modified dissolution by a pore-forming mechanism. Both sodium chloride and sucrose increased dissolution rate by a straightforward pore-forming mechanism. Tetrabutylammonium salts have been used in chromatography to increase the solubility of salicylic acid in organic solvents, and while their addition to the ethylcellulose films was of some benefit, dissolution rate was not greatly enhanced. One feature of these results was that release of salicylic acid was seen to be zero order.

In the area of acrylate coatings, Li *et al.* (1989) have noted that xanthan gum exerts a powerful dissolution enhancing effect on Eudragit NE30D coated theophylline granules.

14.2.4 Insoluble particulate materials

These materials have been traditionally added to modified release coating systems primarily for reasons other than that of altering a particular release profile. Such materials include pigments and anti-tack agents. Some polymers used in modified release coatings are rather sticky on application and their manufacturers have recommended methods to combat this effect. For instance, acrylic type Eudragit E preparations are recommended to be used with talc, magnesium stearate or similar materials.

By their very nature, the aqueous dispersion polymer systems based on ethylcellulose tend to be sticky due to their highly plasticized nature. One of these materials (Surelease) has a quantity of colloidal silicon dioxide built into the formula to decrease this processing problem.

As may be deduced by inspection of Chapter 2, the mechanism by which insoluble particles exert a rate modifying action is one described by Chatfield (1962). At relatively low solid loadings, film permeability, hence dissolution rate of coated actives, would be expected to decrease due to an increased path length encountered by permeating materials. However, at the critical pigment volume concentration insufficient polymer is present to prevent the formation of cracks and fissures, allowing a greatly increased flux of permeating material.

The effect of any one particular insoluble material on a film will be dependent not only on its concentration but also on its particle size, shape and especially how it bonds or interacts with the associated polymer.

These effects are particularly critical when considering the action of solid additives on the aqueous dispersed polymers as the added solid material has the potential to interfere with the coalescence process and hinder film formation. Goodhart et al. (1984) have commented on the addition of talc and magnesium stearate to the ethylcellulose aqueous dispersion products. The effect of kaolin on the release of pellets coated with Eudragit NE30D dispersion has been investigated by Ghebre-Sellassie et al. (1987) and it was shown that as the amount of kaolin in the coating formulation increased, so did the quantity of drug released until the point was achieved when the quantity of kaolin present was sufficient to destroy the retardant property of the film (see Fig. 14.2). In contrast the length of time necessary to initiate release increased as the ratio of kaolin to polymer decreased. It was further seen that kaolin could be replaced in the formulae studied by talc or magnesium trisilicate with no significant quantitative effect.

14.2.5 Pigments

These will, of course, function as insoluble particles as described previously but there are a number of practical issues in addition which concern the aqueous dispersed polymers. Some of the acrylate dispersions are sensitive to electrolyte and will, under certain conditions, irreversibly coagulate. If an inferior grade of aluminium lake, for instance, is used as the pigment, this may well contain an excessive quantity of water-soluble dye unattached to the alumina substrate. As the dye is an electrolyte, this situation could give rise to problems.

Surelease, which is one of the aqueously dispersed ethylcellulose coating systems, has a pH which is sufficiently high so as to de-lake many aluminium lake pigments. These particular colourants should be either avoided with Surelease or reserved for a non-modified release top coat. It should also be remembered that many modified release preparations will be in the form of multiparticulates which will ultimately be filled into hard shell capsules which themselves offer the option of being coloured.

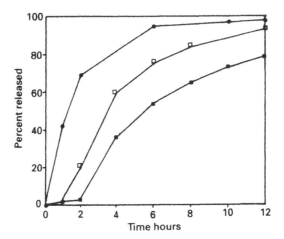

Fig. 14.2   Effect of the relative ratio of Eudragit NE30D resin to kaolin in the final film on release profile. Resin: kaolin ● 3:3, □ 3:2, ■ 3:1

14.2.6   Stabilizing agents

These feature only as additives for certain of the acrylate-based latex products which are susceptible to coagulation by mechanical stirring, etc. Manufacturer's literature recommends the addition of certain materials to help overcome these effects, e.g. PEG, PVP and Tween 60 or 80. It will, of course, be apparent that these materials have effects of their own on films to which they are added.

14.2.7   Miscellaneous additives

These materials feature as manufacturing process aids or stabilizers already present in the commercially available aqueous polymer dispersions. For example, Surelease will contain ammonia and colloidal silica, Aquacoat contains necessary surfactants for stabilization while some of the acrylic latex products need to contain a preservative in order to maintain microbiological integrity. With the acrylate products there is also the question of unreacted monomeric material from the manufacturing process.

These comments are not intended to be exhaustive and the formulator is advised to consult the relevant technical literature on the product concerned.

14.3   THE STRUCTURE AND FORMATION OF MODIFIED RELEASE FILMS AND THE MECHANISM OF DRUG RELEASE

For films produced from true polymer solutions, Porter (1989) has proposed the following sequence of events:

● There is a rapid evaporation of solvent from both the liquid droplets and the surface of the substrate to be coated. While Porter assumed that considerable solvent loss would take place from the droplets of polymer solution during their passage from the spray-gun to the substrate, later studies described in detail in this work (see Chapter 4) indicate that this is not necessarily so.

- There is an increase in polymer concentration in the solution and a contraction in volume of the coating liquid on the substrate.
- Further solvent loss occurs as solvent diffuses to the surface of the coating. The concentration of polymer in the coating increases to the point where the polymer molecules become immobile (defined as the 'solidification point').
- There is a final loss of solvent resulting from diffusion of residual solvent through an essentially 'dry' membrane.

The final step of solvent loss is important in terms of drug release as it is at this point that the film shrinkage so induced gives rise to internal stress within the film. This unrelieved internal stress, if of sufficient magnitude to overcome the ultimate tensile strength of the film, will generate microcracks which will facilitate the diffusion of drug solution from the coated particle. Rowe (1986) has proposed these stress induced cracks as the largest contributing feature in the release of drugs through low molecular weight ethylcellulose membranes. In this study, as the ethylcellulose molecular weight increased, Rowe was able to observe a decrease in release rate up to a limiting value at a molecular weight of 35 000. At this value the increase in tensile strength due to increasing molecular weight was sufficient to overcome the induced stress in the film, hence preventing the generation of cracks and flaws within.

The formation of a film from an aqueous dispersion has been described previously in Chapter 2. Furthermore, Zhang *et al.* (1988, 1989) have suggested that in the initial stages of coating, flaws exist in the coat due to its discontinuous nature such that channels are present connecting the substrate surface with the exterior (see Fig. 14.3). As coating progresses, sufficient material is now applied so that flaws are no longer continuous between the substrate and the exterior. The significance of this point, described as the critical coating level, will be expanded later.

Ghebre-Sellassie *et al.* (1987), working with Eudragit NE30D films, have also produced evidence of the channel-like nature of their applied films. Their visual evidence was augmented with mercury porosimetry studies quantifying the pore structure in the film.

The majority of modified release dosage forms reliant on a film for their functionality will be diffusion controlled. For this, Brossard & Lefort des Ylouses (1984) have identified three activities:

- Penetration of the film by the aqueous environment surrounding the dosage form and the entry of fluid.
- Dissolution of the drug in the fluid entering the dosage form.
- Diffusion of drug solution in the opposite direction across the film.

This diffusion-controlled passage across the film can be defined in its simplest terms by Fick's law;

$$Q = \frac{D}{e} \cdot S(C_1 - C_2)t \tag{14.1}$$

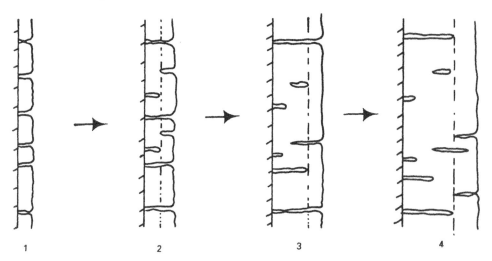

1   2   3   4

Fig. 14.3   Formation of a controlled release membrane as the coating process progresses.

where Q is the quantity of drug diffusing in time t, e is the film thickness, C_1 is the concentration of drug in the dosage form, C_2 is the concentration of drug in the aqueous receptor, D is the diffusion coefficient of the drug and S is the area of diffusion. The rate of diffusion is linked to the solubility of the drug, which may be the limiting factor.

At the beginning of the process the concentration C_2 can be assumed to be negligible and if the rate of dissolution of the drug is greater than the rate of diffusion, then: $C_1 \sim C_0$ and

$$Q = \frac{D}{e} . S . C_0 . t = \text{a constant} \qquad (14.2)$$

It follows, therefore, that in the initial stages release will be zero order. If the rate of dissolution is slower than the rate of diffusion because the drug concentration in the dosage form towards the end of the process will noticeably decrease, then the rate control will become first order.

A number of factors will mitigate against this ideal condition being reached:

● The concentration of drug outside of the membrane may not be negligible, in other words 'sink conditions' will not have been reached.
● The viscosity of the medium immediately surrounding the dosage form may adversely affect the diffusion process.
● The membrane will probably swell or otherwise change its character during the process, hence permeability and dimensional factors may work to vary the diffusion coefficient.

As we accept that the membrane is not homogeneous, an allowance must be made for this factor in our consideration of the diffusion coefficient. Iyer *et al.* (1990) have considered a diffusion coefficient D modified to account for the recognized film structure:

$$D = D_w \frac{e}{t} \tag{14.3}$$

where D_w represents the diffusion coefficient in water and e and t are porosity and tortuosity factors respectively. Ghebre-Sellassie et al. (1987) have suggested that the predominant method of drug release can be expected to be diffusion through water-filled pores and not through the insoluble polymeric membrane. Such systems would be expected to release drug independently of the gastrointestinal fluid provided solubility and pK_a were favourable. This model also implies that the size of the diffusing molecule is less than that of the pore through which it is diffusing.

By the use of pore-forming agents and other suitable additives it is possible to manipulate this modified diffusion coefficient to produce an optimized formulation.

14.3.1 Osmotic effects

While diffusional processes have rightly received the greatest attention when considering drug release from coated multiparticulate systems, Ghebre-Sellassie et al. (1987) suggest that the part played by osmotic effects should not be ignored. This is especially true if it is considered that many bead formulations will contain osmotically active materials such as sugars and electrolytes.

14.3.2 The effect of the nature and quantity of the coating material

Nature of the coating material
For a given substrate it is perhaps reasonable to expect release differences to be observed for changes in the actual coating system employed, and this is what is encountered in practice.

Differences due to polymer constitution can be readily seen: Ghebre-Sellassie et al. (1987, 1988) have shown substantial differences in the dissolution behaviour of diphenhydramine pellets coated with Surelease (Fig. 14.4a) as compared to the acrylic dispersion Eudragit NE30D (Fig. 14.4b).

Significant differences can also be identified in performance between variants of the same polymer type. Iyer et al. (1990), in a comparative study of three forms of ethylcellulose suitable for coating—Aquacoat, Surelease and ethylcellulose from an organic solvent solution—showed that they conferred very different dissolution characteristics on acetaminophen and guaiphenesin pellets. Porter and D'Andrea (1985) have also noted the same phenomenon with ethylcellulose coatings.

In the area of acrylate-based coatings, Lehmann (1986) has coated chlorpheniramine pellets using Eudragit RS polymer in both organic solvent solution and as the aqueous dispersion form. Results showed that on a comparison of T_{50} percent value, rather less of the aqueous presentation was required to achieve an identical dissolution result.

The neutral acrylate latexes, Eudragit RL30D and RS30D differ only in their degree of permeability towards water. The manufacturers recommend blending of the two materials as an effective way of achieving the desired release profile. Lehmann (1989) quotes an example where a 10% coating load of both RL:RS 1:3

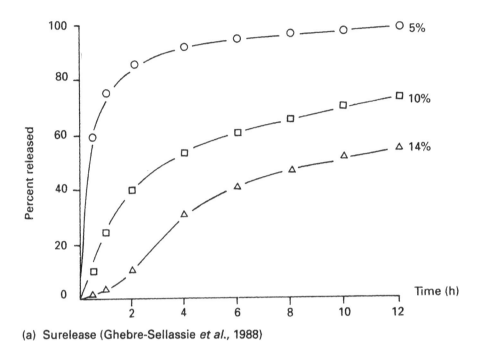

(a) Surelease (Ghebre-Sellassie *et al.*, 1988)

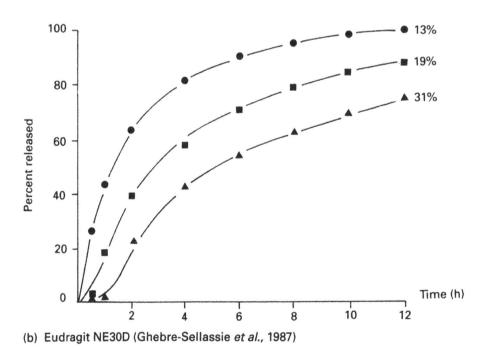

(b) Eudragit NE30D (Ghebre-Sellassie *et al.*, 1987)

Fig. 14.4   Release of diphenyhydramine hydrochloride from pellets coated with an aqueous polymeric dispersion using an Aeromatic strea – 1 coating apparatus.

and RL:RS 1:5 blends have been used to coat theophylline granules, and the results show performance differences between the two formulae.

Quantity of the coating material

For those coated multiparticulates which obey Ficks's law regarding drug release, the quantity of drug diffusing after a given time will be dependent on the thickness of the controlling membrane. It is also empirically well established that one of the most effective measures that can be taken to readily modify the dissolution performance of such a dosage form is to vary the amount of coating material used (see Fig. 14.5). As a further generalization, very water-soluble drugs will require a greater thickness of coating than will relatively water-insoluble drugs.

Since the keen interest shown in modified release dosage forms since the early 1980s the principle of increasing thickness (or, more accurately, increasing coating weight to the multiparticulate mass) leading to decreased dissolution rate, has been amply illustrated. For example, Wouessidjewe *et al.* (1983) showed that TNT release from coated microcapsules was dependent on the quantity of Eudragit employed. Ghebre-Sellassie *et al.* (1988) showed significant dissolution profile differences between diphenhydramine-coated pellets at the 5, 10 and 14% coating level with Surelease, and even at the lowest level coating integrity was preserved. Previously Ghebre-Sellassie *et al.* (1987) had shown a similar effect with the Eudragit NE30D, but on this occasion coating weights of 13–31% were required (Fig. 14.4). Li *et al.* (1991) have shown quantitative differences in release profile for

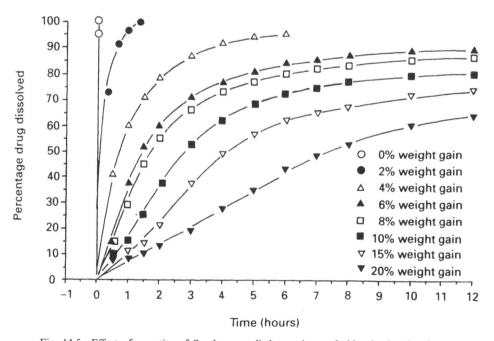

Fig. 14.5 Effect of quantity of Surelease applied on release of chlorpheniramine from nonpareils coated with Surelease.

pseudoephedrine beads coated with between 3 and 8% weight gain of plasticized Eudragit RS.

Shah & Sheth (1972), during their investigations of the passage of dye solution through a mixed membrane of ethylcellulose and HPMC, found that release rate increased as the membrane thickness decreased. Porter (1989) has reported some interesting results where a constant weight gain of 10% of coating material was applied to chlorpheniramine beads of differing mesh sizes; 30–35, 18–20 and 14–18. After coating with Surelease significant differences were seen in the resulting disso-lution profiles. The author was also able to demonstrate similar differences when 'rough' or 'smooth' surface beads were so treated (Fig. 14.6). The practical point here is that for batch to batch reproducibility to be maintained, an adequate control must be exercised on bead size and surface characteristics. This same point is also emphasized by Metha (1986).

Li *et al.* (1988) have also examined the problem of how to ensure a uniform coating. They reject the idea of utilizing only a very narrow size fraction of multi-particulates on the grounds that this practice is wasteful as much of a batch is rejected. Instead they prefer the concept of a fixed weight of polymer for each batch. Experimental work was conducted by coating granules of theophylline with Eudragit NE30D in a Wurster column. The authors suggest that surface area can be related to particle size by plotting particle size versus weight percent oversize from sieve analysis data on log probability paper. The geometric mean can be deter-

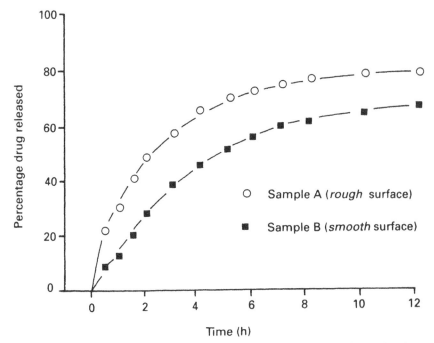

Fig. 14.6 Influence of surface characteristics of substrate on release of chlorpheniramine maleate from beads coated (10% weight gain) with an aqueous ethylcellulose dispersion (Surelease).

mined directly from the plot by determining the particle size which corresponds to the 50% probability value and so leading onto the specific surface area. Using this approach, linearity was achieved on plots of release rate versus the quantity of Eudragit NE30D per unit surface area.

In developing the Fick's law type model for diffusion-controlled drug release from coated multiparticulates, Zhang *et al.* (1991) have attempted to explain the changes occurring as the controlling membrane increases in thickness. Their experimental work was based on an aqueous ethylcellulose system, Aquacoat, which was used on beads comprising 50% acetaminophen and 50% of microcrystalline cellulose. The acetaminophen release was dependent on the level of coating achieved, and the authors suggest a change in mechanism as the change in level progresses:

- At low levels of coating, a square root time relationship exists with respect to the amount of drug released. Furthermore, the release rate constant is linear with respect to coating level. At low levels of coating it is postulated that pores and channels exist so that parts of the substrate are in contact with the exterior.
- Additional coating effectively seals the pores so that drug release becomes zero order and proportional to the reciprocal of the coating level.

14.4 DISSOLUTION RATE CHANGES WITH TIME

Subsequent to the coating of the multiparticulates the ideal state of affairs would be one in which the dissolution performance remained constant with time. However, since the introduction of the aqueous dispersion products for modified release coating, one feature of their performance has been the possibility of such changes, the majority related to an elongation of dissolution time although examples do exist of increasing dissolution rates with time. Commonly these effects are not solely dependent on time but are dependent on a combination of temperature and time.

14.4.1 Decreased dissolution rates

Goodhart *et al.* (1984) demonstrated significant time/temperature changes with phenylpropanolamine beads coated with the aqueous ethylcellulose dispersion product Aquacoat. Interestingly the results also demonstrated the different dissolution profiles obtained with the use of two different plasticizer levels for the Aquacoat system (Fig. 14.7).

Ghebre-Sellassie *et al.* (1988), working with another aqueous ethylcellulose system, Surelease, reports that when this material is coated onto pseudoephedrine pellets, little change is evident up to a temperature of 45°C but that at 60°C the dissolution profile is somewhat slowed. Porter (1989) has also examined Surelease and has found no effect on chlorpheniramine-coated beads even after the rather extreme storage conditions of 144 h at 60°C.

One way of viewing these and similar findings is to consider what is taking place on storage or during an accelerated 'curing' process as a completion of

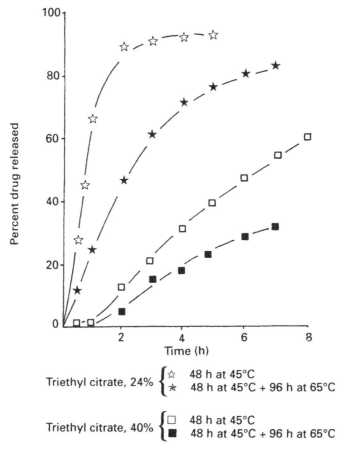

Fig. 14.7 Effect of drying temperature and duration on the release (in water) of phenyl-propanolamine HCl from nonpareils coated with Aquacoat (10% by wt).

the coating process itself. In these instances, for whatever reason, optimal coalescence of the film has not taken place, leaving the necessity to complete the work after the coating activity proper. As has been seen previously, the coalescence process is demanding in the observance of the necessary conditions of moisture presence and minimum temperature to be attained during the coating process. It is therefore not surprising that differences will be found in the examination of individual cases.

As a logical extension of this recognition it is prudent to include a curing step in the early development validation of the dosage form. Should these investigations reveal very large dissolution changes after coating, then the coating process itself should be the subject of further optimization.

14.4.2 Increased dissolution rates
This phenomenon is much less frequent than the previous case and could be due to a variety of causes:

- The drug is preferentially soluble in the rate-controlling membrane but with time may gradually partition away from the bead into the coating, Wald *et al.* (1988) have quoted such an example.
- A combination of circumstances in which a very water-soluble drug in a formulation has been subjected to processing which has left excessive residual water in the particle. On storage, the drug will tend to move with the solvent front and pass through the membrane.
- Physical failure of the rate-controlling membrane.

14.5 ENTERIC COATINGS

14.5.1 Introduction and rationale for use

These coatings form a subgroup of modified release coatings and a simple definition of such a coating would be one that resists the action of stomach acids but rapidly breaks down to release its contents once it has passed into the duodenum. These coatings will come within the definition of 'delayed release forms', as specified in the USP.

Chambliss (1983) has summarized the rationale for the use of enteric coatings:

- Prevention of the drug's destruction by gastric enzymes or by the acidity of the gastric fluid.
- Prevention of nausea and vomiting caused by the drug's irritation of the gastric mucosa.
- Delivering the drug to its local site of action in the intestine.
- Providing a delayed release action.
- Delivering a drug primarily absorbed in the intestine to that site, at the highest possible concentration.

The mechanism by which enteric coating polymers function is by a variable pH solubility profile where the polymer remains intact at a low pH but at a higher pH will undergo dissolution to permit the release of the contents of the dosage form. However, the situation is not as simple as this as there are other critical factors which affect the performance of an enteric-coated dosage form, and these will be examined later. Historically, polymers which produce an enteric effect other than by a differential pH solubility profile have received some attention; for instance, materials which are digestible or susceptible to enzymatic attack. However, these are no longer of commercial interest (Schroeter, 1965).

14.5.2 Gastrointestinal pH and polymer performance

In recent years much more accurate assessments have been made of the pH of various parts of the gastrointestinal tract facilitated by the use of miniature pH electrodes and radiotelemetry.

Healey (1989) states that the pH of the fasting stomach should be considered to be in the region of 0.8 to 2.0 with variations due to food ingestion causing transient rises to pH 4 to 5 or higher. The author also provides values for the proximal jejunum of pH 5.0 to 6.5 and states that the pH slowly rises along the length of the small intestine to reach only 6.0 to 7.0 with most subjects. The caecum and ascending colon are more acid than the small intestine by 0.5 to 1 pH unit but that a higher pH of 6.0 to 7.0 is restored further down the gastrointestinal tract.

A typical feature of more recent determinations of gastrointestinal pH is an awareness that the intestine is not as alkaline as once was thought. For example, Ritschel (1980) quotes values of 6.3 to 7.3 for the jejunum, which should be compared with Healey's data.

All the enteric polymers in current use possess ionizable acid groups, usually a free carboxylic acid from a phthalyl moiety. The equilibrium between unionized insoluble polymer and ionized soluble polymer will be determined by the pH of the medium and the pK_a of the polymer.

$$\text{unionized} \rightleftarrows \text{ionized}$$

The Henderson–Hasselbach equation can be used to predict the ratio of ionized to unionized polymer based on these two parameters, i.e.

$$pH - pK_a = \log \frac{\text{Concentration ionized form}}{\text{Concentration unionized form}} \tag{14.4}$$

For instance, therefore, at a pH level two units below the pK_a of the acid groups of the polymer, just 1% of these groups will be ionized. As the pH is increased and the equilibrium goes towards the right, the ratio of acid groups ionized will increase. For practical purposes there is no sharp cut-off point of solubility. As the pH rises to allow, for instance 10% of acid groups to be ionized, solubility will be considerably enhanced. More recently introduced polymers have pK_a values that take advantage of more recent evaluations of the pH of the gastrointestinal tract distal to the stomach.

Regarding enteric coating polymers in actual use there are formulation considerations which tend to complicate this rather simplistic picture of pH dissolution. Plasticizers and pigments/opacifiers added to the coating will considerably modify the mechanical properties and the permeability characteristics of the film. This may mean in particular that as the pH rises, formulation considerations may hasten the entry of acid through the film compared with the situation where plasticizers and pigments/opacifiers are absent from a film.

14.5.3   Enteric dosage forms in practice

Enteric dosage forms, including enteric-coated tablets, have had a chequered history regarding the esteem and confidence in which they are held. For instance, Chambliss (1983) reports that in the twenty years prior to that year, the number of enteric-coated products has steadily declined and quotes that many hold this dosage form to be the most unreliable on the market. The reasons for this are several-fold. Shellac, which was the mainstay of enteric coating in the past, has repeatedly been shown to be an unreliable polymer. Fundamentally, its pK_a renders it an unsuitable candidate as it dissolves at the relatively high pH of about 7.2.

With better validation of the coating process, and a greater awareness of the fact that a poorly understood non-optimized process is likely to produce non-performing product, enteric failures attributed to the process itself should be eradicated.

A fundamental consideration is the fact, that by their nature, the performance of enteric-coated tablets will be totally subject to the variation imposed by gastric emptying time. No release of active ingredients, of course, will be possible during the tablet's residence within the stomach. As long ago as 1971, Wagner, on considering this problem, observed that the optimum enteric-coated dosage form would be a multiparticulate system. These systems, of course, find much favour today as the coated particles are able to spread themselves down the gastrointestinal tract with much less reliance on gastric emptying time for passage through the stomach.

14.5.4 The performance of enteric coated films

In order to perform adequately, an enteric-coated form should not allow significant release of the drug in the stomach, yet must provide rapid dissolution of the polymer and complete release of the active material once in the environment of intestine. It is a fact, however, that all of the enteric-coating polymers in the hydrated state in the stomach will be permeable to some degree to a given active material. Formulation measures such as variation of the type and concentration of additions to the film will have an important part to play in keeping this permeability within acceptable limits. Manipulation of performance by variation of the quantity of the applied enteric-coating agent has a powerful part to play here. Variation of this parameter has such a powerful influence that there is a temptation to place almost total reliance upon it in the formulation of an enteric-coated product. Instead, due regard should be given to other formula and process considerations in achieving the minimum effective level of enteric-coating agent.

14.5.5 Ideal enteric coatings

An enteric coating must possess the general attributes of a non-functional film coating (see Chapter 2) with suitable modifications regarding the pH solubility requirements. The possession of adequate mechanical strength is particularly important as adverse handling of the tablets may predispose the coating towards chipping or cracking which may lead to a functional failure. A good enteric coating should possess the following qualities.

- pK_a to allow threshold pH of dissolution between pH 5 and 7, ideally between 5 and 6.
- Minimal variation in dissolution due to changes in ionic media and ionic strength of dissolution fluid.
- Rapid dissolution in non-gastric media.
- Low permeability.
- Ability to accept commonly used plasticizers, pigments and other additives without undue loss of function.
- Good response between quantity applied and ability to resist gastric juice.
- Capable of being processed from aqueous media.

- During processing, the material in solution/suspension should be of low viscosity, not subject to coagulation, non-tacky on application and be aesthetically pleasing in its final coating form. Equipment cleaning should not be unduly complicated.
- The enteric-coating material should be stable on storage. Films coated onto tablets or granules should not be subject to performance changes on storage.
- Adhesion between film and substrate should be strong.

Stafford (1982) proposes four 'classic tests' for any satisfactory aqueous enteric-coating material or process, these are summarized as follows:

- Ability to coat fast disintegrating and releasing tablets.
- Ability to coat hydrophilic tablets.
- The coating formulation should release little or no active ingredient in the stomach.
- The ability to coat acid sensitive ingredients.

The formulation of enteric-coated forms in the past has tended to be empirical. One attempt at a more rational approach has been that of Ozturk *et al.* (1988) who presented a model for polymer dissolution and drug release from enteric-coated tablets. They identified certain key parameters in the process:

- The dissolution medium
- The drug
- The polymer
- Mass transfer characteristics of the system.

The authors proposed that their model would be useful in predicting drug release during the polymer disintegration phase and also the time of onset of disintegration for any combination of weekly acidic drug and polymer coating. The model could, therefore, be applied to optimizing the formulation of enteric-coated forms.

14.5.6 The effect of the polymer on enteric performance
Inspection of Chapter 2 will show the variety of enteric-coating polymers available. Because of their differing structure it is to be expected that dissolution behaviour with regard to pH will differ.

Fig. 14.8 shows dissolution rate profiles for four different enteric-coating polymers HPMCP HP-50 and HP-55, PVAP and CAP. The authors (Davis *et al.*, 1986) identified two factors to explain this behaviour: pK_a and polymer backbone structure:

- pK_a; this effect can be illustrated by comparison of the dissolution profile for HP-50 and HP-55. The dissolution rate profile of HP-50 ($pK_a = 4.20$) was found to be shifted 0.3–0.4 units below that of HP-55 ($pK_a = 4.47$).
- The nature of the polymer backbone: HPMCP and PVAP can be viewed as being derived from the water-soluble polymers HPMC and PVA respectively, while CAP is derived from cellulose acetate, an essentially water-insoluble polymer which has water solubility conferred on it at higher pH values by the possession of a phthalyl group.

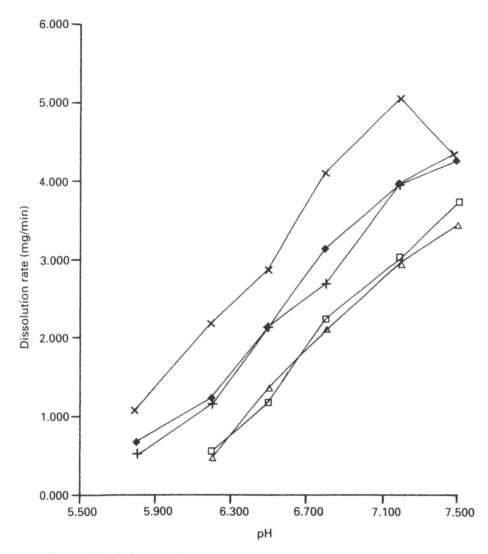

Fig. 14.8   Dissolution rates of the enteric polymers HP-50 lot 28023 (X), HP-55 lot 11232
(+), PVAP lot 44481 (◆), CAP lot 2567 (△) and CAP lot S-2021 (□) in 0.04 M phosphate
buffers at various pH.

In a comprehensive comparison of enteric-coating materials, Chang (1990) has
compared enteric polymer performance in coating theophylline pellets in polymers
from organic solvent solution, aqueous alkaline solutions of polymer and three
commercially available water-dispersible presentations (Aquateric, CAP; Coateric,
PVAP; Eudragit L30D, acrylate derivative).

Under the test conditions, differences in dissolution behaviour in acid were
apparent for organic solvent derived films. The extremes were, zero release over a
4 h period for the Eudragit S100 and 10% release by PVAP.

With the exception of the CAP coating, the ammonium salts showed a much higher loss of the theophylline from their films. The comparison of the polymers in their latex/pseudolatex form showed that Aquateric under these conditions provided no enteric protection while Eudragit L30D was satisfactory and Coateric was intermediate. However, valid comparisons are difficult to draw from this article due to the variations in experimental design.

Nesbitt *et al.* (1985) studied PVAP from two commercial sources, A and B. The polymer characterization profile included molecular weight by membrane osmometry which showed 61 000 and 48 000 for A and B respectively, significant morphological differences were shown between the two materials using scanning electron microscopy. The solubilies of A and B are different in various solvents and their apparent pK_as differ, being a function of their degree of ionization and decrease as the ionic strength of the test solution increases.

However, the neutralization rates of A and B were equivalent and increased with increasing ionic strength. The authors conclude that, despite demonstrated differences in profile, the two materials were functional equivalents. The authors also put forward their test profile as a general evaluation scheme for an enteric-coating excipient.

14.5.7 The effect of formulation of the enteric coating on enteric performance
The effect of formulation factors on the characteristics of a non-functional coating have been previously considered in Chapter 2. The additional features which have a bearing on the enteric performance of the coating will be considered here.

Plasticizers
Thoma & Heckenmuller (1986) have identified something like 19 different plasticisers used in enteric-coated products sampled from the German market. In view of the fact that these materials have a marked effect on film properties it is perhaps not surprising that their manipulation can have an effect on enteric properties.

In a statistically designed experiment, Deshpande & Dongre (1987) described the effect of either 1.5 or 0.6% propylene glycol content on a CAP formula containing talc as the other variable additive in addition to the CAP polymer. The higher plasticizer level was always associated with a marginally faster disintegration time.

On the other hand, Dechesne *et al.* (1982) were unable to distinguish significant differences between plasticizers when a group of six were evaluated for their effect on the disintegration time of Eudragit L30D coated tablets.

Porter & Ridgway (1982) have studied the effect of plasticizer (diethyl phthalate) on the permeability of CAP and PVAP to water vapour and gastric juice. With both diffusing media the same pattern was evident, plasticizer decreased the permeability of CAP yet increased the permeability of PVAP films (see Fig. 14.9). The authors state that the addition of a plasticizer to a film will increase segmental mobility, consequently this should reduce the activation energy for diffusion. While a possible explanation for the PVAP results, it would appear to contradict the CAP findings. Here the authors suggest that due to the possibility of the CAP being a more porous polymer than CAP, the plasticizer will decrease permeability by virtue of the fact that it will act as a solvent for the polymer thus reducing its porosity.

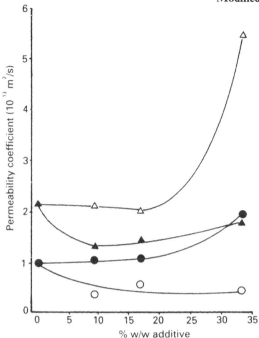

Fig. 14.9 Effect of additives on the permeability to simulated gastric juice of polyvinyl acetate phthalate (PVAP) and cellulose acetate phthalate (CAP) films applied to placebo tablets (points represent a mean of 5 replicates). ● PVAP + plasticizer; ▲ CAP + plasticizer; ○ PVAP + pigment; △CAP + pigment.

Solid inclusions

Just as with non-functional films, enteric film coatings very often contain solid inclusions such as pigments used as colouring agents or talc, etc. used as an anti-tack measure.

In a similar fashion to above, the same authors studied the effect of red iron oxide on the permeability of CAP and PVAP to water vapour and gastric juice. While no effect virtually was seen with PVAP, CAP exhibited an increase in permeability to both water vapour and gastric juice on increasing the addition of red iron oxide pigment (see Fig. 14.9). This was ascribed to a Chatfield effect, as described in Chapter 2. Deshpande & Dongre (1987) also incorporated talc into their previously described study. In contrast to the effect of plasticizer, the effect of increased concentration of talc was to prolong the disintegration time in each case.

14.5.8 The effect of quantity/thickness of the enteric coating on enteric performance

As a general rule, increasing quantities of applied enteric coating material will bring about increasing gastro resistance and an example is provided by Stafford (1982) and described in Table 14.1.

At high application rates, the beneficial effect will be less than at lower concentrations. When carried out to excess, this process is not only economically

Table 14.1 Variation of enteric performance of pindolol cores (as per cent drug released) coated with various amounts of neutralized HPMCP. Film weight is given in terms of amount of HPMCP before neutralization

Time (min)	pH	5.5 mg (%)	8.25 mg (%)	11 mg (%)
5	1.2	0.18	0.19	0.90
15	1.2	0.28	0.28	0.99
30	1.2	0.74	0.37	1.08
60	1.2	4.52	0.93	1.17
90	1.2	8.12	1.85	1.17
120	1.2	10.52	4.26	1.26

unsatisfactory, it may prolong the disintegration/dissolution of the dosage form in the intestinal phase of the test.

In a very comprehensive study Delporte & Jaminet (1976) elucidated the effect of increasing CAP application on acetylsalicylic acid tablets of 500 mg. At both pH 6 and 7 they showed linearity between disintegration time and thickness (expressed as mg per tablet) of coating material. Furthermore, the authors then selected three formulations which at pH 6 showed disintegration times of 9, 26 and 56 min respectively. Compared to the other two, the slow disintegrating formula showed a marked decrease in C_{max} when administered to volunteers for blood level studies (2.75 mg/ml compared with 4.22 and 4.28 mg/ml for the 9 and 26 min disintegrating tablet lots respectively).

Chambliss *et al.* (1984) have applied varying quantities of CAP and PVAP to pencillamine tablet cores. These were then subjected to dissolution testing at both pH 6.0 and 8.0. Increasing quantities of pencillamine remained as the quantity of enteric-coating material was increased. The authors expressed coating quantity as the number of coating applications used, which precludes a more quantitative treatment of their result.

With the acrylate-based material Eudragit L30D, Dechesne *et al.* (1982) have shown that for sodium fluoride tablets there was a need to exceed a given application rate, namely 6 mg/cm^2, in order to achieve a satisfactory coating. Healey (1989) should be consulted for a survey of bioavailability effects of enteric dosage forms in man.

14.5.9 The effect of the stability of the film coating on enteric performance
One of the reasons for the former widespread unease with enteric-coated forms probably stemmed from the recognition of the unstable nature of shellac-coated systems to storage. The literature contains many accounts of how prolonged disintegration times resulted from storage of tablets coated with this once popular enteric-coating agent.

Chambliss (1983), for example, quotes a typical case of shellac-coated dicalcium phosphate tablets which, on storage at ambient conditions for one year, suffered an increase in disintegration time in simulated intestinal fluid from 50 min to greater than 120 min.

More recently, Hoblitzell *et al.* (1985) have examined a marketed product for stability. These aspirin tablets were coated with a 'shellac type enteric coating'. Using a variety of storage conditions and packages, the authors concluded that enteric-coated aspirin tablets should be protected from moderate temperature and humidity in order to maintain an acceptable quality throughout the shelf-life. As would perhaps be expected, the raw material itself is also somewhat unstable and can be shown to undergo solubility changes in various solvents on storage. Its solutions also undergo viscosity changes with time.

In a large study, Thoma *et al.* (1987) examined 181 samples taken from the German marketplace. They found that:

- 15–20% failed either the acid or alkaline phase of the EP enteric disintegration test.
- The percentage was disproportionately high among enteric-coated pancreatin or cardiac glycosides (about 30%).
- 80% of 34 products coated with CAP, HPMCP or polymethacrylic acid ester did not change disintegration time after 2 years' storage at 20°C.
- However, at 40°C this number decreased to 40%.
- After 5 years at 20°C, the number of products which were not stable increased.

Sinko *et al.* (1990) have studied the physical ageing of HPMCP films in relation to the changes observed in the dissolution and mechanical properties of standardized isolated films. Dissolution rate measurements were performed on films which, initially above the glass transition temperature T_g, were quenched to a sub T_g storage temperature. The films were held at that temperature for a period of time and then quenched to 25°C. Depending upon the film former and the formulation, especially plasticizer type and concentration, enteric films on storage may exist as glasses. During the storage periods used, reductions in the dissolution rate to a limiting value were observed. Mechanical test results indicated a change in glass structure and showed that a limiting density was approached. The parallel changes observed in the dissolution study suggest that dissolution rate is at least partly governed by glass density. The susceptibility of CAP to hydrolysis is well known, guidance has been provided to potential users on the storage conditions required and how to assess the remaining enteric potency of a given sample of CAP (Anon., 1986).

In general, hydrolysis of the phthalyl group from the polymer backbone is a feature present to a greater or lesser extent in many of the phthalyl-containing enteric-coating polymers. For instance, 10 day storage at 60°C/75% r.h. demonstrated these results:

Polymer	*phthalyl lost (%)*
CAP	22
HPMCP	8
PVAP	0.3

The effect on mechanical properties of CAP can be demonstrated by the following:

Storage time (months)	Film tensile strength (MPa)		
	Ambient	40°C	60°C
0	77.1	77.1	77.1
2	71.2	62.5	55.3
4	—	41.1	49.0
6	79.8	57.5	39.1

Visual examination of the films showing the greatest losses in tensile strength demonstrated microcracks which almost certainly would lead to enteric failure of these films. Undoubtedly, enteric coatings are somewhat sensitive to storage conditions, and this susceptibility has contributed to the disfavour in which these coated forms were held in the past.

14.5.10   Enteric test criteria

Compendial *in vitro* test methods for enteric-coated products have traditionally relied on a two-stage disintegration type test in order to confirm enteric performance.

As a typical example of such a test, the BP specifies that six tablets are initially treated in a tablet disintegration tester using 0.1 M HCl for 2 h. The tablets must survive this initial stage and are then subject to a further 1 h in mixed phosphate buffer at pH 6.8. In order to pass the test, the tablets must have disintegrated at this point.

In the light of present knowledge, the pH of the buffer in the intestinal phase may be considered too high and Healey (1989) makes the case for a buffer as low as pH 6.0. The comment is also made that instances have been recorded of tablets meeting compendial disintegration standards yet failing to provide adequate bioavailability.

A dissolution-based test is used by the USP. Again this consists of a two part determination, first in simulated gastric fluid, then pH 6.8 buffer. The dissolution results obtained at the end of the respective phases are subjected to acceptance criteria, whereby further tablets are tested beyond the original six should the initial dissolution results exceed specified values.

Within manufacturing companies, 'in house' variations are sometimes made on the compendial disintegration/dissolution testing, frequently to make them more rigorous. Commonly, a greater number of tablets will be tested beyond that specified by the pharmacopoeias.

'In house' tests frequently include a mechanical resistance test in which for example tablets will be subject to a dissolution/disintegration test after a specified time in a tablet friabilator apparatus. This aspect is important as it confirms the ability of the coating to remain intact after mechanical stress, for example, during normal transportation and handling.

14.5.11   The coating process

This was covered in more detail in Chapter 7, suffice it to reinforce the point that the process for applying a functional coating needs to be rigorously validated and controlled. Several points in the process are capable of ruining what would otherwise be a well-formulated product. For instance, the process used must not give rise to any picking or sticking such that the integrity of the coating is impaired. Nor should the process be run at such an excessively high temperature which would give rise to spray drying of the coating medium and poor film formation.

If any aqueous dispersed presentation of an insoluble polymer is being used, the coating conditions should be those specified by the manufacturer unless such changes have again been fully validated.

Lastly, the mixing conditions in the coating equipment, particularly in side-vented cylindrical coating pans, must ensure that individual tablets receive similar quantities of coating material as far as is practically possible.

REFERENCES

Abdul-Razzak, M.H. (1983) Ph.D. Thesis, C.N.A.A, Leicester Polytechnic.

Anon. (1986) *Manuf. Chemist.*, Aug., 35–37.

Bechgaard, H. & Hegermann-Nielsen, G. (1978) *Drug. Dev. Ind. Pharm.* 4, 53–67.

Brossard, C. & Lefort des Ylouses, D. (1984) *Labo-Pharma Probl. Tech.* 32, 857–871.

Chambliss, W.G. (1983) *Pharm. Tech.* 8 (9) 124, 126, 128, 130,132, 138, 140.

Chambliss, W.G., Chambliss, D.A., Cleary, R.W., Jones, A.B., Harland, E.C. & Kibbe, A.H. (1984) *J. Pharm. Sci.* 73, 1215–1219.

Chang, R.K. (1990) *Pharm. Tech.* (10), 62–70.

Chatfield, H.W. (1962) In *The science of surface coatings.* Van Nostrand, New York.

Coletta, V. & Rubin, H. (1964) *J. Pharm. Sci.* 53, 953–955.

Davis, M., Ichikawa, I., Williams, E.J. & Banker, G.S. (1986) *Int. J. Pharm.* 28, 157–166.

Dechesne, J.P., Delporte, J.P., Jaminet, F. & Venturas, K. (1982) *J. Pharm. Belg.* 37, 283–286.

Delporte, J.P. & Jaminet, F. (1976) *J. Pharm. Belg.* 31, 38–50.

Deshpande, S.G. & Dongre, S.A. (1987) *Indian J. Pharm. Sci.* 49, 81–84.

Ghebre-Sellassie, I., Gordon, R.H., Nesbitt, R.U. & Fawzi, M.B. (1987) *Int. J. Pharm.* 37, 211–218.

Ghebre-Sellassie, I., Iyer, U., Kubert, D. & Fawzi, M.B. (1988) *Pharm. Tech.* (9), 96–106.

Goodhart, F.W., Harris, M.R., Murthy, K.S. & Nesbitt, R.U. (1984) *Pharm. Tech.* 8(4), 64–71.

Healey, J.N.C. (1989) in *Drug delivery to the gastrointestinal tract* (eds Hardy, J.G., Davis, S.S. & Wilson, C.G.), Ellis Horwood, 83–96.

Hoblitzell, J.R., Thakker, K.D. & Rhodes, C.T. (1985) *Pharm. Acta. Helv.* 60, 28–32.

Iyer, U., Hong, W-H., Das, N. & Ghebre-Sellassie, I. (1990) *Pharm. Tech.* (9), 68–86.

Kallstrand, G. & Ekman, B. (1983) *J. Pharm. Sci.* 72, 772–775.

Lehmann, K. (1984) *Acta Pharm. Fenn.*, **93**, 55–74.

Lehmann, K. (1989) in *Aqueous polymeric coatings for pharmaceutical dosage forms* (ed. McGinity, J.W.), Marcel Dekker, New York, 153–247.

Lehmann, K. (1986) *Acta Pharm. Tech.* **32**, 146–152.

Li, S.P., Gunvent, N.M., Buehler, J.D., Grim, W.M. & Harwood, R.J. (1988) *Drug Dev. Ind. Pharm.* **14**, 573-585.

Li, S.P., Jhawar, R., Metha, G.N., Harwood, R.J. & Grim, W.M. (1989) *Drug Dev. Ind. Pharm.* **15**, 1231–1242.

Li, S.P., Feld, K.M. & Kowarski, C.R. (1991) *Drug Dev. Ind. Pharm.* **17**, 1655–1683.

Lindholm, T. & Juslin, M. (1982) *Pharm. Ind.* **44**, 937–941.

Lippold, B.C., Lippold, B.H., Sutter, B. & Gunder, W. (1990) *Drug Dev. Ind. Pharm.* **16**, 1725–1747.

Metha, A.M. (1986) *Pharm. Manuf.*, Jan.

Miller, R.A. & Vadas, E.B. (1984) *Drug Dev. Ind. Pharm.* **10**, 1565–1585.

Nesbitt, R.U., Goodhart, F.W. & Gordon, R.H. (1985) *Int. J. Pharm.* **26**, 215–216.

Ozturk, S.S., Palsson, B.O., Donohoe, B. & Dressman, J.B. (1988) *Pharm. Res.* **5**, 550–565.

Porter, S.C. & D'Andrea, L.F (1985) *Proc. 12th Int. Symp. Controlled Release of Bioactive Materials, Geneva.*

Porter, S.C. (1989) *Drug Dev. Ind. Pharm.* **15**, 1495–1521.

Porter, S.C. & Ridgway, K. (1982) *J. Pharm. Pharmacol.* **34**, 5–8.

Ritschel, W.A. (1980) In *Handbook of basic pharmacokinetics* (2nd edn), Drug Intelligence Publications, 71.

Rowe, R.C. (1985) *Pharm. Int.* Jan., 14–17.

Rowe, R.C. (1986) *Int. J. Pharm.* **29**, 37–41.

Sakellariou, P., Rowe, R.C. & White, E.F.T. (1987) *J. Appl. Polym. Sci.*, **34**, 2507–2516.

Schroeter, L.C. (1965) In *Remington's pharmaceutical sciences* (13th edn), Mack Pub. Co.

Shah, N.B. & Sheth, B.B. (1972) *J. Pharm. Sci.* **61**, 412–416.

Sinko, C.M., Yee, A.F. & Amidon, G.L. (1990) *Pharm. Res.* **7**, 648–653.

Stafford, J.W. (1982) *Drug Dev. Ind. Pharm.* **8**, 513–530.

Thoma, K. & Heckenmuller, H. (1986) *Pharmazie* **41**, 328–332.

Thoma, K. and Heckenmuller, H. & Oschmann, R. (1987) *Pharmazie* **42**, 832–836.

Wagner, J.G. (1971) In *Biopharmaceutics and relevant pharmacokinetics*, Drug Intelligence Publications, 158–165.

Wald, R.J., Saddler, S.L. & Amidon, G.F. (1988) *Pharm. Res. (Suppl.)* **5** (10), 5, 115.

Wouessidjewe, D., Brossard, C., Goujon, J.J. & Puisieux, F. (1983) *APGI Congress Proc.*, IV, Paris, 81–89.

Zhang, G., Schwartz, J.B. & Schnaare, R.L. (1988) *Proc. 15th Int. Symp. Controlled Release of Bioactive Materials, Basel.*

Zhang, G., Schwartz, J.B. & Schnaare, R.L. (1989) *Proc. 16th Int. Symp. Controlled Release of Bioactive Materials, Chicago.*

Zhang, G., Schwartz, J.B. & Schnaare, R.L. (1991) *Pharm. Res.* **8**, 331–335.

15

Some common practical questions and suggested answers

During the development of coating formulae and processes, common problems tend to recur. This section brings together a collection of typical queries and provides suggested solutions.

1. **Question:** What major process and formulation parameters do I need to take into account in the change from organic solvent coating to aqueous coating?

    Answer: Looking first of all at the formulation-based parameters, there is a need to increase the solids loading of the coating suspension to something like 12 %w/w if using a typical HPMC-based formula. Maximizing solids will usefully minimize the water content of the suspension but excessively viscous suspension will be difficult to spray. Commonly, organic solvent-based formulae normally contain HPMC viscosity grades of 15 mPa s or even higher. These should be substituted by lower viscosity types such as 5 mPa s. Ethylcellulose is used frequently in organic solvent-based formulae and, of course, will in its simplest form have to be omitted from a totally aqueous formula due to its insolubility. However, use of aqueous dispersions of ethylcellulose (Surelease, Aquacoat) are recommended if a water-insoluble functional coat is required.

    Regarding the tablet core formula, this needs to be more robust to take into account the rather longer spraying times which may be necessary with water-based spraying. Moisture-sensitive actives are not necessarily a problem in a well-controlled process.

    The obvious difficulty from a processing point of view is that water, a liquid with a relatively higher latent heat of evaporation, has to be removed from the process. This necessitates higher process temperatures, additional quantities of drying air and generally lower rates of spray application. The initial application of spray demands extra caution as, unlike organic solvent-based spraying, the core cannot be protected by the initial application of a relatively large quantity of spray material.

As a consequence of changing from organic solvent-based systems to aqueous-based processing, the following phenomena may also be observed.

- A decrease in adhesion of the film for the core. This may be remedied by a formula modification, as described in Chapter 13.
- The coated tablets have a distinctly matt appearance compared with organic solvent-based processing.
- Shade changes, compared with the organic solvent-based process may be observed even when utilizing the same pigments.

2. **Question:** Do I need to stir a coating suspension and for how long can I keep it?
   Answer: A well-milled suspension or a good-quality commercial coating system will need relatively little stirring. However, with formulations containing large quantities of iron oxides and/or talc, stirring should be more or less continuous, especially with talc as a constituent. Cellulosic systems in organic solvents, because of their relatively lower viscosity, will generally settle out more quickly than corresponding aqueous systems.

   Many aqueous-based coating formulae are susceptible to microbial growth. Large quantities of polymer solution made up for incorporation into batches of final coating suspension will need to be preserved. Commercial coating systems can be constituted in small quantities minimizing waste at the end of the processing period and the consequential need to store and preserve suspension. Unpreserved coating suspensions should be discarded at the end of a working shift and certainly within 12 h of make-up to prevent undue microbial growth.

   Note that foam generation either from reconstitution of a commercial system or from milling of an 'in house' mixture should be minimized. Unfortunately foam on coating suspensions is very stable and difficult to remove. Excessive aeration makes for difficult handling of the suspension.

3. **Question:** What quality of water should I be using?
   Answer: Compendial purified water should be used for making coating suspensions of aqueous systems.

4. **Question:** When do I need to add a plasticizer to a coating formula?
   Answer: Generally plasticizers are added to coating formulae to make them more universally applicable and to avoid potential coating problems, e.g. cracking, poor adhesion. Some acrylic systems do not need a plasticizer, e.g. NE30D, due to the specialized nature of the polymer used in this latex preparation.

   For many cellulosic systems, water is a plasticizer but reliance on it is not recommended as it is not permanent within the film and can give rise to problems on storage.

5. **Question:** Are there any detrimental effects caused by using high pigment concentrations?
Answer: Excessively high pigment levels can give rise to brittle films which are rather rough in appearance. However, if moisture vapour permeation is a problem then increasing pigment content slightly will usually be advantageous, but excessive quantities may actually increase permeation through destruction of the integrity of the film. It should be noted that the deleterious effect of pigments, can to some extent, be overcome by the use of good-quality small particle size pigments.

6. **Question:** What is the effect of restrictions in the use of certain organic solvents?
Answer: Legislation in many parts of the world, with environmental and worker protection considerations in mind, has the effect of removing certain solvents from use as process solvents. Frequently, these measures involve chlorinated hydrocarbons which are used as cosolvents with alcohols in solubilizing cellulose ethers.

Obviously consequential changes for the future would be:

● a move to aqueous spraying;
● a move to totally enclosed coating processes with solvent recovery system;
● a move to polymers with different solubility requirements, e.g. the acrylates.

7. **Question:** What problems are there for coating moisture-sensitive tablets or tablets containing water-soluble materials?
Answer: First, attention should be given to the drying conditions in terms of air temperature and quantity. For aqueous processing both of these should be high. As an example, in a Model 120 Accelacota an inlet temperature of 75–80°C coupled with an air volume of 56–60 m^3/min and a low spray rate should be used. With an aqueous system, maximize the solids content to above 12 %w/w if possible so that a low water content is used. The intrinsic permeability of the film should be determined experimentally for a moisture-sensitive core. Adjust pigment and plasticizer levels to minimize moisture vapour transmission.

For particularly troublesome cores, consider a change to non-aqueous coating if this is feasible.

8. **Question:** How do I cure logo bridging on an existing tablet design?
Answer: The aim here should be to increase contact between the tablet core and the film; perhaps the most effective way of doing this is to reduce the internal stress in the film itself. The measures detailed in Chapter 13 should be consulted for appropriate remedial action.

9. **Question:** How can I design the tablet core to avoid logo bridging?
Answer: Bridging of logos can be avoided at the punch logo design stage by paying attention to the angles of cut width and finer points of design. When ordering such tooling, it is imperative to inform the tooling manufacturer that

the tablets will be film coated. Reputable manufacturers have a great deal of experience to offer in this direction and should always be consulted prior to purchase.

10. **Question:** How do I assess tablet core quality for film coating?
Answer: The fundamental point here is that the tablet core should be designed with film coating in prospect. Marginal core quality in terms of capping incidence will never be improved by film coating; it will only serve to make such deficiencies more obvious.

It is difficult to be precise about the normally measured parameters such as diametral crushing strength (DCS) as, to a certain extent, the minimum quantitative values will depend on the coating equipment, its rotational speed or the volume of fluidizing air.

As an example, a normal convex circular tablet 10 mm diameter should have a friability of less than 0.5% and a DCS of at least 100–120 N. Smaller diameter tablets can be allowed to have correspondingly lower DCSs.

11. **Question:** What are the factors to be considered when designing a tablet for coating in terms of size and shape?
Answer: In many ways the circular biconvex tablet is an easy shape to film coat. A number of departures from this should be carefully assessed for their coating efficiency:

- Flat tablet or parallel sided tablets with a deep edge. These will provide flat adherent surfaces which give rise to 'multiple' tablets during the coating process.
- Sharp edges or angular tablets. The apexes of these points will be mechanically weak and especially so if slightly overwetted during an aqueous-based process.
- Inappropriate shaped logos and logos on the crown of the tablet. The crown of the tablet is the area on the tablet face with the least surface hardness yet is exposed to some of the most intensive abrasive forces in the coating process. Ideally the logo should be around the circumference and not on the crown.

It should also be appreciated that the packing density of small tablets is going to be greater than for large tablets. This has the effect that a bed composed of relatively small tablets (and especially pellets) is more resistant to air flow than would occur with large tablets.

12. **Question:** Can I film coat in a conventional pan?
Answer: It must be appreciated that heat and mass transfer in a conventional pan is inherently poor, thus making such equipment a non-ideal choice, especially for aqueous processing.

However, processing is possible under the following conditions. First, the cores should be robust as the process will be lengthy compared with that in a more appropriate piece of equipment. Especially in small pans (about 1 m diameter) there is a certain amount of equipment congestion; air spray gun(s), inlet air duct and exhaust ducts have to be fitted into a small space. Spray 'bounce' tends to make the process messy but an option during solvent-based spraying (if permissible) is to utilize airless atomizing equipment.

Without drying air being able to be drawn completely through the tablet bed, debris from the coating will collect in the pan and may affect the final appearance of the tablets.

13. **Question:** How many spray-guns do I need and what spray shape should I aim for?

Answer: Regarding spray shape, this should be adjusted so that a wide, flattened cone of spray is obtained. However, if very smoothly coated tablets are desired regardless of other factors, then an unmodified cone, as described in Chapter 5, could provide the required results.

With larger equipment there is a general feeling that a gain in quality of coating will result if the spray is spread out between a number of guns, as opposed to being confined through one gun. This is practised to counteract the fall-off in intensity of spray from the centre point of the flattened cone to the edge.

As a guide, in a Manesty 120 Accelacota use four guns, and in a Model 360 use six guns. The use of a multiple gun set-up does impose the need to balance the liquid spray rate evenly between the guns. Overlap should be minimized as this will give rise to localized overwetting. Obviously, avoid spray reaching parts other than the tablet bed.

14. **Question:** What is the best location for the spray-gun in the pan?

Answer: As a general rule in a side-vented pan, the spray should be aimed at the tablet cascade, about a third of the way down the tablet bed. Absolute gun-to-bed distances will be optimized by trial and error but the configuration suggested by the existing placement of fittings should be regarded as a satisfactory starting point.

It should be remembered, especially with large-scale equipment, that increasing the gun-to-bed distance will increase the tendency to spray drying and vice versa on decreasing the distance. This latter action will, of course, lead to a smoother coated surface utilizing the controlled tendency to overwet the tablet bed.

15. **Question:** What spray-gun type should I use?

Answer: One should aim for a purpose-built pharmaceutical spray-gun. These have been made with GMP considerations in mind regarding materials of construction and ease of cleaning. They are generally easier to dismantle than spray-guns from other industries and do not require hand tools for this operation.

16. **Question:** What are the advantages of using liquid delivery by peristaltic pump over the use of a pressure pot?

Answer: Peristaltic pumps give a finer control of liquid flow rate and permit easier stirring of the suspension. They are also, in general, smaller and more self-contained compared with pressurized vessels.

17. **Question:** What pan speed should I be aiming for?
Answer: In some ways pan speed is a compromise between adequate tablet bed mixing and considerations of abrasion of the tablet cores. All manufacturers will give pan speed suggestions for various loadings but occasionally this will have to be modified for a particular need. An example would be a tablet core where edge attrition could be prevented by slowing the pan. This measure can often be helped by increasing spray rate, if that is possible.

18. **Question:** What are the advantages of an airborne over an airless spray?
Answer: Basically an airless spray atomizes a liquid stream by the use of a high hydrostatic pressure through a small orifice nozzle. Its benefits include lack of 'spray bounce'. However, its relatively high throughput and lack of droplet size control make it generally unsuitable for aqueous-based spraying. It also blocks easily. Here the versatility of the airborne spray, where droplet characteristics are more independent of spray rate considerations, is more appropriate with aqueous spraying.

19. **Question:** What can I do about poor mixing in my tablet-coating pan?
Answer: Apart from suspicions arising from observations of the tablets revolving in a pan, this will be apparent from variable colour coverage if a coloured coating is being used. It will also be apparent from intra-batch variability in performance observed with a functional coating.

The tablet bed should flow evenly. Underloading or overloading a pan will cause poor tablet bed rotation and poor mixing.

It is also worth while with old equipment to check the manufacturer's latest recommendation as improvements are often introduced periodically with new models.

Some high solids coating compositions are capable of being applied very rapidly, occasionally so quickly as to 'run ahead' of the mixing ability of the pan. Under these conditions, when coating times are crucial, the mixing ability of the pan must be upgraded with the assistance of the equipment manufacturer.

20. **Question:** How do I know that I have achieved the correct rate of application?
Answer: Within a given set of drying conditions, the 'correct' rate of application will be the one which neither causes overwetting on one hand, nor spray drying on the other. This simplistic picture may be explained further. An excessive spray application rate will be marked by tablet picking and possibly by adherence of tablets to the pan. Spray drying is characterized by an excessively 'dusty' coating process where the window or sight glass is obscured by powder deposits. Any horizontal surfaces such as the gun supports will also tend to collect powder under these conditions.

21. **Question:** Should I expect repeated nozzle blockage with aqueous spray procedures?

Answer: Repeated nozzle blockage should not happen during a coating run. The following should be investigated if this occurs:

- *Coating suspension.* Poorly dispersed pigment agglomerates are a common cause. Also the polymer itself may not have been subject to adequate dispersion to fully solubilize it. When using a commercial latex or pseudolatex dispersion, it should be confirmed that coagulation of the coating suspension is not taking place for some reason. Common causes are excessive temperature (both processing and suspension temperature) and unsuitable additives to the formula, causing polymer coagulation.
- *Process consideration.* The atomizing air pressure may be too low. Alternatively, nozzle blockage may be exacerbated by an unnecessarily small nozzle. A diameter of 1 mm is typical for a standard aqueous process.

22. **Question:** How can film-coated tablets be polished?
    Answer: It is quite feasible to polish film-coated tablets. However, it is also advisable to consider whether this is really necessary. An aqueously coated tablet may appear matt compared with an organic solvent-coated tablet or even a sugar-coated tablet, but nonetheless the final appearance can be aesthetically pleasing.

    On the other hand, if 'house' requirements or marketing dictate a polished appearance, then there are many possibilities. The following should be taken into consideration:

- Acrylic polymer formulations are usually inherently quite shiny but the smoothness of cellulosic systems can be enhanced by a final application of spray suspension without the pigment.
- Attention to process conditions is nearly always capable of producing improvements. Spray conditions should be 'wet' with a relatively low bed temperature and a higher rate of spray than normal. Extreme caution should be exercised in the initial validation of those conditions as they are conducive to overwetting.
- Generally it is possible to use the waxes, polishes and glazes normally utilized for sugar-coated tablets. Nowadays totally aqueous polish mixes are commercially available. Another effective method is to use an aqueous solution of a high molecular weight—PEG, e.g. 20000 grade—sprayed on at the completion of coating. The use of dry carnauba wax added to the completed batch of tablets in a cylindrical pan and rolled for a period until shine develops is also an effective method.

    Should a lustrous appearance be required, the use of talc in the coating formula should be considered. Sometimes, polishing may be completed in the same pan utilized for coating, providing it is not too contaminated with dried spray. The shape of the tablet bed and the change in noise emitted from the pan can be used as indicators as to when polish and shine has been imparted onto the tablets.

23. Question: How can I cure variable dissolution results with controlled release coatings?

Answer: Assuming that the dissolution methodology and analytical testing are satisfactory, the process should be examined with regard to the following features:

- Is the pan design and product loading appropriate to enable sufficient mixing to take place?
- Is the process constant and optimal regarding overwetting or spray drying of coating material?
- Has sufficient coating been applied?
- In particular with an aqueous dispersed commercial coating for modified release, have the manufacturer's recommendations regarding processing been followed?

The coating formula should be examined to see if it is appropriate for the task, e.g. ethylcellulose will not give an enteric effect. Is the quality of the materials adequate?

If changes in dissolution performance of, for instance, modified release coated beads alters on storage then the coating itself is 'maturing' or possibly there are interactions between the coat and the core material (see Chapters 2 and 14 for explanation and remedial action).

24. Question: How can I cure metallic marks on white-coated tablets?

Answer: This is a problem most often seen with new pans and is especially noticeable with white or pale-coloured tablets. First, the pan should be thoroughly cleaned. If necessary a thin application of spray material to the pan itself will cure the problem. Ensuring that unduly dry spray conditions are not used will also aid the resolution of the problem.

25. Question: How can I optimize the smoothness of a film coating?

Answer: Occasionally smoothness and elegance of a film coating is of paramount importance over other factors such as speed of operation and batch throughput. The viscosity of the coating suspension has a major part to play since, generally, smoother coatings result from low-viscosity suspensions/solutions. Chapter 4 should be consulted in detail where recommendations are made on certain types of spray-gun, which can also be a contributing factor to the overall effect. Other process parameters of importance are:

- reduction of the gun-to-bed distance
- increase in atomizing air pressure
- use of an unmodified spray cone.

These measures will combine to produce a 'controlled overwetting'.

16

Bibliography

Michael E. Aulton

A PHARMACEUTICAL FILM COATING PUBLICATIONS BIBLIOGRAPHY

This chapter contains a comprehensive listing of research papers, reviews, book chapters and theses covering the subject of pharmaceutical film coating. Coating is a very extensive subject and so this bibliography is restricted to those publications of direct pharmaceutical relevance or authorship. Non-pharmaceutical polymer science or coating processes of other industries are not included.

While the listing is extensive, it is by no means exhaustive. Indeed, the author would welcome notification of any missing articles in order that this work can be included in the next edition. Similarly, notification of any errors in these listings would be welcomed.

For convenience, the published work is categorized into the following subjects; some papers fall into more than one category.

- General
- Film-coating materials (polymers, additives, formulation—including solutions and suspension properties)
- Physicochemical properties of coating systems (including interactions of polymers and additives, and thermomechanical properties)
- Coating processes
- Wetting and adhesion
- Mechanical properties
- Quality of coats (including defects, gloss, surface roughness and colour)
- Permeability (to gases and water vapour)
- Drug release characteristics
- Stability
- Miscellaneous pharmaceutical coating publications: Bioadhesion; Coating of hard gelatin capsules.

General

Banker, G.S. (1966) Film coating theory and practice. *J. Pharm. Sci.* **55(1)**, 81–89.

Banker, G.S., Peck, G., Jan, S., Pirakitikulr, P. & Taylor, D. (1981) Evaluation of hydroxypropyl cellulose and hydroxypropyl methyl cellulose as aqueous based film coatings. *Drug Dev. Ind. Pharm.* **7(6)**, 693–716.

Ellis, J.R., Prillig, E.B. & Endicott, C.J. (1970) Tablet coating. In Lachman, L. (ed.), *The theory and practice of industrial pharmacy*, Lea and Fabinger, Philadelphia, PA, USA, chap. 10, 197–225.

Hogan, J.E. (1978) Aqueous cellulosic film coating of tablets. *J. Pharm. Pharmacol.* **30** Suppl., 88P.

Hogan, J.E. (1988) Tablet coating. In *Pharmaceutics: the science of dosage form design* (ed. Aulton, M.E.), Churchill-Livingstone, Edinburgh.

McGinity, J.W. (ed.) (1989) *Aqueous polymeric coatings for pharmaceutical dosage forms*, Marcel Dekker, New York, 424pp.

Onions, A. (1986) Films from water-based colloidal dispersions. *Manuf. Chem.* **57(3)**, 55–59.

Onions, A. (1986) Films from water-based colloidal dispersions. *Manuf. Chem.* **57(4)**, 66–67.

Pickard, J.F. & Rees, J.E. (1972) Modern trends in pharmaceutical coating. *Pharm. Ind.* **34(11)**, 833–839.

Pickard, J.F. & Rees, J.E. (1974) Film coating: 1 Formulation and process considerations in film coating. *Manuf. Chem.* **54(4)**, 19–22.

Porter, S.C. (1978) Aqueous film coating: an overview. *Pharm. Technol.* **3(9)**, 55–59.

Porter, S.C. (1981) Tablet coating I. *Drug Cosmet. Ind.* **129(5)**, 46–53, 86–93.

Porter, S.C. (1981) Tablet coating II. *Drug Cosmet. Ind.* **129**.

Porter, S.C. (1981) Tablet coating III. *Drug Cosmet. Ind.* **129(8)**, 40–44, 87–88.

Porter, S.C. (1981) Tablet coating IV. *Drug Cosmet. Ind.* **129(9)**, 50–58.

Porter, S.C. & Hogan, J.E. (1984) Tablet film-coating. *Pharm. Int.* **5(5)**, 122–127.

Tondachi, M., Hoshi, N. & Sekigawa, F. (1977) Tablet coating in an aqueous system. *Drug Dev. Ind. Pharm.* **3(3)**, 227–240.

Film coating materials (polymers, additives, formulation—including solutions and suspension properties)

Banker, G.S. & Peck, G.E. (1981) The new, water-based colloidal dispersions. *Pharm. Technol.* **5(4)**.

Banker, G.S., Peck, G.E., Jan, S., Pirakitikulr, P. & Taylor, D. (1981) Evaluation of hydroxypropyl cellulose and hydroxypropyl methyl cellulose as aqueous based film coatings. *Drug Dev. Ind. Pharm.* **7(6)**, 693–716.

Banker, G.S., Peck, G.E., Williams, E., Taylor, D. & Pirakitikulr, P. (1982) Microbiological considerations of polymer solutions used in aqueous film coating. *Drug Dev. Ind. Pharm.* **8(1)**, 41–51.

Benita, S. (1987) Cellulose hydrogen phthalate. A coating polymer in controlled release dosage forms. *Pharm. Acta Helv.* **62**, 255–261.

Bergisadi, N. (1986) Two new derivatives of alginic acid for tablet coating. *S.T.P. Pharma* **2(18)**, 620–622.

Bindschaedler, C., Gurny, R. & Doelker, E. (1983) Notions theoriques sur la formation des films obtenus a partir de microdispersions aqueuses et application a l'enrobage. *Labo-Pharma Probl. Tech.* **31(331)**, 389–394.

Bodmeier, R. & Paeratakul, O. (1989) Evaluation of drug-containing polymer films prepared from aqueous latexes. *Pharm. Res.* **6(8)**, 725–730.

Chang, R.-K. (1990) Preparation and evaluation of shellac pseudolatex as an aqueous enteric coating system for pellets. *Int. J. Pharmaceut.* **60**, 171–173.

Chang, R.-K. (1990) A comparison of rheological and enteric properties among organic solutions, ammonium salt aqueous solutions and latex systems. *Pharm. Technol.* **14(10)**, 62–70.

Chopra, S.K. & Tawashi, R. (1982) Tack behavior of coating solutions I. *J. Pharm. Sci.*,**71(8)**, 907–911.

Chopra, S.K. & Tawashi, R. (1984) Tack behavior of coating solutions II. *J. Pharm. Sci.* **73(4)**, 477–481.

Chopra, S.K & Tawashi, R. (1985) Tack behavior of coating solutions III. *J. Pharm. Sci.* **74(7)**, 746–749.

Delonca, H. (1989) Étude de films à base d'hydroxypropylméthylcellulose phtalate (HP55). I: Films isolés. *J. Pharm. Belg.* **44**, 17–35.

Delonca, H. (1989) Étude de films à base d'hydroxypropylméthylcellulose phtalate (HP55). II: Films appliqués. *J. Pharm. Belg.* **44**, 101–108.

Eskilsson, C., Appelgren, C. & Bogentoft, C. (1976) A note on the properties of ethylcellulose–propylene glycol membranes. *Acta Pharm. Suec.* **13**, 285–288.

Gumowski, F., Doelker, E. & Gurny, R. (1987) The use of a new redispersible aqueous enteric coating material. *Pharm. Technol.* **11**, 26–32.

Hogan, J.E. (1983) Additive effects on aqueous film coatings. *Manuf. Chem.* **54(4)**, 43–47.

Joachim, J. (1990) Études comparative de deux filmogènes: acétophtalate de cellulose et l'Aquatéric. *Pharm. Acta Helv.* **65**, 311–314.

Kanig, J.L. & Goodman, H. (1962) Evaluative procedures for film-forming materials used in pharmaceutical applications. *J. Pharm. Sci.* **51**, 77–82.

Kent, D.J. & Rowe, R.C. (1978) Solubility studies on ethyl cellulose used in film coating. *J. Pharm. Pharmacol.* **30**, 808–810.

Kovács, B. & Merényi, G. (1990) Evaluation of tack behaviour of coating solutions. *Drug Dev. Ind. Pharm.* **16(15)**, 2303–2323.

Kumar, V. & Banker, G.S. (1993) Chemically-modified cellulosic polymers. *Drug Dev. Ind. Pharm.* **19(1 and 2)**, 1–31.

Lehmann, K. (1986) Mischbarkheit wässriger Poly(meth)acrylat-Dispersionen für Arzneimittelüberzüge. *Pharm. Ind.* **48**, 1182–1183.

Lehmann, K. (1989) Chemistry and application properties of polymethacrylate coating systems. In McGinity, J.W. (ed.), *Aqueous polymeric coatings for pharmaceutical dosage forms*, Marcel Dekker, New York, 153–245.

Lejeune, B. (1987) Emploi du rouge de betterave pour la coloration de comprimés pelliculés. *S.T.P. Pharma.* **3**, 400–406.

Lindholm, T. (1982) Controlled release tablets. Part 3: Ethylcellulose coats containing surfactant and powdered matter. *Pharm. Ind.* **44**, 937–941.

Lindholm, T., Huhtikangas, A. & Saarikivi, P. (1984) Organic solvent residues in free ethyl cellulose films. *Int. J. Pharmaceut.* **21**, 119–121.

Munden, B.J., DeKay, H.G. & Banker, G.S. (1964) Evaluation of polymeric materials I: Screening of selected polymers as film coating agents. *J. Pharm. Sci.* **53**, 395–401.

Okor, R.S. (1982) Influence of hydrophilic character of plasticizer and polymer on certain film properties. *Int. J. Pharmaceut.* **11**, 1–9.

Okor, R.S. (1991) Thixotropic phenomenon in flocculated aqueous dispersions of acrylate methacrylate copolymers. *J. Pharm. Pharmacol.* **43**, 198–200.

Opota, O. (1988) Comportement rhéologique des solutions aqueuses d'hydroxy-propylcellulose. Influence de la concentration et de la masse moléculaire. *Pharm. Acta Helv.* **63**, 26–32.

Osterwald, H.P. (1982) Wirkungsweise und Optimierungsmöglichkeiten der Anwendung von Weichmachern in Filmüberzügen. *Acta Pharm. Technol.* **28**, 34–43.

Osterwald, H.P. (1985) Properties of film-formers and their use in aqueous systems. *Pharm. Res.* **2(1)**, 14–18.

Pathak, Y.V. (1985) Study of rosin and rosin esters as coating materials. *Int. J. Pharmaceut.* **24**, 351–354.

Pillai, J.C., Babar, A. & Plakogiannis, F.M. (1988) Polymers in cosmetic and pharmaceutical industries. *Pharm. Acta Helv.* **63(2)**, 46–53.

Plaizer-Vercammen, J.A. (1991) Evaluation of aqueous dispersions of Eudragit L100–55 for their enteric coating properties. *S.T.P. Pharma Sci.* **1**, 267–271.

Porter, S.C. (1980) The effect of additives on the properties of an aqueous film coating. *Pharm. Technol.* **4(3)**, 66–75.

Prillig, E.B. (1969) Effect of colorants on the solubility of modified cellulose polymers. *J. Pharm. Sci.* **50(10)**, 1245–1249.

Reiland, T.L. & Eber, A.C. (1986) Aqueous gloss solutions: formula and process variables effects on the surface texture of film coated tablets. *Drug Dev. Ind. Pharm.* **12(3)**, 231–245.

Rosoff, M. & Sheen, P.C. (1983) Abrasion and polymorphism of titanium dioxide in coating suspensions. *J. Pharm. Sci.* **72(12)**, 1485.

Rowe, R.C. (1980) The molecular weight and molecular weight distribution of hydroxypropyl methylcellulose used in film coating of tablets. *J. Pharm. Pharmacol.* **32**, 116–119.

Rowe, R.C. (1982) Molecular weight studies on ethyl cellulose used in film coating. *Acta Pharm. Suec.* **19**, 157–160.

Rowe, R.C. (1982) Molecular weight studies on hydroxypropyl methylcellulose phthalate (HP55) *Acta Pharm. Technol.* **28(2)**, 127–130.

Rowe, R.C. (1982) Some fundamental properties of polymeric materials and their application in film coating formulations—a review. *Int. J. Pharm. Tech. Prod. Mfr* **3(1)**, 3–8.

Rowe, R.C. (1983) The orientation and alignment of particles in tablet film coatings. *J. Pharm. Pharmacol.* **35**, 43–44.

Rowe, R.C. (1984) Materials used in the film coating of oral dosage forms. In

Florence, A.T. (ed.), *Materials used in pharmaceutical formulation. Critical Reports in Applied Chemistry* **6**, 1–36.

Rowe, R.C. (1988) Characterisation of the structure of filled polymer film coating using ion beam etching. *Int. J. Pharmaceut.* **47**, 205–208.

Rowe, R.C. (1992) Molecular weight dependence of the properties of ethyl cellulose and hydroxypropyl methylcellulose films. *Int. J. Pharmaceut.* **88**, 405–408.

Rowe, R.C. & Forse, S.F. (1983) The refractive indices of polymer film formers, pigments and additives used in tablet film coating: their significance and practical application. *J. Pharm. Pharmacol.* **35**, 205–207.

Spitael, J. & Kinget, R. (1980) Influence of solvent composition upon film-coating. *Pharm. Acta Helv.* **55**, 157–160.

Tardieu, M. (1992) Étude comparative de dispersions aqueuses de polymerès gastrorésistants entérosolubles. *Pharm. Acta Helv.* **67**, 29–32.

Thoennes, C.J. & McCurdy, V.E. (1989) Evaluation of a rapidly disintegrating, moisture resistant lacquer film coating. *Drug Dev. Ind. Pharm.* **15(2)**, 165–185.

Utsumi, I., Ida, T., Takahashi, S. & Sugimoto, N. (1961) Studies on protective coatings IX: polyvinylpyridine derivatives. *J. Pharm. Sci.* **50**, 592–597.

Venkateswarlu, V., Kokate, C.K., Rambhau, D. & Veeresham, C. (1993) Pharmaceutical investigations of a film forming material isolated from roots of *salacia macrosperma*. *Drug Dev. Ind. Pharm.* **19(4)**, 461–472.

Wan, L.S.C. (1991) A simple method to assess the tack of coating formulations. *S.T.P. Pharma* **2**, 174–180.

Wan, L.S.C. (1991) An application of tack measurement to fluidized bed coating. *S.T.P. Pharma* **2**, 404–410.

Physicochemical properties of coating systems (including interactions of polymers and additives, and thermomechanical properties)

Arwidsson, H. & Johansson, B. (1991) Application of intrinsic viscosity and interaction constant as a formulation tool for film coating. III: Mechanical studies on free ethylcellulose films cast from organic solvents. *Int. J. Pharmaceut.* **76**, 91–97.

Arwidsson, H. & Nicklasson, M. (1989) Application of intrinsic viscosity and interaction constant as a formulation tool for film coating. I. Studies on ethyl cellulose 10cps in organic solvents. *Int. J. Pharmaceut.* **56**, 187–193.

Arwidsson, H. & Nicklasson, M. (1990) Application of intrinsic viscosity and interaction constant as a formulation tool for film coating. II. Studies on different grades of ethyl cellulose in organic solvent systems. *Int. J. Pharmaceut.* **58**, 73–77.

Aulton, M.E., Houghton, R.J. & Wells, J.I. (1985) Compatibility of polymeric binders and potential plasticisers. *J. Pharm. Pharmacol.* **37**, 113P.

Bommel, E.M.G.van, Fokkens, J.G. & Crommelin, D.J.A. (1989) Effects of additives on the physico-chemical properties of sprayed ethylcellulose films. *Acta Pharm. Technol.* **35(4)**, 232–237.

Davies, M.C., Wilding, I.R., Short, R.D., Khan, M.A. Watts, J.F. & Melia, C.D. (1989) An analysis of the surface chemical structure of polymethacrylate (Eudragit) film coating polymers by XPS. *Int. J. Pharmaceut.* **57**, 183–187.

Davies, M.C., Wilding, I.R., Short, R.D., Melia, C.D. & Rowe, R.C. (1990) The *in situ* chemical analysis of polymer film coatings using static secondary ion mass spectrometry (SSIMS) *Int. J. Pharmaceut.* **62**, 97–103.

Dechesne, J.P. (1984) Influence des plastifiants sur la temperature de transition vitreuse de filmogenes gastrorésistants entérosolubles. *J. Pharm. Belg.* **39**, 341–347.

Delporte, J.P. (1979) Effects of ageing on physico-chemical properties of free cellulose acetate phthalate films. *Pharm. Ind.* **41(10)**, 984–990.

Devereux, C. (1988) Physicochemical properties of some methacrylate polymer films prepared from aqueous dispersions. M.Phil. Thesis, University of Bradford.

Dittgen, M. & Jensch, H.-P. (1988) Influence of the physico-chemical properties of the drug on its release from acrylic films. *Acta Pharm. Jugosl.* **38**, 315–320.

Gibson, S.H.M., Rowe, R.C. & White, E.F.T. (1988) Characterisation of the structure of filled polymer film coatings using ion beam etching. *Int. J. Pharmaceut.* **47**, 205–208.

Gibson, S.H.M., Rowe, R.C. & White, E.F.T. (1988) Quantitative assessment of additive–polymer interaction in pigmented hydroxypropyl methylcellulose formulations using immersion calorimetry. *Int. J. Pharmaceut.* **48**, 113–117.

Humeke-Bogner, R., Liu, J.-C. & Chien, Y.W. (1988) Methods for determining partial solubility parameters of potential film-coating polymers. *Int. J. Pharmaceut.* **42**, 199–209.

Jacobsson, S. & Hagman, A. (1990) Characterization of polymers used as pharmaceutical excipients by dynamic headspace gas chromatography-mass spectrometry. *Drug Dev. Ind. Pharm.* **16(17)**, 2547–2560.

Jenquin, M.R., Leibowitz, S.M., Sarabia, R.E. & McGinity, J.W. (1990) Physical and chemical factors influencing the release of drugs from acrylic resin films. *J. Pharm. Sci.* **79**, 811–816.

Kararli, T.T., Hurebut, J.B. & Needham, T.E. (1990) Glass-rubber transitions of cellulosic polymers by dynamic mechanical analysis. *J. Pharm. Sci.* **79**, 845–848.

Kratochvil, P. & Sundelöf, L.-O. (1986) Interactions in polymer solutions. *Acta Pharm. Suec.* **23**, 31–46

Lafferty, S.V., Summers, M.P., Mackey, R. & Newton, J.M. (1990) The application of dynamic mechanical thermal analysis to study the physical properties of free polymeric films. *J. Pharm. Pharmacol.* **42** Suppl., 25P.

Lehmann, K. (1989) Chemistry and application properties of polymethacrylate coating systems. In McGinity, J.W. (ed.), *Aqueous polymeric coatings for pharmaceutical dosage forms*, Marcel Dekker, New York, 153–245.

Lippold, B.C., Lippold, B.H., Sutter, B.K. & Gunder, W. (1990) Properties of aqueous, plasticizer-containing ethyl cellulose dispersions and prepared films in respect to the production of oral extended release formulations. *Drug Dev. Ind. Pharm.* **16**, 1725–1747.

Liron, Z., Srebrenik, S., Martin, A. & Cohen, S. (1986) Theoretical derivation of solute–solvent interaction parameter in binary solution: Case of the deviation from Raoult's law. *J. Pharm. Sci.* **75**, 463–468.

Masilungan, F.C. & Lordi, N.G. (1984) Evaluation of film coating compositions by thermomechanical analysis. I. Penetration mode. *Int. J. Pharmaceut.* **20**, 295–305.

Okhamafe, A.O. & York, P. (1983) Polymer-polymer interactions in some representative aqueous-based film coating systems. *Proc. 3rd Int. Conf., Pharm. Technol. APGI, Paris, France* **3**, 136–144.

Okhamafe, A.O. & York, P. (1984) Effect of solids-polymer interactions on the properties of some aqueous-based tablet film coating formulations. I. Moisture permeability. *Int. J. Pharmaceut.* **22**, 265–272.

Okhamafe, A.O. & York, P. (1984) Effect of solid–polymer interactions on the properties of some aqueous-based tablet film coating formulations. II. Mechanical characteristics. *Int. J. Pharmaceut.* **22**, 273–281.

Okhamafe, A.O. & York, P. (1984/85) The glass transition in some pigmented polymer systems used for tablet coating. *J. Macromol. Sci.-Phys* **B23**, 373–382.

Okhamafe, A.O. & York, P. (1985) Characterization of moisture interactions in some aqueous-based tablet film coating formulations. *J. Pharm. Pharmacol.* **37**, 385–390.

Okhamafe, A.O. & York, P. (1985) Interaction phenomena in some aqueous-based tablet film coating polymer systems. *Pharm. Res.* **2**, 19–23.

Okhamafe, A.O. & York, P. (1987) Interaction phenomena in pharmaceutical film coatings and testing methods. *Int. J. Pharmaceut.* **39**, 1–21.

Okhamafe, A.O. & York, P. (1988) Studies of interaction phenomena in aqueous-based film coatings containing soluble additives using thermal analysis techniques. *J. Pharm. Sci.* **77(5)**, 438–443.

Okhamafe, A.O. & York, P. (1989) Thermal characterisation of drug/polymer and excipient/polymer interactions in some film coating formulations. *J.Pharm. Pharmacol.* **41**, 1–6.

Oksanen, C.A. & Zografi, G. (1990) The relationship between Tg and water vapour absorption by poly(vinyl pyrrolidone) *Pharm. Res.* **7(6)**, 654–657.

Porter, S.C. & Ridgway, K. (1983) An evaluation of the properties of enteric coating polymers: measurement of glass transition temperature. *J. Pharm. Pharmacol.* **35**, 341–344.

Rosilio, V., Roblot-Trepel, L., de Lourdes Costa, M. & Baskin, A. (1988) Physico-chemical characterization of ethylcellulose drug-loaded cast films. *J. Controlled Release* **7**, 171–190.

Rowe, R.C. (1986) The prediction of compatibility/incompatibility in blends of ethyl-cellulose with hydroxypropyl methylcellulose or hydroxy-propyl cellulose using 2-dimensional solubility parameter maps. *J. Pharm. Pharmacol.* **38**, 214–215.

Rowe, R.C. (1988) Quantitative assessment of additive–polymer interaction in pigmented hydroxypropylmethylcellulose formulations using immersion calorimetry. *Int. J. Pharmaceut.* **48**, 113–117.

Sakellariou, P., Rowe, R.C. & White, E.F.T. (1985) The thermomechanical properties and glass transition temperatures of some cellulose derivatives used in film coating. *Int. J. Pharmaceut.* **27**, 267–277.

Sakellariou, P., Rowe, R.C. & White, E.F.T. (1986) An evaluation of the interaction and plasticizing efficiency of the polyethylene glycols in ethyl cellulose and hydroxypropyl methylcellulose films using the torsional braid pendulum. *Int. J. Pharmaceut.* **31**, 55–64.

Sakellariou, P., Rowe, R.C. & White, E.F.T. (1986) The solubility parameters of some cellulose derivatives and polyethylene glycols used in tablet film coating. *Int. J. Pharmaceut.* **31**, 175–177.

Sakellariou, P., Rowe, R.C. & White, E.F.T. (1986) Polymer/polymer interaction in blends of ethyl cellulose with both cellulose derivatives and polyethylene glycol 6000. *Int. J. Pharmaceut.* **34**, 93–103.

Sakellariou, P., Rowe, R.C. & White, E.F.T. (1987) The interactions and partitioning of low molecular weight polyethylene glycols and diethyl phthalate in ethylcellulose/hydroxypropyl methylcellulose blends. *J. Appl. Polym. Sci.* **34**, 2507–2516.

Schwartz, J.B. & Alvino, T.P. (1976) Effect of thermal gelation on dissolution from coated tablets. *J. Pharm. Sci.* **65(4)**, 572–575.

Tuffnell, K.J., May, G. & Meakin, B.J. (1983) Physico-chemical properties of some commercial hydroxypropylmethyl cellulose film forming materials. *Proc. 3rd Int. Conf. Pharm. Technol., APGI, Paris, France* V, 111–118.

Coating processes

Abdul-Razzak, M.H. & Aulton, M.E. (1982) Fluidised bed coating of tablets. Part 1: An introduction and review. *Iraqi J. Pharm. Sci.* **1(2)**, 7–11.

Abdul-Razzak, M.H. & Aulton, M.E. (1983) Fluidised bed coating of tablets. Part 2: An investigation into the effect of process variables on the quality of the coat. *Iraqi J. Pharm. Sci.* **2(1)**, 83–97.

Alcorn, G.J., Closs, G.H., Timko, R.J., Rosenberg, H.A., Hall, J. & Shatwell, J. (1988) Comparison of coating efficiency between a Vector Hicoater and a Manesty Accela-Cota. *Drug Dev. Ind. Pharm.* **14(12)**, 1699–1711.

Arwidsson, H. & Nicklasson, M. (1987) Evaluation of a rapid technique for the preparation of ethylcellulose films. *Proc. F.I.P. Congress, Amsterdam, The Netherlands.*

Aulton, M.E., Twitchell, A.M. & Hogan, J.E. (1985) Factors affecting the atomisation of tablet coating solutions. *J. Pharm. Pharmacol.* **37** Suppl., 114P.

Aulton, M.E., Twitchell, A.M. & Hogan, J.E. (1986) The influence of solution properties and atomisation parameters on the droplet size of HPMC film-coating solutions. *Proc. 4th Int. Conf. Pharm. Tech., APGI, Paris, France* V, 133–140.

Baveja, S.K., Ranga, K.V. & Rao, A.S. (1983) Design and evaluation of a miniature air-suspension coating apparatus. *J. Pharm. Pharmacol.* **35**, 475–476.

Bodmeier, R. (1991) Process and formulation variables affecting the drug release from chlorpheniramine maleate loaded beads coated with commercial and self-prepared aqueous ethylcellulose pseudolatexes. *Int. J. Pharmaceut.* **70**, 59–68.

Bodmeier, R. & Paeratakul, O. (1991) Formulation and process variables affecting the coating with aqueous polymer dispersions. *Proc. Pharm. Technol. Conf., New Brunswick, NJ, USA*, 439–449.

Bommel, E.M.G. van, Fokkens, J.G. & Crommelin, D.J.A. (1989) Production of a spherical Gradient Matrix System with zero-order release kinetics. *Proc. Int.*

Symp. Controlled Release Bioactive Mater. **16**, 324–325.

Bommel, E.M.G. van, Fokkens, J.G. & Crommelin, D.J.A. (1989) Development of a Gradient Matrix System with different geometries. *Proc. 8th Pharm. Technol. Conf.*, 59–68.

Bommel, E.M.G. van, Fokkens, J.G. & Crommelin, D.J.A. (1990) Production and evaluation of *in vitro* release characteristics of spherical Gradient Matrix Systems. *Acta Pharm. Technol.* **36(2)**, 74–78.

Boymond, C. (1983) Enrobage gastrorésistant de gélules au moyen de résines acryliques: Techniques d'enrobage et essais *in vivo*. *Pharm. Acta Helv.* **58**, 266–269.

Braeckman, P. (1983) A new small scale apparatus for enteric coating of hard gelatin capsules. *Acta Pharm. Technol.* **29**, 25–27.

Buri, P. (1989) A novel laboratory model for the film coating of microparticles. *Acta Pharm. Technol.* **35**, 256–257.

Chang, R.-K., Hsiao, C.H. & Robinson, J.R. (1987) A review of aqueous coating techniques and preliminary data on release from a theofylline product. *Pharm. Technol.* **11**, 56–68.

Chéhadé, J., Gurny, R., Doelker, E. & Buri, P. (1982) Aqueous coating with the laboratory apparatus Hi-Coater® HCT-20 Mini. *Acta Pharm. Technol.* **28(2)**, 141–148.

Cole, G.C., May, G., Neale, P.J., Olver, M.C. & Ridgway, K. (1983) The design and performance of an instrumentation system for aqueous film coating in an industrial tablet coating machine. *Drug Dev. Ind. Pharm.* **9(6)**, 909–944.

Cole, G.C., Neale, P.J. & Wilde, J.S. (1980) The measurement of droplet size and velocity in an atomised film-coating spray. *J. Pharm. Pharmacol.* **32** Suppl, 92P.

Dansereau, R., Brock, M & Redman-Furey, N. (1993) The solubilization of drug and excipient into a hydroxypropyl methyl cellulose (HPMC)-based film coating as a function for the coating parameters in a 24" Accela-Cota. *Drug Dev. Ind. Pharm.* **19(7)**, 793–808.

Dechesne, J.P. (1982) Etude des conditions d'application des enrobages gastrorésistants entérosolubles à base d'Eudragit L30D. *J. Pharm. Belg.* **37**, 273–282.

de Jong, S.W. (1993) Control of automated coating processes for the production of controlled-release pellets. *Pharm. Technol. Int.* **5(2)**, 34–36.

Delporte, J.P., De Seille, J.M. & Jaminet, F. (1981) Appareillages et condition d'application d'un enrobage d'hydroxypropylméthylcellulose de basse viscosité en milieu aqueux à l'échelle de laboratoire. *J. Pharm. Belg.* **36(5)**, 337–347.

Dietrich, R. (1991) Pharmazeutisch-technologische Gegenüberstellung moderner Trommel-Coater. *Pharm. Ind.* **54**, 459–464.

Dietrich, R. & Brausse, R. (1988) Validation of the pellet coating process used for a new sustained-release theophylline formulation. *Arzneim.-Forsch./Drug Res.* **38**, 1210–1219.

Ebey, G.C. (1987) A thermodynamic model for aqueous film-coating. *Pharm. Technol.* **11(4)**, 41–50.

Ehrhardt, L. (1982) Einsatz einer Ruckgewinnungsanlage für Lösungsmittel beim Filmcoating. *Pharm. Ind.* **44**, 1161–1165.

Farina, J.B. (1987) Sustained release pharmaceutical oral dosage forms. Review of patented manufacturing processes registered in the US Patent Office (1970/1985) *S.T.P. Pharma* **3**, 505–509.

Faroongsarng, D. & Peck, G.E. (1991) The swelling of core tablets during aqueous coating I: A simple model describing extent of swelling and water penetration for insoluble tablets containing a superdisintegrant. *Drug Dev. Ind. Pharm.* **17(18)**, 2439–2455.

Faroongsarng, D. & Peck, G.E. (1992) The swelling of core tablets during aqueous coating II: An application of the model describing extent of swelling and water penetration for insoluble tablets. *Drug Dev. Ind. Pharm.* **18(14)**, 1527–1534.

Flaig, E. (1983) Ein- oder Zweistoffsprühen, eine Alternative im Filmcoating. *Acta Pharm. Technol.* **29**, 51–61.

Franz, R.M. & Doonan, G.W. (1983) Measuring the surface temperature of tablet beds using infrared thermometry. *Pharm. Technol.* **7(3)**, 54–67.

Fricke, H. (1982) Trocknungstechnik beim Dragieren. Eine vergleichende Beurteilung verschiedener Systeme in konventionellen Dragierkesseln. *Pharm. Ind.* **44**, 1088–1093.

Ghebre-Sellassie, I. (1990) The effect of product bed temperature on the microstructure of Aquacoat-based controlled-release coatings. *Int. J. Pharmaceut.* **60**, 109–124.

Graf, E. (1983) Studies on the direct compression of pharmaceuticals. 12-Pancreatin g) Film coating. *Pharm. Ind.* **45**, 295–299.

Groppenbacher, G. (1985) PIK AS—zur wirtschaftlichen Herstellung von Filmtabletten. *Pharm. Ind.* **47**, 73–76.

Gross, H.M. & Endicott, C.J. (1960) Transformulation to film coating. *Drug and Cosmetic Industry* **86**, 170–264.

Harris, M.R., Ghebre-Sellassie, I. & Nesbitt, R.U. (1986) A water-based coating process for sustained release. *Pharm. Technol.* **10(3)**, 102–107.

Harrison, J.J., Lafferty, I., Moore, W.D., Rawlins, D.A., Rissen, N.R. & Thwaites, P.M. (1991) Titanium determination as a method of quantifying film-coat application on to tablets. *Drug Dev. Ind. Pharm.* **17(1)**, 149–155.

Heyd, A. (1973) Variables involved in an automated tablet-coating system. *J. Pharm. Sci.* **62(5)**, 818–820.

Heyd, A. & Kanig, J.L. (1970) Improved self-programming automated tablet-coating system. *J. Pharm. Sci.* **59**, 1171–1174.

Hogan, J.E. (1982) Aqueous versus organic solvent film coating. *Int. J. Pharm. Tech. Prod. Mfr* **3(1)**, 17–20.

Horváth, E. & Ormós, Z. (1989) Film coating of dragée seeds by fluidized bed spraying. *Acta Pharm. Technol.* **35**, 90–96.

Hossain, M. & Ayers, J.W. (1990) Variables that influence coat integrity in a laboratory spray coater. *Pharm. Technol.* **14(10)**, 72–82.

Johansson, M.E., Ringberg, A. & Nicklasson, M. (1987) Optimization of a fluid bed spray coating process using reduced factorial design. *J. Microencap.* **4**, 217–222.

Jones, D.M. (1991) Fluidized bed hot melt coating for modified release products. *Proc. Pharm Tech Conf., New Brunswick, NJ, USA*, 450–457.

Joshi, H.N., Kral, M.A. & Topp, E.M. (1989) Microwave drying of aqueous tablet film coatings; a study on free films. *Int. J. Pharmaceut.* **51**, 19–25.

Kala, H. (1983) Aufbau, Arbeitsweise und erste Erfahrungen mit einem Laborgerät zum Überziehen von Partikeln in der Wirbelschicht. *Die Pharm.* **38**, 879–881.

Kara, M.A.K., Leaver, T.M. & Rowe, R.C. (1982) Material carryover and process efficiency during tablet film coating in a side-vented perforated drum (Accela-Cota) *J. Pharm. Pharmacol.* **34**, 469–470.

Kim, S., Mankad, A. & Sheen, P. (1986) The effect of application rate of coating suspension on the incidence of the bridging of monograms on aqueous film-coated tablets. *Drug Dev. Ind. Pharm.* **12(6)**, 801–809.

Köblitz, T. (1988) Filmcoating unter Produktionsbedingungen mit Lösungs-mittelrück-gewinnungs-Anlage und im geschlossenen Gaskreislauf. *Pharm. Ind.* **50**, 81–91.

Kovács, B. (1982) Optimierung der Verfahrensparameter bei der Herstellung von Filmüberzugen auf Grund eines Mehrfaktoren-Versuchsplanes. *Pharm. Ind.* **44**, 830–833.

Kräuchi, E. (1983) Eignung einer Anlage mit perforierter Dragiertrommel zur Lösung spezieller Probleme der Zuckerdragierung. *Acta Pharm. Technol.* **29**, 47–50.

Lachman, L. & Cooper, J. (1963) A programmed automated film-coating process. *J. Pharm. Sci.* **52(5)**, 490–496.

Lantz, R.J., Bailey, A. & Robinson, M.J. (1970) Monitoring volatile coating solution applications in a coating pan. *J. Pharm. Sci.* **59(8)**, 1174–1177.

Leaver, T.M., Shannon, H.D. & Rowe, R.C. (1985) A photometric analysis of tablet movement in a side-vented perforated drum (Accela-Cota) *J. Pharm. Pharmacol.* **37**, 17–21.

Lehmann, K. (1981) Coating of tablets and small particles with acrylic resins by fluidized bed technology. *Int. J. Pharm. Tech. Prod. Mfr* **2**, 31–43.

Li, S.P., Mehta, G.N., Buehler, J.D., Grim, W.M. & Harwood, R.J. (1988) A method of coating non-uniform granular particles. *Drug Dev. Ind. Pharm.* **14(4)**, 573–585.

Lindberg, N.-O. & Jönsson, E. (1972) Film coating by hydroxypropyl cellulose in an automatic process. I. Influence of solvent on tablet bed temperature. *Acta Pharm. Suec.* **9**, 581–588.

Lindberg, N.-O. & Jönsson, E. (1972) Film coating by hydroxypropyl cellulose in an automatic process. II. Evaluation of coating solutions. *Acta Pharm. Suec.* **9**, 589–594.

List, P.H. (1982) Über die Wasserdampf– und Sauerstoffdurchlässigkeit verschiedener Tablettenüberzüge. *Acta Pharm. Technol.* **28**, 21–33.

MacLaren, D.D. & Hollenbeck, R.G. (1987) A high performance liquid chromatographic method for the determination of the amount of hydroxypropyl methyl-cellulose applied to tablets during an aqueous film coating operation. *Drug Dev. Ind. Pharm.* **13(12)**, 2179–2197.

Mathur, L.K., Forbes, St J. & Yelvigi, M. (1984) Characterization techniques for the aqueous film coating process. *Pharm. Technol.* **8(10)**, 42–54.

Meakin, B.J. & May, G. (1986) The use of potassium bromide to determine variations in tablet film coat weights. *Proc. 4th Int. Conf. Pharm. Technol., APGI,
Paris, France* **V**, 145–153.

Mehta, A.M., Valazza, M.J. & Abele, S.E. (1986) Evaluation of fluid-bed processes
for enteric coating systems. *Pharm. Technol.* **10**, 46–56.

Message, S.R. (1987) Towards automated tablet film coating. *Manuf. Chem.* **58(5)**,
85–87.

Mody, D.S., Scott, M.W. & Lieberman, H.A. (1964) Development of a simple automated film-coating procedure. *J. Pharm. Sci.* **53(8)**, 949–952.

Montel, J.-L. & Cotty, J. (1977) Enrobage de comprimés pharmaceutiques par films
cellulosiques en solution aqueuse. *Labo-Pharm—Problémes et Techniques* **261**,
51–55.

Okutgen, E. (1991) Dimensional changes and internal stress predictions in film
coated tablets. Ph.D. Thesis, De Montfort University Leicester, UK.

Okutgen, E., Hogan, J.E. & Aulton, M.E. (1991) Effects of tablet core dimensional
instability, during and after a film coating process, on the generation of internal
stresses within film coats. *Proc. 10th Pharm. Technol. Conf., Bologna, Italy* **3**,
52–57.

Okutgen, E., Hogan, J.E. & Aulton, M.E. (1991) Effects of tablet core dimensional
instability on the generation of internal stresses within film coats. Part I:
Influence of temperature changes during the film coating process. *Drug Dev. Ind.
Pharm.* **17(9)**, 1177–1189.

Okutgen, E., Hogan, J.E. & Aulton, M.E. (1991) Effects of tablet core dimensional
instability on the generation of internal stresses within film coats. Part III:
Exposure to temperatures and relative humidities which mimic the film coating
process. *Drug Dev. Ind. Pharm.* **17(14)**, 2005–2016.

Okutgen, E., Hogan, J.E. & Aulton, M.E. (1991) Quantitative evaluation of internal stress development in aqueous HPMC film coats. *Pharm. Res.* **8(10)**, S-90.

Okutgen, E., Jordan, M., Hogan, J.E. & Aulton, M.E. (1991) Effects of tablet core
dimensional instability on the generation of internal stresses within film coats.
Part II: Temperature and relative humidity variation within a tablet bed during
aqueous film coating in an Accela-Cota. *Drug Dev. Ind. Pharm.* **17(9)**, 1191–1199.

Okutgen, E., Travers, D.N., Hogan, J.E. & Aulton, M.E. (1989) Dimensional changes
occurring in tablet cores exposed to temperatures that mimic the film coating
process. *Proc. 5th Int. Conf. Pharm. Technol., APGI, Paris, France* **II**, 15–22.

Parikh, N.H., Porter, S.C. & Rohera, B. D. (1993) Aqueous ethylcellulose dispersion of ethylcellulose I: Evaluation of coating process variables. *Pharm. Res.*
10(4), 525–534.

Pickard, J.F. & Rees, J.E. (1972) Modern trends in pharmaceutical coating. *Pharm.
Ind.* **34(11)**, 833–839.

Pickard, J.F. & Rees, J.E. (1974) Film coating: 2 Processing equipment. *Manuf.
Chem.* **45(5)**, 42–45.

Pondell, R.E. (1984) From solvent to aqueous coatings. *Drug Dev. Ind. Pharm.*
10(2), 191–202.

Pondell, R.E. (1985) Scale-up of film coating processes. *Pharm. Technol.* **9(6)**, 68–70.

Porter, S.C. (1982) Film coating equipment. *Int. J. Pharm. Tech Prod. Mfr* **3(1)**, 27–32.

Porter, S.C. & Saraceni, K. (1988) Opportunities for cost containment in aqueous film coating. *Pharm. Technol.* **12(9)**, 62–75.

Porter, S.C. & Saraceni, K. (1989) Opportunities for cost containment in aqueous film coating. *Pharm. Technol.* **13(7/8)**, 20–27.

Prater, D.A., Wilde, J.S. & Meakin, B.J. (1980) A model system for the production of aqueous tablet film coatings for laboratory evaluation. *J. Pharm. Pharmacol.* **32** Suppl., 90P.

Reiland, T.L. & Eber, A.C. (1986) Aqueous gloss solutions: formula and process variables effects on the surface texture of film coated tablets. *Drug Dev. Ind. Pharm.* **12(3)**, 231–245.

Reiland, T.L., Seitz, J.A., Yeager, J.L. & Brusenback, R.A. (1983) Aqueous film-coating vaporization efficiency. *Drug Dev. Ind. Pharm.* **9**(6), 945–948.

Rekhi, G.S., Mendes, R.W., Porter, S.C. & Jambhekar, S.S. (1989) Aqueous polymeric dispersions for controlled drug delivery—Wurster process. *Pharm. Technol.* **13(3)**, 112–125.

Rowe, R.C. (1980) The expansion and contraction of tablets during film coating— a possible contributory factor in the creation of stresses within the film? *J. Pharm. Pharmacol.* **32**, 851.

Rowe, R.C. (1985) A photometric analysis of tablet movement in a side-vented perforated drum (Accela-Cota) *J. Pharm. Pharmacol.* **37**, 17–21.

Rowe, R.C. (1988) Tablet–tablet contact and mutual rubbing within a coating drum—an important factor governing the properties and appearance of tablet film coatings. *Int. J. Pharmaceut.* **43**, 155–159

Rowe, R.C. (1988) Monitoring production scale film coating using surface roughness measurements. *S.T.P. Pharma* **4**, 28–30.

Rowe, R.C. & Forse, S.F. (1982) The effect of process conditions on the incidence of bridging of the intagliations and edge splitting and peeling on film coated tablets. *Acta Pharm. Technol.* **28(3)**, 207–210.

Schmidt, P.C. & Niemann, F. (1992) The miniWid-Coater: II. Comparison of acid resistance of enteric-coated bisacodyl pellets coated with different polymers. *Drug Dev. Ind. Pharm.* **18(18)**, 1969–1979.

Seager, H., Rue, P.J., Burt, I., Ryder, J., Warrack, J.K. & Gamlen, M.J. (1985) Choice of method for the manufacture of tablets suitable for film coating. *Int. J. Pharm. Tech. Prod. Mfr* **6(1)**, 1–20.

Skultety, P.F., Rivera, D., Dunleavy, J. & Lin, C.T. (1988) Quantitation of the amount and uniformity of aqueous film coating applied to tablets in a 24" Accela-Cota. *Drug Dev. Ind Pharm.* **14(5)**, 617–631.

Stafford, J.W. & Lenkeit, D. (1984) The effect of film coating formulation on product quality when coating in different types of film coating equipment. *Pharm. Ind.* **46(10)**, 1062–1067.

Stetsko, G., Banker, G.S. & Peck, G.E. (1983) Mathematical modeling of an aqueous film coating process. *Pharm. Technol.* **7(11)**, 50–62.

Story, M.J. (1981) Granulation and film coating in the fluidized bed. *Int. J. Pharm. Tech. Prod. Mfr* **2**, 19–23.

Thoma, K. (1986) Herstellung von Filmüberzügen bei Arzneimittelentwicklung. I: Prinzip und Anwendung eines Laborsprühgeräts mit rotieren der Wirbelschicht. *Acta Pharma. Technol.* **32**, 146–152.

Trudelle, F., Rowe, R.C. & Witkowski, A.R. (1988) Monitoring production scale film coating using surface roughness measurements. *S.T.P. Pharma* **4(1)**, 28–30.

Turkoglu, M. & Sakr, A. (1992) Mathematical modelling and optimization of a rotary fluidized-bed coating process. *Int. J. Pharmaceut.* **88**, 75–87.

Twitchell, A.M. (1990) Studies on the role of atomisation in aqueous tablet film coating. Ph.D. Thesis, De Montfort University Leicester, UK.

Twitchell, A.M., Hogan, J.E. & Aulton, M.E. (1986) Estimated surface tensions of atomised droplets in aqueous film coating. *J. Pharm. Pharmacol.* **38** Suppl., 75P.

Twitchell, A.M., Hogan, J.E. & Aulton, M.E. (1987) The effect of atomisation conditions on the surface roughness of aqueous film-coated tablets. *J. Pharm. Pharmacol.* **39** Suppl., 128P.

Wan, L.S.C. (1991) Preparation of coated particles using a spray drying process with an aqueous system. *Int. J. Pharmaceut.* **77**, 183–191.

Wehrle, K. (1982) Vakuum–Filmcoating–Anlagen. System Dr Stellmach mit Lösungsmittel rückgewinnung. *Pharm. Ind.* **44**, 83–86.

Wesdyk, R. (1990) The effect of size and mass on the film thickness of beads coated in fluidized bed equipment. *Int. J. Pharmaceut.* **65**, 69–76.

Wou, L.L.S. (1988) Effect of dispersion on the coloring properties of aluminium dye lakes. *J. Pharm. Sci.* **77**, 866–871.

Yang, S.T. (1992) The effect of spray mode and chamber geometry of fluid-bed coating equipment and other parameters on an aqueous-based ethylcellulose coating. *Int. J. Pharmaceut.* **86**, 247–257.

Yang, S.T. & Ghebre-Sellassie, I. (1990) The effect of product bed temperature on the microstructure of Aquacoat-based controlled-release coatings. *Int. J. Pharmaceut.* **60**, 109–124.

Yoakam, D.A. & Campbell, R.J. (1984) Modeling of a film coating system for computer automation. *Pharm. Technol.* **8(1)**, 38–44.

Zaro, J.J. & Smith, W.E. (1972) Technique for preparing simulated coated dosage forms and preliminary evaluation of sprayed and cast films. *J. Pharm. Sci.* **61(5)**, 814–815.

Wetting and adhesion

Bauer, K.H. (1989) Auswahl und Optimierung von Antiklebmitteln für Umhüllungszubereitungen durch kontinuierliche Klebraftmessungen. *Pharm. Ind.* **51**, 203–209.

Fisher, D.G. & Rowe, R.C. (1976) The adhesion of film coatings to tablet surfaces—instrumentation and preliminary evaluation. *J. Pharm. Pharmacol.* **28**, 886–889.

Fung, R.M. & Parrott, E.L. (1980) Measurement of film-coating adhesiveness. *J. Pharm. Sci.* **69**, 439–441.

Gamlen, M.J. (1983) Preparing tablet cores for film coating. *Manuf. Chem.* **54(4)**, 38–41.

Harder, S.W., Zuck, D.A. & Wood, J.A. (1970) Characterization of tablet surfaces by their critical surface-tension values. *J. Pharm. Sci.* **59(12)**, 1787–1792.

Harder, S.W., Zuck, D.A. & Wood, J.A. (1971) An investigation of the forces responsible for the adhesive process in the film coating of tablets. *Canadian J. Pharm. Sci.* **6(3)**, 63–70.

Johnson, B.A. & Zografi, G. (1986) Adhesion of hydroxypropyl cellulose films to low energy solid substrates. *J. Pharm. Sci.* **75(6)**, 529–533.

Kulvanich, P. & Stewart, P.J. (1988) Influence of relative humidity on the adhesive properties of a model interactive system. *J. Pharm. Pharmacol.* **40**, 453–458.

Nadkarni, P.D., Kildsig, D.O., Kramer, P.A. & Banker, G.S. (1975) Effect of surface roughness and coating solvent on film adhesion to tablets. *J. Pharm. Sci.* **64(9)**, 1554–1557.

Okhamafe, A.O. & York, P. (1984) Effect of ageing on the adhesion of film coatings to aspirin tablets. *J. Pharm. Pharmacol.* **36**, Suppl., 1P.

Okhamafe, A.O. & York, P. (1985) The adhesion characteristics of some pigmented and unpigmented aqueous-based film coatings applied to aspirin tablets. *J. Pharm. Pharmacol.* **37**, 849–853.

Rowe, R.C. (1977) The adhesion of film coatings to tablets surfaces—measurement on biconvex tablets. *J. Pharm. Pharmacol.* **29**, 58–59.

Rowe, R.C. (1977) The adhesion of film coatings to tablet surfaces—the effect of some direct compression excipients and lubricants. *J. Pharm. Pharmacol.* **29**, 723–726.

Rowe, R.C. (1978) The measurement of the adhesion of film coatings to tablet surfaces: the effect of tablet porosity, surface roughness and film thickness. *J. Pharm. Pharmacol.* **30**, 343–346.

Rowe, R.C. (1981) The adhesion of tablet film coatings to tablet surfaces—a problem of stress distribution. *J. Pharm. Pharmacol.* **33**, 610–612.

Rowe, R.C. (1982) Material carryover and process efficiency during tablet film coating in a side-vented perforated drum (Accela-Cota) *J. Pharm. Pharmacol.* **34**, 469–470.

Rowe, R.C. (1983) The coating of tablet surfaces by lubricants as determined by a film/tablet adhesion measurement. *Acta Pharm. Suec.* **20**, 77–80.

Rowe, R.C. (1988) Adhesion of film coatings to tablets surfaces—a theoretical approach based on solubility parameters. *Int. J. Pharmaceut.* **41**, 219–222.

Twitchell, A.M., Hogan, J.E. & Aulton, M.E. (1986) Estimated surface tensions of atomised droplets in aqueous film coating. *J. Pharm. Pharmacol.* **38** Suppl., 75P.

Twitchell, A.M., Hogan, J.E. & Aulton, M.E. (1993) Contact angles formed by film coating formulations on uncoated and coated tablets. *Proc. 12th Pharm. Technol. Conf., Helsingør, Denmark* **1**, 246–257.

Wood, J.A. & Harder, S.W. (1970) The adhesion of film coatings to the surfaces of compressed tablets. *Canadian J. Pharm. Sci.* **5(1)**, 18–23.

Zografi, G. & Johnson, B. (1984) Effects of surface roughness on advancing and receding contact angles. *Int. J. Pharmaceut.* **22**, 159–176.

Mechanical properties

Abdul-Razzak, M.H. (1980) The mechanical properties of hydroxypropylmethyl-cellulose films derived from aqueous systems. M.Phil. Thesis, De Montfort University Leicester, UK.

Allen, D.J., DeMarco, J.D. & Kwan, K.C. (1972) Free films I: Apparatus and preliminary evaluation. *J. Pharm Sci.* **61(1)**, 106–109.

Arwidsson, H. & Johansson, B. (1991) Application of intrinsic viscosity and interaction constant as a formulation tool for film coating. III: Mechanical studies on free ethylcellulose films cast from organic solvents. *Int. J. Pharmaceut.* **76**, 91–97.

Aulton, M.E. (1977) Microindentation tests for pharmaceuticals. *Manuf. Chem.* **48(5)**, 28–37.

Aulton, M.E. (1982) Assessment of the mechanical properties of film coating materials. *Int. J. Pharm. Tech. Prod. Mfr* **3(1)**, 9–16.

Aulton, M.E., Abdul-Razzak, M.H. & Hogan, J.E. (1980) The mechanical properties of hydroxypropylmethylcellulose films derived from aqueous systems. *Proc. 2nd Int. Conf. Pharm. Technol., APGI, Paris, France* **V**, 16–25.

Aulton, M.E., Abdul-Razzak, M.H. & Hogan, J.E. (1981) The influence of solid inclusions on the mechanical properties of hydroxypropylmethylcellulose films. *Proc. 41st Int. Congr. Pharm. Sci. F.I.P., Vienna, Austria*, 150.

Aulton, M.E., Abdul-Razzak, M.H. & Hogan, J.E. (1981) The mechanical properties of hydroxypropylmethylcellulose films derived from aqueous systems. Part 1: The influence of plasticizers. *Drug Dev. Ind. Pharm.* **7(6)**, 649–668.

Aulton, M.E., Abdul-Razzak, M.H. & Hogan, J.E. (1984) The mechanical properties of hydroxypropylmethylcellulose films derived from aqueous systems. Part 2: The influence of solid inclusions. *Drug Dev. Ind. Pharm.* **10(4)**, 541–561.

Benita, S. (1986) Permeability and mechanical properties of a new polymer: cellulose hydrogenphthalate. *Int. J. Pharmaceut.* **33**, 71–80.

Bindschaedler, C., Gurny, R. & Doelker, E. (1987) Mechanically strong films produced from cellulose acetate latexes. *J. Pharm. Pharmacol.* **39**, 335–338.

Bommel, E.M.G. van, Fokkens, J.G. & Crommelin, D.J.A. (1989) Effects of additives on the physico-chemical properties of sprayed ethylcellulose films. *Acta Pharm. Technol.* **35(4)**, 232–237.

Bommel, E.M.G. van, Fokkens, J.G. & Crommelin, D.J.A. (1989) Physical characterization of drug-containing ethylcellulose films. *Proc. 5th Int. Conf. Pharm. Technol., APGI, Paris, France* 39–45.

Crawford, R.R. & Esmerian, O.K. (1971) Effect of plasticisers on some physical properties of cellulose acetate phthalate films. *J.Pharm. Sci.* **60(2)**, 312–314.

Dechesne, J.P. (1982) Étude de l'influence des plastifiants sur les caractéristiques des films appliqués d'Eudragit L30D. *J. Pharm. Belg.* **37**, 283–286.

Dechesne, J.P. & Jaminet, F. (1985) Influence de quelques plastifiants sur les propriétés de résistance mécanique de films isolés d'acetylphtalate de cellulose. *J. Pharm. Belg.* **40(1)**, 5–13.

Dechesne, J.P. & Jaminet, F. (1985) Influence de quelques plastifiants sur les propriétés mécaniques des films isolés de phtalate d'hydroxypropylmethylcellulose (HP55) *J. Pharm. Belg.* **40(3)**, 139–146.

Delonca, H. (1989) Étude de films à base d'hydroxypropylméthylcellulose phtalate (HP55) I: Films isolés. *J. Pharm. Belg.* **44**, 17–35.

Delonca, H. (1989) Étude de films à base d'hydroxypropylméthylcellulose phtalate (HP55) II: Films appliqués. *J. Pharm. Belg.* **44**, 101–108.

Delporte, J.P. (1980) *Proc. 2nd Int. Conf. Pharm. Technol., APGI, Paris, France* **V**, 6–15.

Delporte, J.P. (1980) Étude de quelques propriétés physiques de deux hydroxypropylméthylcellusoses de basse viscosité proposées pour l'enrobage de formes pharmaceutiques en milieu aqueux. *J. Pharm. Belg.* **35(6)**, 417–426.

Delporte, J.P. (1981) Influence de quelques additifs sur les propriétés de résistance mécanique de films isolés d'hydroxypropylméthylcellulose de basse viscosité. *J. Pharm. Belg.* **36(1)**, 27–37.

Dittgen, M. (1985) Relationship between film properties and drug release from acrylic films. *Drug Dev. Ind. Pharm.* **11**, 269–279.

Eerikäinen, S. (1991) Effects of spheronization on some properties of uncoated and coated granules containing different kinds of fillers. *Int. J. Pharmaceut.* **77**, 89–106.

Entwistle, C.A. & Rowe, R.C. (1978) Plasticization of cellulose ethers used in the film coating of tablets—the effect of plasticizer molecular weight. *J. Pharm. Pharmacol.* **30** Suppl., 27P.

Entwistle, C.A. & Rowe, R.C. (1979) Plasticization of cellulose ethers used in the film coating of tablets. *J. Pharm. Pharmacol.* **31**, 269–272.

Fell, J.T., Rowe, R.C. & Newton, J.M. (1979) The mechanical strength of film-coated tablets. *J. Pharm. Pharmacol.* **31**, 69–72.

Gibson, S.H.M., Rowe, R.C. & White, E.F.T. (1988) Mechanical properties of pigmented tablet coating formulations and their resistance to cracking. I. Static mechanical measurement. *Int. J. Pharmaceut.* **48**, 63–77.

Gibson, S.H.M., Rowe, R.C. & White, E.F.T. (1989) The mechanical properties of pigmented tablet coating formulations and their resistance to cracking II. Dynamic mechanical measurement. *Int. J. Pharmaceut.* **50**, 163–173.

Guo, J,-H., Robertson, R.E. & Amidon, G.L. (1991) Influence of physical ageing on mechanical properties of polymer free films: The prediction of long term ageing effects on the water permeability and dissolution rate of polymer film-coated tablets. *Pharm. Res.* **8(12)**, 1500–1504.

Gutierrez-Rocca, J.C. & McGinity, J.W. (1993) Influence of ageing on the physical-mechanical properties of acrylic resin films cast from aqueous dispersions and organic solutions. *Drug Dev. Ind. Pharm.* **19(3)**, 315–332.

Hawes, M.R. (1978) The effect of some commonly used excipients on the physical properties of film formers used in aqueous coatings of pharmaceutical tablets. R.P. Scherer Award report, Roy. Pharm. Soc. G.B., London, UK.

Hjärtstam, J., Borg, K. & Lindstedt, B. (1990) The effect of tensile stress on permeability of free films of ethyl cellulose containing hydroxypropyl methylcellulose. *Int. J. Pharmaceut.* **61**, 101–107.

Johnson, K. (1991) Effect of triacetin and polyethylene glycol 400 on some physical properties of HPMC free films. *Int. J. Pharmaceut.* **73**, 197–208.

Kovács, B., Gyarmathy, M. & Racz, I. (1986) The influence of some additives on the elasticity of polymer films. *Proc. 4th Int. Conf. Pharm. Technol. APGI, Paris, France* V, 99–102.

Lindholm, T. (1986) Controlled release tablets. Part 5: Some release and mechanical properties of ethyl cellulose tablet coats containing surfactant. *Pharm. Ind.* **48**, 1075–1078.

Lindholm, T., Juslin, M., Lindholm, B.-Å., Poikala, M., Tiilikainen, S. & Varis, H. (1986) Properties of free ethyl cellulose films containing surfactant and particulate matter. *Pharm. Ind.* **49**, 740–746.

Majeed, S.S. (1984) The influence of surfactant addition on the properties of hydroxypropylmethylcellulose in tablet film coating. M.Phil. Thesis, De Montfort University Leicester, UK.

Mortada, S.A.M. (1990) Systematic evaluation of polymer films. Part 1: Effect of solvent composition on the physical properties of fresh and aged films of *n*-propyl and *n*-butyl half ester of PVM/MA. *Pharm. Ind.* **52**, 107–112.

Mortada, S.A.M. (1990) Systematic evaluation of polymer films. Part 2: Effect of solvent composition, plasticizer type and concentration on mechanical characteristics of aged films of *n*-propyl and *n*-butyl half ester of PVM/MA. *Pharm. Ind.* **52**, 233–237.

Okhamafe, A.O. & York, P. (1983) Analysis of the permeation and mechanical characteristics of some aqueous-based film coating systems. *J. Pharm. Pharmacol.* **35**, 409–415.

Okhamafe, A.O. & York, P. (1984) Effect of solid–polymer interactions on the properties of some aqueous-based tablet film coating formulations. II. Mechanical characteristics. *Int. J. Pharmaceut.* **22**, 273–281.

Okhamafe, A.O. & York, P. (1985) Tensile anisotropy of some pigmented tablet film coating systems. *J. Pharm. Pharmacol.* **37**, 492–493.

Okhamafe, A.O. & York, P. (1986) Mechanical properties of some pigmented and unpigmented aqueous-based film coating formulations applied to aspirin tablets. *J. Pharm. Pharmacol.* **38**, 414–419.

Ononokopono, O.E. and Spring, M.S. (1988) The influence of binder film thickness on the mechanical properties of binder films in tension. *J. Pharm. Pharmacol.* **40**, 126–128.

Ononokopono, O.E. and Spring, M.S. (1988) The effects of inclusions and conditions of storage on the mechanical properties of maize starch and methylcellulose films. *J. Pharm. Pharmacol.* **40**, 313–319.

Ostewald, H.P., Eisenbach, C.D. & Bauer, K.H. (1982) Wirkungsweise und Optimierungsmöglichkeiten der Anwendung von Weichmachern in Filmüberzüger. *Acta Pharm. Technol.* **28(1)**, 34–43.

Pickard, J.F., Elworthy, P. & Sucker, H. (1975) A comparison of the properties of film coatings prepared from water- and organic solvent-based solutions. *J. Pharm. Pharmacol.* **27** Suppl., 6P.

Pilpel, N. (1986) The plasto-elasticity and compressibility of coated powders and the tensile strengths of their tablets. *J. Pharm. Pharmacol.* **38**, 1–7.

Porter, S.C. (1982) The practical significance of the permeability and mechanical properties of polymer films used for the coating of pharmaceutical dosage forms. *Int. J. Pharm. Tech. Prod. Mfr* **3(1)**, 21–25.

Radebaugh, G.W. (1988) Methods for evaluating the puncture and shear properties of pharmaceutical polymer films. *Int. J. Pharmaceut.* **45**, 39–46.

Rowe, R.C. (1976) Microindentation—a method for measuring the elastic properties and hardness of films on conventionally coated tablets. *J. Pharm. Pharmacol.* **28**, 310–311.

Rowe, R.C. (1976) The effect of molecular weight on the properties of films prepared from hydroxypropyl methylcellulose. *Pharm. Acta Helv.* **51(11)**, 330–334.

Rowe, R.C. (1982) Modulus enhancement in pigmented film coating formulations. *Int. J. Pharmaceut.* **12**, 175–179.

Rowe, R.C. (1983) Correlations between the in-situ performance of tablet film coating formulations based on hydroxypropyl methylcellulose and data obtained from the tensile testing of free films. *Acta Pharm. Technol.* **29(3)**, 205–207.

Rowe, R.C. (1983) Modulus enhancement in pigmented tablet film coating formulations. *Int. J. Pharmaceut.* **14**, 355–359.

Rowe, R.C. (1984) An evaluation of the plasticizing efficiency of the dialkyl phthalates in ethylcellulose films using the torsional braid pendulum. *Int. J. Pharmaceut.* **22**, 57–62.

Rowe, R.C. (1988) Mechanical properties of pigmented tablet coating formulations and their resistance to cracking. I: Static mechanical measurement. *Int. J. Pharmaceut.* **48**, 63–77.

Rowe, R.C. (1989) The mechanical properties of pigmented tablet coating formulations and their resistance to cracking. II: Dynamic mechanical measurement. *Int. J. Pharmaceut.* **50**, 163–173.

Rowe, R.C., Kotaras, A.D. & White, E.F.T. (1984) An evaluation of the plasticizing efficiency of the dialkyl phthalates in ethyl cellulose films using the torsional braid pendulum. *Int. J. Pharmaceut.* **22**, 57–62.

Shah, P.S. & Zatz, J.L. (1992) Plasticization of cellulose esters used in the coating of sustained release solid dosage forms. *Drug Dev. Ind. Pharm.* **18(16)**, 1759–1772.

Sina, A., El-Aziz, S.A.M., El-Sourady, H.A. & Hafez, E. (1978) Effect of casting solvent on some properties of ethylcellulose films. *Egypt. J. Pharm. Sci.* **19**, 97–105.

Sinko, C.M. & Amidon, G.L. (1989) Plasticizer-induced changes in the mechanical rate of response of film coatings: an approach to quantitating plasticizer effectiveness. *Int. J. Pharmaceut.* **55**, 247–256.

Spang, R. (1982) Teilbarkeit von Tabletten und Filmdragées. *Pharm. Acta Helv.* **57**, 99–111.

Stanley, P., Rowe, R.C. & Newton, J.M. (1981) Theoretical considerations of the influence of polymer film coatings on the mechanical strength of tablets. *J. Pharm. Pharmacol.* **33**, 557–560.

Stern, P.W. (1976) Effects of film coatings on tablet hardness. *J. Pharm. Sci.* **65(9)**, 1291–1295.

Topham, J.D. (1981) Indenter to evaluate the viscoelastic properties of tablets and tablet coatings. *J. Pharm. Pharmacol.* 33 Suppl., 115P.

Vemba, T., Gillard, J. & Roland, M. (1980) Influence des solvents et des plastifiants sur la perméabilité et la tension de rupture de films d'ethylcellulose. *Pharm. Acta Helv.* **55(3)**, 65–71.

Quality of coats (including defects, gloss, surface roughness and colour)

Breech, J.A., Lucisano, L.J. & Franz, R.M. (1988) Investigation into substrate cracking of a film-coated bilayered tablet. *J. Pharm. Pharmacol.* **40**, 282–283.

Down, G.R.B. (1982) An alternative mechanism responsible for the bridging of intagliations on film-coated tablets. *J. Pharm. Pharmacol.* **34**, 281–282.

Down, G.R.B. (1991) The etiology of pinhole and bubble defects in enteric and controlled-release film coatings. *Drug Dev. Ind. Pharm.* **17(2)**, 309–315.

Gibson, S.H.M., Rowe, R.C. & White, E.F.T. (1988) Determination of the critical pigment volume concentrations of pigmented film coating formulations using gloss measurements. *Int. J. Pharmaceut.* **45**, 245–248.

Hossain, M. & Ayers, J.W. (1990) Variables that influence coat integrity in a laboratory spray coater. *Pharm. Technol.* **14(10)**, 72–82.

Kim, S., Mankad, A. & Sheen, P. (1986) The effect of application rate of coating suspension on the incidence of the bridging of monograms on aqueous film-coated tablets. *Drug Dev. Ind. Pharm.* **12(6)**, 801–809.

Masilungan, F.C., Carabba, C.D. & Bohidar, N.R. (1991) Application of simplex and statistical analysis for correction of pitting in aqueous film coated tablets. *Drug Dev. Ind. Pharm.* **17(4)**, 609–615.

Mehta, A.M. & Jones, D.M. (1985) Coated pellets under the microscope. *Pharm. Technol.* **9(6)**, 52–60.

Nadkarni, P.D., Kildsig, D.O., Kramer, P.A. & Banker, G.S. (1975) Effect of surface roughness and coating solvent on film adhesion to tablets. *J. Pharm. Sci.* **64(9)**, 1554–1557.

Okhamafe, A.O. & York, P. (1985) Stress crack resistance of some pigmented and unpigmented tablet film coating systems. *J. Pharm. Pharmacol.* **37**, 449–454.

Okutgen, E. (1991) Dimensional changes and internal stress predictions in film coated tablets. Ph.D. Thesis, De Montfort University Leicester, UK.

Okutgen, E., Hogan, J.E. & Aulton, M.E. (1991) Effects of tablet core dimensional instability, during and after a film coating process, on the generation of internal stresses within film coats. *Proc. 10th Pharm. Technol. Conf., Bologna, Italy* **3**, 52–57.

Okutgen, E., Hogan, J.E. & Aulton, M.E. (1991) Effects of tablet core dimensional instability on the generation of internal stresses within film coats. Part I: Influence of temperature changes during the film coating process. *Drug Dev. Ind. Pharm.* **17(9)**, 1177–1189.

Okutgen, E., Hogan, J.E. & Aulton, M.E. (1991) Effects of tablet core dimensional instability on the generation of internal stresses within film coats. Part III:

Exposure to temperatures and relative humidities which mimic the film coating process. *Drug Dev. Ind. Pharm.* **17(14)**, 2005–2016.

Okutgen, E., Hogan, J.E. & Aulton, M.E. (1991) Quantitative evaluation of internal stress development in aqueous HPMC film coats. *Pharm. Res.* **8(10)**, S-90.

Okutgen, E., Jordan, M., Hogan, J.E. & Aulton, M.E. (1991) Effects of tablet core dimensional instability on the generation of internal stresses within film coats. Part II: Temperature and relative humidity variation within a tablet bed during aqueous film coating in an Accela-Cota. *Drug Dev. Ind. Pharm.* **17(9)**, 1191–1199.

Prater, D.A., Meakin, B.J., Rowe, R.C. & Wilde, J.S. (1981) A technique for investigating changes in the surface roughness of tablets during film coating. *J. Pharm. Pharmacol.* **33**, 666–668.

Reiland, T.L. & Eber, A.C. (1986) Aqueous gloss solutions: formula and process variables effects on the surface texture of film coated tablets. *Drug Dev. Ind. Pharm.* **12(3)**, 231–245.

Rowe, R.C. (1978) The effect of some formulation and process variables on the surface roughness of film coated tablets. *J. Pharm. Pharmacol.* **30**, 669–672.

Rowe, R.C. (1979) Surface roughness measurements on both uncoated and film-coated tablets. *J. Pharm. Pharmacol.* **31**, 473–474.

Rowe, R.C. (1980) The expansion and contraction of tablets during film coating—a possible contributory factor in the creation of stresses within the film? *J. Pharm. Pharmacol.* **32**, 851.

Rowe, R.C. (1981) The effect of the particle size of an inert additive on the surface roughness of a film-coated tablet. *J. Pharm. Pharmacol.* **33**, 1–4.

Rowe, R.C. (1981) The cracking of film coatings on film-coated tablets—a theoretical approach with practical implications. *J. Pharm. Pharmacol.* **33**, 423–426.

Rowe, R.C. (1982) A comment on the localised cracking around pigment particles in film coatings applied to tablets. *Int. J. Pharm. Tech. Prod, Mfr* **3(2)**, 67–68.

Rowe, R.C. (1982) Bridging of the intagliations on film coated tablets. *J. Pharm. Pharmacol.* **34**, 282.

Rowe, R.C. (1982) The effect of pigment type and concentration on the incidence of edge splitting on film-coated tablets. *Pharm. Acta Helv.* **57(8)**, 221–225.

Rowe, R.C. (1983) A reappraisal of the equations used to predict the internal stresses in film coatings applied to tablet substrates. *J. Pharm. Pharmacol.* **35**, 112–113.

Rowe, R.C. (1983) Coating defects—causes and cures. *Manuf. Chem.* **54(4)**, 49–50.

Rowe, R.C. (1983) Film coating: the ideal process for enhancing tablet identity. *Pharm. Int.* **4(7)**, 173–175.

Rowe, R.C. (1984) The effect of white extender pigments on the incidence of edge splitting on film coated tablets. *Acta Pharm. Technol.* **30(3)**, 235–238.

Rowe, R.C. (1984) Quantitative opacity measurements on tablet film coatings containing titanium dioxide. *Int. J. Pharmaceut.* **22**, 17–23.

Rowe, R.C. (1984) The opacity of tablet film coatings. *J. Pharm. Pharmacol.* **36**, 569–572.

Rowe, R.C. (1985) Gloss measurement on film coated tablets. *J. Pharm. Pharmacol.* **37**, 761–765.

Rowe, R.C. (1985) The effect of the particle size of synthetic red iron oxide on the appearance of tablet film coating. *Pharm. Acta Helv.* **60**, 157–161.

Rowe, R.C. (1985) Appearance measurements on tablets. *Pharm. Int.* **6**, 225–230.

Rowe, R.C. (1986) Localized cracking around pigment particles in tablet film coatings: a theoretical approach. *J. Pharm. Pharmacol.* **38**, 529–530.

Rowe, R.C. (1986) A scientific approach to the solution of film splitting and bridging of the intagliations on film coated tablets. *S.T.P. Pharma* **2(16)**, 416–421.

Rowe, R.C. (1988) Determination of the critical pigment volume concentrations of pigmented film coating formulations using gloss measurement. *Int. J. Pharmaceut.* **45**, 245–248.

Rowe, R.C. (1988) Monitoring production scale film coating using surface roughness measurements. *S.T.P. Pharma* **4**, 28–30.

Rowe, R.C. (1992) Defects in film-coated tablets: aetiology and solutions. In Ganderton, D. & Jones, T.M. (eds), *Advances in pharmaceutical sciences*, vol. 6, Academic Press, London.

Rowe, R.C. (1992) The effect of some formulation variables on crack propagation in pigmented tablet film coatings using computer simulation. *Int. J. Pharmaceut.* **86**, 49–58.

Rowe, R.C. & Forse, S.F. (1974) A preliminary evaluation of a mercury intrusion method for assessing film continuity on coated tablets. *J. Pharm. Pharmacol.* **26** Suppl., 61P–62P.

Rowe, R.C. & Forse, S.F. (1980) The effect of polymer molecular weight on the incidence of film cracking and splitting on film coated tablets. *J. Pharm. Pharmacol.* **32**, 583–584.

Rowe, R.C. & Forse, S.F. (1980) The effect of film thickness on the incidence of the defect bridging of intagliations on film coated tablets. *J. Pharm. Pharmacol.* **32**, 647–648.

Rowe, R.C. & Forse, S.F. (1981) The effect of plasticizer type and concentration on the incidence of bridging of intagliations on film-coated tablets. *J. Pharm. Pharmacol.* **33**, 174–175.

Rowe, R.C. & Force, S.F. (1981) The effect of intagliation shape on the incidence of bridging on film-coated tablets. *J. Pharm. Pharmacol.* **33**, 412.

Rowe, R.C. & Forse, S.F. (1982) The effect of process conditions on the incidence of bridging of the intagliations and edge splitting and peeling on film coated tablets. *Acta Pharm. Technol.* **28(3)**, 207–210.

Rowe, R.C. & Forse, S.F. (1982) Bridging of intagliations on film coated tablets. *J. Pharm. Pharmacol.* **34**, 282.

Rowe, R.C. & Force, S.F. (1983) Pitting—a defect on film-coated tablets. *Int. J. Pharmaceut.* **17**, 347–349.

Rowe, R.C. & Roberts, R.J. (1992) Simulation of crack propagation in tablet film coatings containing pigments. *Int. J. Pharmaceut.* **78**, 49–57.

Rowe, R.C. & Roberts, R.J. (1992) The effect of some formulation variables on crack propagation in pigmented tablet film coatings using computer simulation. *Int. J. Pharmaceut.* **86**, 49–58.

Simpkin, G.T., Johnson, M.C.R. & Bell, J.H. (1983) The influence of drug solubility on the quality of film coated tablets. *Proc. 3rd Int. Conf. Pharm. Technol., APGI, Paris, France* **III**, 163–169.

Stafford, J.W. & Lenkeit, D. (1984) The effect of film coating formulation on product quality when coating in different types of film coating equipment. *Pharm. Ind.* **46(10)**, 1062–1067.

Toyoshima, K., Yasumura, M., Ohnishi, N. & Ueda, Y. (1988) Quantitative evaluation of tablet sticking by surface roughness measurement. *Int. J. Pharmaceut.* **46**, 211–215.

Trudelle, F., Rowe, R.C. & Witkowski, A.R. (1988) Monitoring production scale film coating using surface roughness measurements. *S.T.P. Pharma* **4(1)**, 28–30.

Twitchell, A.M. (1990) Studies on the role of atomisation in aqueous tablet film coating. Ph.D. Thesis, De Montfort University Leicester, UK.

Twitchell, A.M., Hogan, J.E. & Aulton, M.E. (1987) The effect of atomisation conditions on the surface roughness of aqueous film-coated tablets. *J. Pharm. Pharmacol.* **39** Suppl., 128P.

Twitchell, A.M., Hogan, J.E. & Aulton, M.E. (1993) Contact angles formed by film coating formulations on uncoated and coated tablets. *Proc. 12th Pharm. Technol. Conf., Helsingør, Denmark*, **1**, 246–257.

Twitchell, A.M., Hogan, J.E. & Aulton, M.E. (1994) Assessment of the thickness variation and roughness of aqueous film-coated tablets using a light section microscope. *Proc. 13th Pharm. Technol. Conf., Strasbourg, France* **1**, 660–671.

Wou, L.L.S. (1988) Effect of dispersion on the coloring properties of aluminium dye lakes. *J. Pharm. Sci.* **77**, 866–871.

Permeability (to gases and water vapour)

Amann, A.H., Lindstrom, R.E. & Swarbrick, J. (1974) Factors affecting water vapour transmission through polymer films applied to solid surfaces. *J. Pharm. Sci.* **63(6)**, 931–933.

Banker, G.S., Gore, A.Y. & Swarbrick, J. (1966) Water vapour transmission properties of free polymer films. *J. Pharm. Pharmacol.* **18**, 457–466.

Banker, G.S., Gore, A.Y. & Swarbrick, J. (1966) Water vapour transmission properties of applied polymer films. *J. Pharm. Pharmacol.* **18**, Suppl., 205S–211S.

Benita, S. (1986) Permeability and mechanical properties of a new polymer: cellulose hydrogenphthalate. *Int. J. Pharmaceut.* **33**, 71–80.

Bindschaedler, C., Gurny, R. & Doelker, E. (1986) Osmotically controlled drug delivery systems produced from organic solutions and aqueous dispersions of cellulose acetate. *J. Controlled Release* **4**, 203–212.

Bindschaedler, C., Gurny, R. & Doelker, E. (1987) Osmotic water transport through cellulose acetate membranes produced from a latex system. *J. Pharm. Sci.* **76**, 455–460.

Bond, J.R., York, P & Woodhead, P.J. (1989) Water vapour permeability of cellulose acetate films. *J. Pharm. Pharmacol.* **41**, 16P.

Faroongsarng, D. & Peck, G.E. (1991) The swelling of core tablets during aqueous coating I: A simple model describing extent of swelling and water penetration for insoluble tablets containing a superdisintegrant. *Drug Dev. Ind. Pharm.* **17(18)**, 2439–2455.

Faroongsarng, D. & Peck, G.E. (1992) The swelling of core tablets during aqueous coating II: An application of the model describing extent of swelling and water penetration for insoluble tablets. *Drug Dev. Ind. Pharm.* **18(14)**, 1527–1534.

Guo, J,-H., Robertson, R.E. & Amidon, G.L. (1991) Influence of physical ageing on mechanical properties of polymer free films: The prediction of long term ageing effects on the water permeability and dissolution rate of polymer film-coated tablets. *Pharm. Res.* **8(12)**, 1500–1504.

Hjärtstam, J., Borg, K. & Lindstedt, B. (1990) The effect of tensile stress on permeability of free films of ethyl cellulose containing hydroxypropyl methylcellulose. *Int. J. Pharmaceut.* **61**, 101–107.

Kala, H. (1986) Einfluss von Weichmachern auf die Permeabilität von Polymethacrylatüberzügen (Eudragit® RS) *Die Pharm.* **41**, 335–338.

Kala, H. (1987) Einsatz von Polyäthylenglycol zur Steuerung der Permeabilität von Poly(meth)acrylatüberzügen. *Die Pharm.* **42**, 26–28.

Kildsig, D.O., Nedich, R.L. & Banker, G.S. (1970) Theoretical justification of reciprocal rate plots in studies of water vapour transmission through films. *J. Pharm. Sci.* **59(11)**, 1634–1637.

Kolbe, I. & List, P.H. (1982) Untersuchungen über die Wasserdampfdurchlässigkeit von Ethylcellulose-Filmen aus wäßriger Dispersion. *Pharm. Ind.* **44**, 619–621.

Kuriyama, T., Nobutoki, M. & Nakanishi, M. (1970) Permeability of double-layer films. I. *J. Pharm. Sci.* **59(9)**, 1341–1343.

Kuriyama, T., Nobutoki, M. & Nakanishi, M. (1970) Permeability of double-layer films. II., *J. Pharm. Sci.* **59(9)**, 1344–.

Lachman, L. & Drubulis, A. (1964) Factors influencing the properties of films used for tablet coating I. Effects of plasticizers on the water vapor transmission of cellulose acetate phthalate films. *J. Pharm. Sci.* **53(6)**, 639–643.

Lehmann, K. (1986) In Wasser dispergierbare, hydrophile Acrylharze mit abgestufter Permeabilität für diffusionsgesteuerte Wirkstoffabgabe aus Arzneiformen. *Acta Pharm. Technol.* **32**, 146–152.

Lindholm, T. (1982) Controlled release tablets. Part 3: Ethylcellulose coats containing surfactant and powdered matter. *Pharm. Ind.* **44**, 937–941.

Lindholm, T., Juslin, M., Lindholm, B.-Å., Poikala, M., Tiilikainen, S. & Varis, H. (1986) Properties of free ethyl cellulose films containing surfactant and particulate matter. *Pharm. Ind.* **49**, 740–746.

List, P.H. (1981) Eine kontinuierliche, selbsregistrierende Methode zur Bestimmung der Wasserdampfdurchlässigkeit von freitragenden Tablettenüberzügen. *Acta Pharm. Technol.* **27**, 211–214.

List, P.H. (1982) Über die Wasserdampf- und Sauerstoffdurchlässigkeit verschiedener Tablettenüberzüge. *Acta Pharm. Technol.* **28**, 21–33.

Okhamafe, A.O. & Iwebor, H.U. (1986) Moisture permeability mechanisms of some aqueous-based tablet film coatings containing soluble additives. *Proc 4th Int. Conf. Pharm. Technol., APGI, Paris, France* **V**, 103–110.

Okhamafe, A.O. & York, P. (1983) Analysis of the permeation and mechanical characteristics of some aqueous-based film coating systems. *J. Pharm. Pharmacol.* **35**, 409–415.

Okhamafe, A.O. & York, P. (1984) Effect of solids–polymer interactions on the properties of some aqueous-based tablet film coating formulations. I. Moisture permeability. *Int. J. Pharmaceut.* **22**, 265–272.

Okhamafe, A.O. & York, P. (1985) Studies on the moisture permeation process in some pigmented aqueous-based tablet film coats. *Pharm. Acta Helv.* **60(3)**, 92–96.

Okhamafe, A.O. & York, P. (1987) Moisture permeability mechanisms of some aqueous-based tablet film coatings containing soluble additives. *Die Pharm.* **42**, 611–613.

Okor, R.S. (1982) Effects of polymer cation content on certain film properties. *J. Pharm. Pharmacol.* **34**, 83–86.

Okor, R.S. (1989) Solute adsorption and concentration dependent permeability in certain polymer films. *J. Pharm. Pharmacol.* **41**, 483–484.

Okor, R.S. & Anderson, W. (1986) Swellability of cast films of an acrylate-methacrylate copolymer in aqueous solutions of certain permeants and concentration-dependent permeability. *J. Macromol. Sci.-Phys.* **B25(4)**, 505–513.

Oksanen, C.A. & Zografi, G. (1990) The relationship between Tg and water vapour absorption by poly(vinyl pyrrolidone) *Pharm. Res.* **7(6)**, 654–657.

Parker, J.W., Peck, G.E. & Banker, G.S. (1974) Effects of solids loading on moisture permeability coefficients of free films. *J. Pharm. Sci.* **63(1)**, 119–125.

Patel, M., Patel, J.M. & Lemberger, A.P. (1964) Water vapor permeation of selected cellulose ester films. *J. Pharm. Sci.* **53(3)**, 286–290.

Pickard, J.F., Rees, J.E. & Elworthy, P.H. (1972) Water vapour permeability of poured and sprayed polymer films. *J. Pharm. Pharmacol.* **24** Suppl., 139P.

Porter, S.C. (1982) The practical significance of the permeability and mechanical properties of polymer films used for the coating of pharmaceutical dosage forms. *Int. J. Pharm. Tech. Prod. Mfr* **3(1)**, 21–25.

Porter, S.C. & Ridgway, K. (1982) The permeability of enteric coatings and the dissolution rates of coated tablets. *J. Pharm. Pharmacol.* **34**, 5–8.

Prater, D.A., Meakin, B.J. & Wilde, J.S. (1982) A mass spectrometric technique for the determination of gas and vapour permeabilities of thin pharmaceutical films. *Int. J. Pharm. Tech. Prod. Mfr* **3(2)**, 33–41.

Prater, D.A., Wilde, J.S. & Meakin, B.J. (1981) The effect of titanium dioxide on the oxygen permeability of hydroxypropylmethyl cellulose (HPMC) films. *J. Pharm. Pharmacol.* **33**, 26P.

Sprockel, O.L., Prapaitrakul, W. & Shivanand, P. (1990) Permeability of cellulose polymers: water vapour transmission rates. *J. Pharm. Pharmacol.* **42**, 152–157.

Swarbrick, J. & Amann, A.H. (1968) Moisture permeation through polymer films. *J. Pharm. Pharmacol.* **20**, 886–888.

Swarbrick, J., Amann, A.H. & Lindstrom, R.E. (1972) Factors affecting water vapor transmission through free polymer films. *J. Pharm. Sci.* **61(10)**, 1645–1647.

Thoma, K. (1991) Untersuchungen zur Säurepermeabilität magensaftresistenter Überzüge. 5. Mitteilung: Pharmazeutische-technologisches und analytische Untersuchungen an magensaftresistenten Darreichungsformen. *Die Pharm.* **46**, 278–282.

Vemba, T., Gillard, J. & Roland, M. (1980) Influence des solvents et des plastifiants sur la perméabilité et la tension de rupture de films d'ethylcellulose. *Pharm. Acta Helv.* **55(3)**, 65–71.

Woodruff, C.W., Peck, G.E. & Banker, G.S. (1972) Effect of environmental conditions and polymer ratio on water vapour transmission through free plasticized cellulose films. *J. Pharm. Sci.* **61(12)**, 1956–1959.

Drug release characteristics

Arwidsson, H. (1991) Properties of ethyl cellulose films for extended release. I. Influence of process factors when using organic solutions. *Acta Pharm. Nord.* **3(1)**, 25–30.

Azoury, R., Elkayam, R. & Friedman, M. (1988) Nuclear magnetic resonance study of an ethyl cellulose sustained-release delivery system. I: Effect of casting solvent on hydration properties. *J. Pharm. Sci.* **77**, 425–427.

Azoury, R., Elkayam, R. & Friedman, M. (1988) Nuclear magnetic resonance study of an ethyl cellulose sustained-release delivery system. II: Release rate behavior of tetracyline. *J. Pharm. Sci.* **77**, 428–431.

Béchard, S.R. & Leroux, J.C. (1992) Coated pelletized dosage form: effect of compaction on drug release. *Drug Dev. Ind. Pharm.* **18(18)**, 1927–1944.

Bechgaard, H. (1982) Mathematical model for *in-vitro* drug release from controlled release dosage forms applied to propoxyphene hydrochloride pellets. *J. Pharm. Sci.* **71**, 694–699.

Benita, S. (1987) Cellulose hydrogen phthalate. A coating polymer in controlled release dosage forms. *Pharm. Acta Helv.* **62**, 255–261.

Biachini, R., Resciniti, M. & Vecchio, C. (1989) Aqueous-based enteric film coatings containing insoluble additives. *Proc. 5th Int. Conf. Pharm. Tech., APGI, Paris, France* **V**, 416–425.

Bindschaedler, C., Gurny, R. & Doelker, E. (1986) Osmotically controlled drug delivery systems produced from organic solutions and aqueous dispersions of cellulose acetate. *J. Controlled Release* **4**, 203–212.

Bindschaedler, C., Gurny, R. & Doelker, E. (1986) Osmotic water transport through cellulose acetate membranes produced from a latex system. *J. Pharm. Sci.* **76(6)**, 455–460.

Blanchon, S., Couarraze, G., Rieg-Falson, F., Cohen, G. & Puisieux, F. (1991) Permeability of progesterone and synthetic progestin through methacrylic films. *Int. J. Pharmaceut.* **72**, 1–10.

Bodmeier, R. (1991) Process and formulation variables affecting the drug release from chlorpheniramine maleate loaded beads coated with commercial and self-prepared aqueous ethylcellulose pseudolatexes. *Int. J. Pharmaceut.* **70**, 59–68.

Bodmeier, R. & Paeratakul, O. (1989) Drug release from laminated polymeric films prepared from aqueous latexes. *J. Pharm. Sci.* **79(1)**, 32–36.

Bodmeier, R. & Paeratakul, O. (1989) Evaluation of drug-containing polymer films prepared from aqueous latexes. *Pharm. Res.* **6(8)**, 725–730.

Bodmeier, R. & Paeratakul, O. (1990) Propranolol hydrochloride release from acrylic films prepared from aqueous latexes. *Int. J. Pharmaceut.* **59**, 197–204.

Bodmeier, R. & Paeratakul, O. (1990) Theophylline tablets coated with aqueous latexes containing dispersed pore formers. *J. Pharm. Sci.* **79**, 925–928.

Bommel, E.M.G. van, Dezentjé, R.F.R., Fokkens, J.G. & Crommelin, D.J.A. (1991) Drug release kinetics from the Gradient Matrix System: Mathematical modelling. *Int. J. Pharmaceut.* **72**, 19–27.

Bommel, E.M.G. van & Fokkens, J.G. (1988) Release from a Gradient Matrix System. *Proc. Int. Symp. Controlled Release Bioactive Mater.* **15**, 316–317.

Bommel, E.M.G. van, Fokkens, J.G. & Crommelin, D.J.A. (1989) A Gradient Matrix System as a controlled release device. Release from a slab model system. *J. Controlled Release* **10**, 283–292.

Bommel, E.M.G. van, Fokkens, J.G. & Crommelin, D.J.A. (1990) Production and evaluation of *in vitro* release characteristics of spherical Gradient Matrix Systems. *Acta Pharm. Technol.* **36(2)**, 74–78.

Borodkin, S. & Tucker, F.E. (1974) Drug release from hydroxypropyl cellulose-polyvinyl acetate films. *J. Pharm. Sci.* **63(9)**, 1359–1364.

Boymond, C. (1983) Enrobage gastrorésistant de gélules au moyer de résines acryliques: Techniques d'enrobage et essais *in vivo*. *Pharm. Acta Helv.* **58**, 266–269.

Byron, P.R. (1987) Effects of heat treatment on the permeability of polyvinyl alcohol films to a hydrophilic solute. *J. Pharm Sci.* **76**, 65–67.

Chang, R.-K. (1990) Preparation and evaluation of shellac pseudolatex as an aqueous enteric coating system for pellets. *Int. J. Pharmaceut.* **60**, 171–173.

Chang, R.-K. (1990) A comparison of rheological and enteric properties among organic solutions, ammonium salt aqueous solutions and latex systems. *Pharm. Technol.* **14(10)**, 62–70.

Chang, R.-K. & Hsiao, C.M. (1989) Eudragit RL and RS pseudolatices: properties and performance in pharmaceutical coating as a controlled release membrane for theophylline pellets. *Drug Dev. Ind. Pharm.* **15(2)**, 187–196.

Chang, R.-K., Hsiao, C.H. & Robinson, J.R. (1987) A review of aqueous coating techniques and preliminary data on release from a theofylline product. *Pharm. Technol.* **11**, 56–68.

Chang, R.-K., Price, J.C. & Hsiao, C. (1989) Preparation and preliminary evaluation of Eudragit RL & RS pseudolatices for controlled drug release. *Drug Dev. Ind. Pharm.* **15(3)**, 361–372.

Chang, R.-K. & Rudnic, E.M. (1991) The effect of various polymeric coating systems on the dissolution and tableting properties of potassium chloride microcapsules. *Int. J. Pharmaceut.* **70**, 261–270.

Couarraze, G. (1992) Influence of size polydispersity on drug release from coated pellets. *Int. J. Pharmaceut.* **86**, 113–121.

Curatolo, W. (1988) Perforated coated tablets for controlled-release of drugs at a constant rate. *J. Pharm. Sci.* **77**, 322–324.

Danscreau, R. (1989) Development of a new coated-bead dosage form of sodium iodide I[131]. *Int. J. Pharmaceut.* **49**, 115–119.

Davis, M.B. (1986) Comparison and evaluation of enteric polymer properties in aqueous solutions. *Int. J. Pharmaceut.* **28**, 157–166.

Dechesne, J.P. (1982) Étude des conditions d'application des enrobages gastrorésistants entérosolubles à base d'Eudragit L 30 D. *J. Pharm. Belg.* **37**, 273–282.

Dechesne, J.P. (1987) A new enteric tablet of acetylsalicylic acid. I: Technological aspects. *Int. J. Pharmaceut.* **37**, 203–209.

Dechesne, J.P. (1987) A new enteric tablet of acetylsalicylic acid. II: Biopharmaceutical aspects. *Int. J. Pharmaceut.* **34**, 259–262.

de Jong, S.W. (1993) Control of automated coating processes for the production of controlled-release pellets. *Pharm. Technol. Int.* **5(2)**, 34–36.

Deshpande, S.G. & Dongre, S.A. (1987) Mathematical model for enteric coated tablets using cellulose acetate phthalate. *Indian J. Pharm. Sci.* **49(3)**, 81–84.

Dietrich, R. & Brausse, R. (1988) Validation of the pellet coating process used for a new sustained-release theophylline formulation. *Arzneim.-Forsch./Drug Res.* **38**, 1210–1219.

Dittgen, M. (1985) Relationship between film properties and drug release from acrylic films. *Drug Dev. Ind. Pharm.* **11**, 269–279.

Dittgen, M. & Jensch, H.-P. (1988) Influence of the physico-chemical properties of the drug on its release from acrylic films. *Acta Pharm. Jugosl.* **38**, 315–320.

Donbrow, M. & Friedmann, M. (1975) Enhancement of permeability of ethylcellulose films for drug penetration. *J. Pharm. Pharmacol.* **27**, 633–646.

Dor, P., Benita, S. & Levesque, G. (1987) Cellulose hydrogen phthalate. A coating polymer in controlled release dosage forms. *Pharm. Acta Helv.* **62(9)**, 255–261.

Dyer, A.M. (1992) Design and study of a drug delivery system comprising polymer-coated pellets. Ph.D. Thesis, De Montfort University Leicester, UK.

Dyer, A.M., Khan, K.A. & Aulton, M.E. (1992) Design of an oral sustained release drug delivery system comprising polymer coated pellets compacted into tablets. *Proc. 11th Pharm. Technol. Conf., Manchester* **2**, 37–53.

Ekman, B. (1983) Membrane-coated tablets: A system for the controlled release of drugs. *J. Pharm. Sci.* **72**, 772–775.

El-Egakey, M.A. (1982) Drug release from films of polyalkylcyanoacrylates. *Acta Pharm. Technol.* **28**, 103–109.

Eerikäinen, S. (1991) The behaviour of the sodium salt of indomethacin in the cores of film-coated granules containing various fillers. *Int. J. Pharmaceut.* **71**, 201–211.

Frömming, K.H. (1983) Magensaftresistente Filmüberzüge auf Tabletten aus Wässsriger Lösung mit einem Copolymer aus Vinylacetat und Crotonsaure. 3 Mitt: Röntgenologische Untersuchungen. *Pharm. Ind.* **45**, 199–202.

Frömming, K.H. (1984) Über die In-vivo-Stabilität magensaftresistenter Tabletten bei erhölten Magen-pH-Werten. *Pharm. Ind.* **46**, 180–183.

Ghebre-Sellassie, I. (1986) A unique application and characterization of Eudragit E 30 D film coatings in sustained release formulations. *Int. J. Pharmaceut.* **31**, 43–54.

Ghebre-Sellassie, I. (1987) Evaluation of acrylic-based modified-release film coatings. *Int. J. Pharmaceut.* **37**, 211–218.

Ghebre-Sellassie, I. (1990) The effect of product bed temperature on the microstructure of Aquacoat-based controlled-release coatings. *Int. J. Pharmaceut.* **60**, 109–124.

Ghebre-Sellassie, I., Iyer, U., Kubert, D. & Fawzi, M.B. (1988) Characterization of a new water-based coating for modified-release preparations. *Pharm. Technol.* **12**, 96–106.

Gilligan, C.A. & Li, Wan Po A. (1991) Factors affecting drug release from a pellet system coated with an aqueous colloidal dispersion. *Int. J. Pharmaceut.* **73**, 51–68.

Goodhart, F.W., Harris, M.R., Murthy, K.S. & Nesbitt, R.U. (1984) An evaluation of aqueous film-forming dispersions for controlled release. *Pharm. Technol.* **8(4)**, 64–71.

Green, P.G., Hadgraft, J. & Wolff, M. (1989) Measurement of diffusion rates across fragile polymeric films. *Int. J. Pharmaceut.* **54**, R1–R3.

Guo, J,-H., Robertson, R.E. & Amidon, G.L. (1991) Influence of physical ageing on mechanical properties of polymer free films: The prediction of long term ageing effects on the water permeability and dissolution rate of polymer film-coated tablets. *Pharm. Res.* **8(12)**, 1500–1504.

Hannula, A.-M. (1988) Coating of gelatin capsules. *Acta Pharm. Technol.* **34**, 234–236.

Harris, M.R., Ghebre-Sellassie, I. & Nesbitt, R.U. (1986) A water-based coating process for sustained release. *Pharm. Technol.* **10(3)**, 102–107.

Heliová, M., Rak, J. & Chalabala, M. (1986) Filme und Membranen für kontrollierte Wirkstoff freigabe. *Acta Fac. Pharm.* **40**, 163–176.

Iyer, U., Hong, W., Das, N. & Ghebre-Selassie, I. (1990) Comparative evaluation of three organic solvent and dispersion-based ethylcellulose coating formulations. *Pharm. Technol.* **14**, 68–86.

Jenquin, M.R. (1992) Relationship of film properties to drug release from monolithic films containing adjuvants. *J. Pharm. Sci.* **81**, 983–989.

Jenquin, M.R., Leibowitz, S.M., Sarabia, R.E. & McGinity, J.W. (1990) Physical and chemical factors influencing the release of drugs from acrylic resin films. *J. Pharm. Sci.* **79**, 811–816.

Joachim, J. (1988) Étude galénique et spectrale du sulfathiazol sodique enrobé à l'Aquatéric. *J. Pharm. Belg.* **43**, 349–358.

Källstrand, G. & Ekman, B. (1983) Membrane-coated tablets: A system for the controlled release of drugs. *J. Pharm. Sci.* **72**, 772–775.

Kassem, M.A. (1986) Effect of formulation variables on the permeation of dexamethasone through different polymeric films. I: Effect of different polymer types and plasticizers. *S.T.P. Pharma* **2**, 34–37.

Kassem, M.A. (1986) Effect of formulation variables on the permeation of dexamethasone through different polymeric films. II: Effect of different surfactants. *S.T.P. Pharma* **2**, 106–109.

Kent, D.J. & Rowe, R.C. (1978) Solubility studies on ethyl cellulose used in film coating. *J. Pharm. Pharmacol.* **30**, 808–810.

Korsatko-Wabnegg, B. (1990) Entwicklung von Manteltabletten mit 'Controlled Release'. Effeckt auf der Basis von Poly-D-(—)-3-hydroxybuttersäure. *Die Pharm.* **45**, 842–844.

Laakso, R. (1991) Effects of core components on indomethacin release from film-coated granules. *Int. J. Pharmaceut.* **67**, 79–88.

Li, L.C. & Peck, G.E. (1989) Water based silicone elastomer controlled release tablet film coating I: Free film evaluation. *Drug Dev. Ind. Pharm.* **15(1)**, 65–95.

Li, L.C. & Peck, G.E. (1989) Water based silicone elastomer controlled release tablet film coating II: Formulation considerations and coating evaluation. *Drug Dev. Ind. Pharm.* **15(4)**, 499–531.

Li, L.C. & Peck, G.E. (1989) Water based silicone elastomer controlled release tablet film coating III: Drug release mechanisms. *Drug Dev. Ind. Pharm.* **15(12)**, 1943–1968.

Li, L.C. & Peck, G.E. (1990) Water based silicone elastomer controlled release tablet film coating IV: Process evaluation. *Drug Dev. Ind. Pharm.* **16(3)**, 415–435.

Li, S.P., Feld, K.M. & Kowarski, C.R. (1991) Preparation and evaluation of Eudragit® acrylic resin for controlled drug release of pseudoephedrine hydrochloride. *Drug Dev. Ind. Pharm.* **17(12)**, 1655–1683.

Li, S.P., Jhawar, R., Mehta, G.N., Harwood, R.J. & Grim, W.M. (1989) Preparation and *in vitro* evaluation of a controlled release drug delivery system of theophylline using an aqueous acrylic resin dispersion. *Drug Dev. Ind. Pharm.* **15**, 1231–1242.

Li, S.P., Mehta, G.N., Buehler, J.D., Grim, W.M. & Harwood, R.J. (1990) The effect of film-coating additives on the *in vitro* dissolution release rate of ethyl cellulose-coated theophylline granules. *Pharm. Technol.* **14**, 20–24.

Lin, S.-Y. & Kawashima, Y. (1987) Drug release from tablets containing cellulose acetate phthalate as an additive or enteric-coating material. *Pharm. Res.* **4(1)**, 70–74.

Lindholm, T. (1985) Controlled release tablets. Part 4: Sodium salicylate tablets with ethylcellulose coats containing surfactant and particular matter. *Pharm. Ind.* **47**, 1093–1098.

Lindholm, T. (1986) Controlled release tablets. Part 5: Some release and mechanical properties of ethyl cellulose tablet coats containing surfactant. *Pharm. Ind.* **48**, 1075–1078.

Lindholm, T., Lindholm, B.-Å., Niskanen, M. & Koskiniemi, J. (1986) Polysorbate 20 as a drug release regulator in ethyl cellulose film coatings. *J. Pharm. Pharmacol.* **38**, 686–688.

Lindstedt, B., Ragnarsson, G. & Hjärtstam, J., (1989) Osmotic pumping as a release mechanism for membrane-coated drug formulations. *Int. J. Pharmaceut.* **56**, 261–268.

Lippold, B.C. (1988) Polymerfilme als Diffusionsbarrieren für perorale Retardarzneiformen unter besonderer Berücksichtigung wässriger Dispersionen. *Acta Pharm. Technol.* **34**, 179–188.

Lippold, B.C., Lippold, B.H., Sutter, B.K. & Gunder, W. (1990) Properties of aqueous, plasticizer-containing ethyl cellulose dispersions and prepared films in respect to the production of oral extended release formulations. *Drug Dev. Ind. Pharm.* **16**, 1725–1747.

Lippold, B.H., Sutter, B.K. & Lippold, B.C. (1989) Parameters controlling drug release from pellets coated with aqueous ethyl cellulose dispersion. *Int. J. Pharmaceut.* **54**, 15–25.

Mehta, A.M., Valazza, M.J. & Abele, S.E. (1986) Evaluation of fluid-bed processes for enteric coating systems. *Pharm. Technol.* **10**, 46–56.

Mortada, S.A.M. (1990) Systematic evaluation of polymer films. Part 3: Drug release from *n*-propyl and *n*-butyl half ester of PVM/MA. *Pharm. Ind.* **52**, 352–356.

Munday, D.L. & Fassihi, A.R. (1989) Controlled release delivery: effect of coating composition on release characteristics of mini-tablets. *Int. J. Pharmaceut.* **52**, 109–114.

Munday, D.L. & Fassihi, A.R. (1989) Dissolution of theophylline from film-coated slow release mini-tablets in various dissolution media. *J. Pharm. Pharmacol.* **41**, 369–372.

Munday, D.L. & Fassihi, A.R. (1991) Changes in drug release rate: effect of stress storage conditions on film coated mini-tablets. *Drug Dev. Ind. Pharm.* **17(15)**, 2135–2143.

Murthy, K.S., Enders, N.A., Mahjour, M. & Fawzi, M.B. (1986) A comparative evaluation of aqueous enteric polymers in capsule coatings. *Pharm. Technol.* **10(10)**, 36–46.

Nesbitt, R.U. (1991) Mechanism of drug release from coated dosage forms. *Proc. Pharm Tech Conf., New Brunswick, N.J., USA*, 458–463.

Okor, R.S. & Anderson, W. (1979) Variation of polymer film composition and solute permeability. *J. Pharm. Pharmacol.* **31** Suppl., 31P.

Okor, R.S. & Anderson, W. (1987) Casting solvent effects on the permeability of polymer films with differing quaternary ammonium (cation) content. *J. Pharm. Pharmacol.* **39**, 547–548.

Okor, R.S. & Obi, C.E. (1990) Drug release through aqueous-based film coatings of acrylate-methacrylate, a water-insoluble copolymer. *Int. J. Pharmaceut.* **58**, 89–91.

Ozturk, A.G., Ozturk, S.S., Palsson, B.O., Wheatley, T.A. & Dressman, J.B. (1990) Mechanism of release from pellets coated with an ethylcellulose-based film. *J. Controlled Release* **14**, 203–213.

Plaizer-Vercammen, J.A. (1991) Evaluation of aqueous dispersions of Eudragit L 100–55 for their enteric coating properties. *S.T.P. Pharma Sci.* **1**, 267–271.

Plaizer-Vercammen, J.A. (1991) Evaluation of Aquateric, a pseudolatex of cellulose acetate phthalate, for its enteric coating properties on tablets. *S.T.P. Pharma Sci.* **1**, 307–312.

Plaizer-Vercammen, J.A. (1992) Enteric coating properties of Eudragit®, Aquateric®, and cellulose acetate trimellitate applied to capsules. *Eur. J. Pharm. Biopharm.* **38**, 145–149.

Plaizer-Vercammen, J.A. (1992) Evaluation of a water dispersion of Aquateric for its enteric coating properties of hard gelatin capsules manufactured with a fluidized bed technique. *Pharm. Acta Helv.* **67**, 227–230.

Plaizer-Vercammen, J.A. (1992) Evaluation of enteric coated capsules coated with ammoniated water solutions of cellulose acetate phthalate and cellulose acetate trimellitate. *Pharm. Ind.* **54**, 1050–1052.

Porter, S.C. (1989) The use of Opadry, Coateric and Surelease in the aqueous film coating of pharmaceutical oral dosage forms. In McGinity, J.W. (ed.), *Aqueous polymeric coatings for pharmaceutical dosage forms*, Marcel Dekker, New York, Chap. 8, 317–362.

Porter, S.C. (1989) Controlled-release film coatings based on ethyl cellulose. *Drug Dev. Ind. Pharm.* **15(10)**, 1495–1521.

Porter, S.C. & Ridgway, K. (1977) The properties of enteric tablet coatings made from polyvinyl acetate-phthalate and cellulose acetate-phthalate. *J. Pharm. Pharmacol.* **29** Suppl., 42P.

Porter, S.C. & Ridgway, K. (1983) An evaluation of the properties of enteric coating polymers: measurement of glass transition temperature. *J. Pharm. Pharmacol.* **35**, 341–344.

Ragnarsson, G. & Johansson, M.O. (1988) Coated drug cores in multiple unit preparations: influence of particle size. *Drug Dev. Ind. Pharm.* **14(15–17)**, 2285–2297.

Rekhi, G.S., Mendes, R.W., Porter, S.C. & Jambhekar, S.S. (1989) Aqueous polymeric dispersions for controlled drug delivery—Wurster process. *Pharm. Technol.*, **13(3)**, 112–125.

Rekkas, D.M. (1986) *In vitro* study of dissolution rate of diphylline tablets. *Pharm. Acta Helv.* **61**, 164–166.

Ritschel, W.A. (1987) Drug release mechanisms from matrix and barrier coated tablets prepared with acrylic resin, with and without addition of channeling agents. *Pharm. Ind.* **49**, 734–739.

Rowe, R.C. (1985) Film coating—the ideal process for the production of modified-release oral dosage forms. *Pharm. Int.* **6(1)**, 14–17.

Rowe, R.C. (1986) The effect of the molecular weight of ethylcellulose on the drug release properties of mixed films of ethylcellulose and hydroxypropyl methylcellulose. *Int. J. Pharmaceut.* **29**, 37–41.

Samuelov, Y., Donbrow, M. & Friedmann, M. (1979) Sustained release of drugs from ethylcellulose–polyethylene glycol films and kinetics of drug release. *J. Pharm. Sci.* **68**, 325–329.

Schepky, G. & Thoma, K. (1991) Influence of enteric coating of drug delivery and absorption of fusidic acid film-coated tablets. *Pharm. Ind.* **53**, 1135–1139.

Schmidt, P.C. & Niemann, F. (1992) The miniWid-Coater: II. Comparison of acid resistance of enteric-coated bisacodyl pellets coated with different polymers. *Drug Dev. Ind. Pharm.* **18(18)**, 1969–1979.

Shah, N.B. & Sheth, B.B. (1972) A method for study of timed-release films. *J. Pharm. Sci.* **61(3)**, 412–415.

Shah, P.S. & Zatz, J.L. (1992) Plasticization of cellulose esters used in the coating of sustained release solid dosage forms. *Drug Dev. Ind. Pharm.* **18(16)**, 1759–1772.

Sheen, P.-C., Sabol, P.J., Alcorn, G.J. & Feld, K.M. (1992) Aqueous film coating studies of sustained release nicotinic acid pellets: an *in-vitro* evaluation. *Drug Dev. Ind. Pharm.* **18(8)**, 851–860.

Sinko, C.M., Yee, A.F. & Amidon, G.L. (1990) The effect of physical ageing on the dissolution rate of anionic polyelectrolytes. *Pharm. Res.* **7(6)**, 648–653.

Sinko, C.M., Yee, A.F. & Amidon, G.L. (1991) Prediction of physical ageing in controlled-release coatings: The application of the relaxation coupling model to glassy cellulose acetate. *Pharm. Res.* **8(6)**, 696–705.

Stafford, J.W. (1982) Enteric film coating using completely aqueous dissolved hydroxypropyl methyl cellulose phthalate spray solutions. *Drug Dev. Ind. Pharm.* **8(4)**, 513–530.

Steuernagel, C.R. (1989) Latex emulsions for controlled drug delivery. In McGinity, J.W. (ed.), *Aqueous polymeric coatings for pharmaceutical dosage forms*, Marcel Dekker, New York, Chap. 1, 1–61.

Sutter, B.K., Lippold, B.H. & Lippold, B.C. (1988) Polymerfilme als Diffusionsbarrieren für perorale Retardarzneiformen unter besonderer Berücksichtigung wäßriger Dispersionen. *Acta Pharm. Technol.* **34**, 179–188.

Tan, E.L., Liu, J.C. & Chien, Y.W. (1988) Controlled drug release from silicone coated tablets: preliminary evaluation of coating techniques and characterization of membrane permeation kinetics. *Int. J. Pharmaceut.* **42**, 161–169.

Tardieu, M. (1992) Étude comparative de dispersions aqueuses de polymerès gastrorésistants entérosolubles. *Pharm. Acta Helv.* **67**, 29–32.

Thoma, K. (1991) Retardierung schwach basischer Arzneistoffe. 3. Mitteilung: Verbesserung der Verfügbarkeit von Phenothiazin. Neuroleptika aus tabletten mit Diffusionsüberzügen. *Pharm. Ind.* **53**, 69–73.

Thoma, K. (1991) Retardierung schwach basischer Arzneistoffe. 4. Mitteilung: Behebung der Verfügbarkeitsprobleme von Vincamin aus Diffusions-Depotarzneiformen. *Pharm. Ind.* **53**, 595–600.

Thoma, K. (1991) Retardierung schwach basischer Arzneistoffen 6. Mitteilung: Verbesserung der Freisetzung und Verfügbarkeit von Dihydroergotaminmethansulfonat mit Hilfe magensaftresistenter Filmüberzüge. *Pharm. Ind.* **53**, 778–785.

Vasavada, R.C. (1985) Evaluation of propylene glycol monostearate—ethoxylated stearyl alcohol films and kinetics of cortisol release. *Int. J. Pharmaceut.* **25**, 199–206.

Vergnaud, J.M. (1985) Model for matter transfers between sodium salicylate–Eudragit matrix and gastric liquid. *Int. J. Pharmaceut.* **27**, 233–243.

Vergnaud, J.M. (1986) Effect of pH on drug release between sodium salicylate–Eudragit compound and gastric liquid: modelling of the process. *Int. J. Pharmaceut.* **32**, 143–150.

Voigt, R. (1985) Spruhfilmcoating von sphärischen Mikroformlingen mit nichtwassrigen Lackrezepturen. *Die Pharm.* **40**, 772–776.

Voigt, R. (1986) Prufüng der Arzneistoffliberation aus filmpellets unter besonderer Berücksichtigung der Polymerschichtdicke. *Die Pharm.* **41**, 114–117.

Wan, L.S.C. (1991) Factors affecting drug release from drug-coated granules prepared by fluidized-bed coating. *Int. J. Pharmaceut.* **72**, 163–174.

Wan, L.S.C. (1992) Multilayer drug-coated cores: A system for controlling drug release. *Int. J. Pharmaceut.* **81**, 75–88.

Wouessidjewe, D., Devissaguet, J.P. & Carstensen, J.T. (1991) Effect of multiple film coverage in sustained release pellets. *Drug Dev. Ind. Pharm.* **17(1)**, 7–25.

Yuen, K.H. (1993) Development and *in vitro* evaluation of a multiparticulate sustained-release theophylline formulation. *Drug Dev. Ind. Pharm.* **19**, 855–874.

Zhang, G., Schwartz, J.B., Schnaare, R.L., Wigent, R.J. & Sugita, E.T. (1991) Bead Coating: II. Effect of spheronization technique on drug release from coated spheres. *Drug Dev. Ind. Pharm.* **17(6)**, 817–830.

Stability

Abdul-Razzak, M.H. (1983) Studies on the migration of drugs between polymeric film coats and tablet cores. Ph.D. Thesis, De Montfort University Leicester, UK.

Aulton, M.E., Richards, J.H., Abdul-Razzak, M.H. & Hogan, J.E. (1983) Migration of active ingredient between film coats and tablet cores. *Proc. 3rd Int. Conf. Pharm. Technol., APGI, Paris, France* **III**, 154–162.

Béchard, S.R., Quraishi, O. & Kwong, E. (1992) Film coating: effect of titanium dioxide concentration and film thickness on the photostability of nifedipine. *Int. J. Pharmaceut.* **87**, 133–139.

Bodmeier, R. & Paeratakul, O. (1992) Leaching of water-soluble plasticizers from polymeric films prepared from aqueous colloidal polymer dispersions. *Drug Dev. Ind. Pharm.* **18(17)**, 1865–1882.

Bommel, E.M.G. van (1991) Handling properties and stability on storage of the Gradient Matrix System. *Eur. J. Pharm. Biopharm.* **37(1)**, 3–6.

Charro, D. (1993) Ageing of sustained-release formulations of amoxycillin and Gelucire 64/02. *Drug Dev. Ind. Pharm.* **19**, 473–482.

Chowhan, Z.T., Amaro, A.A. & Li-Hua Chi (1982) Comparative evaluations of aqueous film coated tablet formulations by high humidity ageing. *Drug Dev. Ind. Pharm.* **8(5)**, 713–737.

Davis, M.B., Peck, G.E. & Banker, G.S. (1986) Preparation and stability of aqueous-based enteric polymer dispersions. *Drug Dev. Ind. Pharm.* **12(10)**, 1419–1448.

Gürsoy, A. (1986) Film-coated zinc sulphate tablets and the effect of humidity on tablet properties. *Die Pharm.* **41**, 575–578.

Gutierrez-Rocca, J.C. & McGinity, J.W. (1993) Influence of ageing on the physical-mechanical properties of acrylic resin films cast from aqueous dispersions and organic solutions. *Drug Dev. Ind. Pharm.* **19(3)**, 315–332.

Miller, R.A. & Vadas, E.B. (1984) The physical stability of tablets coated using an aqueous dispersion of ethylcellulose. *Drug Dev. Ind. Pharm.* **10**, 1565–1585.

Mortada, S.A.M. (1990) Systematic evaluation of polymer films. Part 1: Effect of solvent composition on the physical properties of fresh and aged films of *n*-propyl and *n*-butyl half ester of PVM/MA. *Pharm. Ind.* **52**, 107–112.

Mortada, S.A.M. (1990) Systematic evaluation of polymer films. Part 2: Effect of solvent composition, plasticizer type and concentration on mechanical characteristics of aged films of *n*-propyl and *n*-butyl half ester of PVM/MA. *Pharm. Ind.*

52, 233–237.

Nyqvist, H., Nicklasson, M. & Lundgren, P. (1982) Studies on the physical properties of tablets and tablet excipients. V. Film coating for protection of a light sensitive tablet formulation. *Acta Pharm. Suec.* **19**, 223–228.

Ononokopono, O.E. & Spring, M.S. (1988) The effects of inclusions and conditions of storage on the mechanical properties of maize starch and methylcellulose films. *J. Pharm. Pharmacol.* **40**, 313–319.

Saarnivaara, K. & Kahela, P. (1985) Effect of storage on the properties of acetylsalicylic acid tablets coated with aqueous hydroxypropyl methylcellulose dispersion. *Drug Dev. Ind. Pharm.* **11(2 and 3)**, 481–492.

Skultety, P.F. & Sims, S.M. (1987) Evaluation of the loss of propylene glycol during aqueous film coating. *Drug Dev. Ind. Pharm.* **13(12)**, 2209–2219.

Teraoka, R., Matsuda, Y. & Sugimoto, I. (1989) Quantitative design for photostabilization of nifedipine by using titanium dioxide and/or tartrazine as colorants in model film coating systems. *J. Pharm. Pharmacol.* **41**, 293–297.

Thoma, K. (1987) Resistenz- und Zerfallsverhalten magensaftresistenter Fertigarzneimittel. 3 und 4. Mitt.: Pharmazeutisch-technologische und analytische Untersuchungen an magensaftresistenten Darreichsungsformen. Einfluss von Filmbildern und Weichmachern auf die Stabilität des Resistenz- und Zerfallsverhaltens. *Die Pharm.* **42**, 832–841.

Thoma, K. (1991) Untersuchungen zur Säurepermeabilität magensaftresistenter Überzüge. 5. Mitteilung: Pharmazeutische-technologisches und analytische Untersuchungen an magensaftresistenten Darreichungsformen. *Die Pharm.* **46**, 278–282.

Thoma, K. (1991) Nachweis lagerungsbedingter Alterungsvorgänge bei magensaftresistenten Filmen durch gesteuerte Pyrolyse und IR-spektoskopische Untersuchungen. 7. Mitteilung: Über pharmazeutisch-technologische und analytische Untersuchungen an magensaftresistenten Darreichungsformen. *Die Pharm.* **47**, 355–362.

Thoma, K. (1992) Einflussfaktoren auf die Lagerstabilität magensaftresistenter Fertigarzneimittel unter Temperatur belastung. 8. Mitteilung : Über pharmazeutisch technologische und analytische Untersuchungen an magensaftresistenten Darreichungsformen. *Die Pharm.* **47**, 595–601.

Yuen, K.H. (1993) Development and *in vitro* evaluation of a multiparticulate sustained-release theophylline formulation. *Drug. Dev. Ind. Pharm.* **19**, 855–874.

Miscellaneous pharmaceutical coating publications

Bioadhesion

Al-Dulaili, H. Florence, A.T. & Salole, E.G. (1986) *In vitro* assessment of the adhesiveness of film-coated tablets. *Int. J. Pharmaceut.* **34**, 67–74.

Duchêne, D. (1988) Méthodes d'évaluation de la bioadhésion et facteurs influenants. *S.T.P. Pharma* **4**, 688–697.

Florence, A.T. (1986) The adhesiveness of proprietary tablets and capsules to porcine oesophageal tissue. *Int. J. Pharmaceut.* **34**, 75–79.

Marvola, M. (1983) Effect of dosage form and formulation factors on the adherence of drugs to the esophagus. *J. Pharm. Sci.* **72**, 1034–1036.

Marvola, M. (1982) Development of a method for study of the tendency of drug products to adhere to the esophagus. *J. Pharm. Sci.* **71**, 975–977.

Peppas, N.A. (1989) Experimental methods for determination of bioadhesive bond strength of polymers with mucus. *S.T.P. Pharma* **5**, 187–191.

Sam, A.P. (1992) Mucoadhesion of the film-forming and non-film-forming polymeric materials as evaluated with the Wilhelmy plate method. *Int. J. Pharmaceut.* **79**, 97–105.

Coating of hard gelatin capsules

Braeckman, P. (1983) A new small scale apparatus for enteric coating of hard gelatin capsules. *Acta Pharm. Technol.* **29**, 25–27.

Hannula, A.-M. (1986) Evaluation of a gliding coat for rectal hard gelatin capsules. *Acta Pharm. Technol.* **32**, 26–28.

Hannula, A.-M. (1988) Coating of gelatin capsules. *Acta Pharm. Technol.* **34**, 234–236.

Index

Printed and bound by CPI Group (UK) Ltd, Croydon, CR0 4YY

23/10/2024

01778230-0004